Chemokines

Chemical Immunology

Vol. 72

KARGER

Basel · Freiburg · Paris · London · New York ·
New Delhi · Bangkok · Singapore · Tokyo · Sydney

....

Chemokines

Volume Editor *Alberto Mantovani*, Milan/Brescia

31 figures, 3 in color, and 14 tables, 1999

KARGER Basel · Freiburg · Paris · London · New York ·
New Delhi · Bangkok · Singapore · Tokyo · Sydney

Chemical Immunology

Formerly published as 'Progress in Allergy'
Founded 1939 by Paul Kallos

Prof. Alberto Mantovani

Istituto di Ricerche Farmacologiche 'Mario Negri', Milano
and University of Brescia, Italy

Bibliographic Indices. This publication is listed in bibliographic services, including Current Contents® and Index Medicus.

Drug Dosage. The authors and the publisher have exerted every effort to ensure that drug selection and dosage set forth in this text are in accord with current recommendations and practice at the time of publication. However, in view of ongoing research, changes in government regulations, and the constant flow of information relating to drug therapy and drug reactions, the reader is urged to check the package insert for each drug for any change in indications and dosage and for added warnings and precautions. This is particularly important when the recommended agent is a new and/or infrequently employed drug.

www.karger.com
Printed in Switzerland on acid-free paper by Reinhardt Druck, Basel
ISBN 3–8055–6861–4

Contents

Preface

Directional movement of leukocytes in any aspect of their activities, such as development, homeostatic circulation and inflammatory response, is controlled by chemotactic cytokines, the chemokines. IL-8, the first chemokine to be defined, was formally identified just over 10 years ago. Since then, the field has rapidly matured: some 40 chemokines and their receptors have so far been characterized, their nomenclature has been rationalized, chemokine- and chemokine receptor-deficient mice have been generated. These tools make it possible to ask important biological questions on the function and regulation of the chemokine network, which are well covered in the present volume. Eventually, the answers will provide a coherent picture, allowing for the integration of the chemokine network within the many facets of the immune system, from T cell development to leukocyte migration and APC trafficking, and also to more distant systems like angiogenesis. The interest in the chemokine network undoubtedly also stems from its relevance in pathological states, from inflammation to autoimmunity and viral infection to tumorigenesis. The control of inflammation and other pathological processes with chemokine receptor antagonists has been achieved in preclinical models and will soon be tested in clinical trials. Indeed, the structure of chemokine receptors, which are all seven transmembrane domain G-protein-coupled receptors, makes the development of receptor antagonists chemically tractable and promising as potential drugs, provided that issues related to in vivo pleiotropy and redundancy of the chemokine system are taken care of.

The impressive progress in chemokine research is reviewed in this volume by leading scientists who have made substantial contributions to its development. This makes the reading even more stimulating and vividly conveys the state of the art as well as the breadth of the intricate connections yet to be deciphered.

Luciano Adorini, Milan

Mantovani A (ed): Chemokines.
Chem Immunol. Basel, Karger, 1999, vol 72, pp 1–6

Introduction and Overview

Alberto Mantovani

Istituto di Ricerche Farmacologiche 'Mario Negri', Milan, and
University of Brescia, Brescia, Italy

Chemokine research is an area of intense efforts, rapid progress and high expectations in terms of therapeutic results. This book offers a series of assays on some of the most challenging aspects of chemokine research, ranging from viral infections to the design of inhibitors. This preface contains an overview of some of the general features of chemokines, with the aim to avoid repetitious general introductions in individual chapters and to provide the unaccustomed reader with essential tools.

Several independent lines of work lead to the identification of chemokines such as discussed here for monocyte chemotactic protein-1 (MCP-1). Already in the early 1970s it had been noted that supernatants of activated blood mononuclear cells contained attractants active on monocytes and neutrophils [1]. Subsequently a chemotactic factor active on monocytes was identified in culture supernatants of mouse [2] and human [3, 4] tumor lines and called tumor-derived chemotactic factor (TDCF) [3–5]. TDCF was at the time rather unique in that it was active on monocytes but not on neutrophils [4] and had a low (12 kDa) molecular weight [3, 4]. Moreover, correlative evidence suggested its involvement in the regulation of macrophage infiltration in murine and human tumors [3, 4, 6]. A molecule with similar cellular specificity and physicochemical properties was independently identified in the culture supernatant of smooth muscle cells (SMDCF) [7]. The JE gene had been identifed as an immediate-early PDGF-inducible gene in fibroblasts [8, 9]. Thus, in the mid 1980s a gene (JE) was in search of function and a monocyte-specific attractant was waiting for molecular definition. In 1989, MCP-1 was successfully purified from supernatants of a human glioma [10], a human monocytic leukemia [11] and a human sarcoma [12–14]: sequencing and molecular cloning revealed its relationship with the long known JE gene [15–17].

Chemokines are a superfamily of small proteins which play a crucial role in immune and inflammatory reactions and in viral infection [18–20]. Most

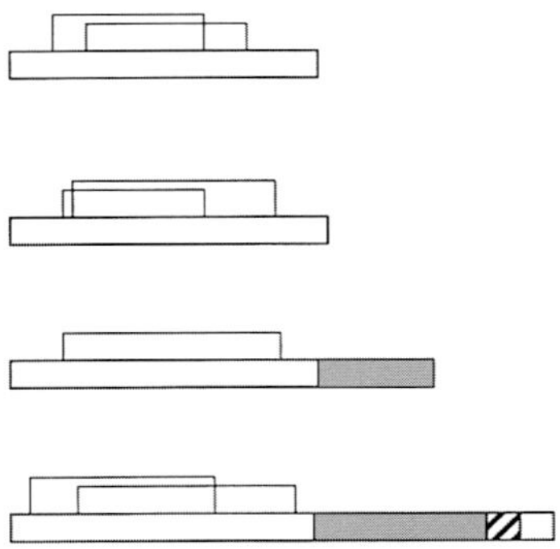

Fig. 1. Chemokine families: a schematic, simplified view. Acronyms and chromosomes refer to man. Only prototypic molecules or family of molecules and main cellular targets are shown. Clusters of related molecules are identified as monocyte chemotactic proteins (MCPs, 1 through 4), macrophage inflammatory proteins (MIPs), molecules with a 6-Cys motif (6 CCK). Certain molecules are bigger (lymphotactin, fractalkine), with a C terminal, mucin-like domain (dotted part). Fractalkine is expressed as a membrane molecule, with a transmembrane domain, on activated endothelial cells. The chromosomal localization is shown in parentheses and receptors are in the right-hand column. Mo = Monocytes; Neu = neutrophils; Eo = eosinophils; Ba = basophils; DC = dendritic cells.

chemokines cause chemotactic migration of leukocytes, but these molecules also affect other functions such as angiogenesis, collagen production, the proliferation of hematopoietic precursors and the ontogeny of the central nervous system. Based on a cysteine motif, a CXC, CC, C and CX3C family have been identified (fig. 1). The chemokine scaffold consists of an N-terminal loop connected via Cys bonds to the more structured core of the molecule (3 β sheets) with a C terminal α helix. About 50 human chemokines have been identified.

Chemokines interact with seven transmembrane domain, G protein-coupled receptors. Nine CC (CCR1 through 9), 5 CXC (CXCR1 through 5) and 1 CX3C (CX3CR1) receptors have been identified. Receptor expression is a crucial determinant of the spectrum of action of chemokines. For instance, recent results indicate that polarized Th1 and Th2 populations show differential receptor expression and responsiveness to chemokines [21–23]. Emerging evidence shows that regulation of receptor expression during activation or deactivation of monocytes is as important as regulation of chemokine production for tuning the chemokine system [24, 25].

The major eponymous function of chemokines is chemotaxis for leukocytes. Schematically (fig. 1), CXC (or α) chemokines are active on neutrophils

Table 1. Expression of chemokine receptors in human leukocyte populations

Receptor	Main ligands	Main cells
CCR1	MCP-3, RANTES, MIP-1α	Mo, T, NK, DC, PMN
CCR2 B/A	MCP-s (1–4)	Mo, T (act.), NK (act.)
CCR3	Eotaxin, MCP-3, RANTES	Eo, Ba, T (Th2)
CCR4	TARC, MDC	T (Th2, Tc2), NK, DC
CCR5	MIP-1β, MIP-1α, RANTES	Mo, T (Th1, Tc1), DC
CCR6	MIP-3α/LARC/Exodus	T, DC (CD34)
CCR7	ELC, SLC	T, Mo
CCR8	I309, TARC	T (Th2), Mo
CCR9	TECK	T, Mo, DC
CXCR1	IL-8	PMN
CXCR2	IL-8, gro, NAP-2	PMN
CXCR3	IP10, MIG	T (Th1)
CXCR4	SDF-1	Widely expressed
CXCR5	BCA-1	B
CX3CR1	Fractalkine	Mo, NK, T

Mo = Monocytes; DC = dendritic cells; DC (CD34) = DC-derived from CD34 cells in vitro; PMN = neutrophils; Eo = eosinophils; Ba = basophils; Th = T helper; Tc = T cytotoxic; (act.) = activated.

(PMN) and T lymphocytes while CC (or β) chemokines exert their action on multiple leukocyte subtypes, including monocytes, basophils, eosinophils, T lymphocytes, dendritic cells and NK cells, but they are generally inactive on PMN. Eotaxins (CC) represent the chemokines with the most restricted spectrum of action being selectively active on eosinophilic and basophilic granulocytes [18, 26–28]. Lymphotactin and fractalkine are the only proteins so far described with a C and CX3C motif, respectively [29–31]. They both act on lymphoid cells (T lymphocytes and NK cells) and fractalkine is also active on monocytes and PMN [29–32, and Sozzani et al., unpubl. data].

Chemokines are redundant in their action on target cells (table 1). No chemokine is active only on one leukocyte population and usually a given leukocyte population has receptors for and responds to different molecules (table 1). Interestingly, mononuclear phagocytes, the most evolutionary ancient cell type of innate immunity, respond to the widest range of chemokines. These include most CC chemokines, fractalkine (CX3C) and certain CXC molecules (e.g. SDF1 and, under certain conditions, IL-8).

The interaction of chemokines with their receptors is characterized by considerable promiscuity. Most known receptors have been reported to interact

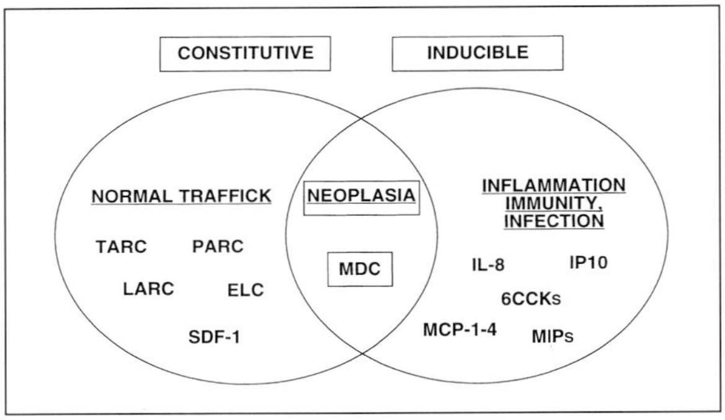

Fig. 2. Two general modes of chemokine production. Inflammatory/inducible cytokines are induced by immune and inflammatory stimuli and mediate recruitment on demand. Other chemokines are produced constitutively and play a role in regulating the basal trafficking of leukocytes. Molecules such as MDC are produced both in a tonic (e.g. the thymus) and in an inducible way. Moreover, cancer cells produce in a constitutive way, inducible cytokines such as MCP-1. Only a few molecules are mentioned.

with multiple ligands and most ligands interact with more than one receptor. For instance, all four monocyte chemotactic proteins (MCPs) interact with CCR2, and at least MCP-2, MCP-3 and MCP-4 also recognize other receptors (CCR1 and CCR3).

Probably all cell types can produce chemokines under appropriate conditions. Two general modes of chemokine production can be defined (fig. 2). Molecules such as SDF1 or MDC are produced constitutively either by specialized cells and organs (macrophages, dendritic cells; thymus and lymphoid organs for MDC) or in a more diffuse way as for SDF1. Most chemokines however are produced upon cell activation. Interestingly, chemokines are also produced in a redundant way (polyspeirism, πολνσ, many, σπειρω, make). Usually the same cell produces many chemokines concomitantly in response to the same stimulus. Again, polyspeirism is particularly striking for mononuclear phagocytes and endothelial cells exposed to bacterial products or primary inflammatory cytokines. In these cells, bacterial lipopolysaccharide, interleukin-1 and tumor necrosis factor elicit production of MCPs, MIPs, RANTES (CC), fractalkine (CX3C) and various CXC molecules [26–28, 33, 34].

G protein-coupled receptors are a classic target in pharmacology. Given the role of chemokines in diverse human diseases, ranging from HIV infection to allergy, their pharmacology is a prime target for research. Although redundancy is a formidable stumbling block (see table 1), available information suggests that blocking one agonist or one receptor can be beneficial in certain disease models as demonstrated for MCP-1 and its receptor CCR2 for monocytes and for eotaxins and their receptor CCR3 for eosinophils and basophils. Therefore, simple chemicals with chemokine antagonistic properties or with selective inhibitory activity on chemokine production are a holy grail in present-day cytokine pharmacology.

References

1 Ward PA, Remold HG, David JR: The production by antigen-stimulated lymphocytes of a lekotactic factor distinct from migration inhibitory factor. Cell Immunol 1970;1:162–174.

2 Meltzer MS, Stevenson MM, Leonard EJ: Characterization of macrophage chemotaxis in tumor cell cultures and comparison with lymphocyte-derived chemotactic factors. Cancer Res 1977;37: 721–725.

3 Bottazzi B, Polentarutti N, Acero R, Balsari A, Boraschi D, Ghezzi P, Salmona M, Mantovani A: Regulation of the macrophage content of neoplasms by chemoattractants. Science 1983;220: 210–212.

4 Bottazzi B, Polentarutti N, Balsari A, Boraschi D, Ghezzi P, Salmona M, Mantovani A: Chemotactic activity for mononuclear phagocytes of culture supernatants from murine and human tumor cells: Evidence for a role in the regulation of the macrophage content of neoplastic tissues. Int J Cancer 1983;31:55–63.

5 Bottazzi B, Ghezzi P, Taraboletti G, Salmona M, Colombo N, Bonazzi C, Mangioni C, Mantovani A: Tumor-derived chemotactic factor(s) from human ovarian carcinoma: Evidence for a role in the regulation of macrophage content of neoplastic tissues. Int J Cancer 1985;36:167–173.

6 Mantovani A, Bottazzi B, Colotta F, Sozzani S, Ruco L: The origin and function of tumor-associated macrophages. Immunol Today 1992;13:265–270.

7 Valente AJ, Fowler SR, Sprague EA, Kelley JL, Suenram CA, Schwartz CJ: Initial characterization of a peripheral blood mononuclear cell chemoattractant derived from cultured arterial smooth muscle cells. Am J Pathol 1984;117:409–417.

8 Zullo JN, Cochran BH, Huang AS, Stiles CD: Platelet-derived growth factor and double-stranded ribonucleic acids stimulate expression of the same genes in 3T3 cells. Cell 1985;43:793–800.

9 Rollins BJ, Morrison ED, Stiles CD: Cloning and expression of JE, a gene inducible by platelet-derived growth factor and whose product has cytokine-like properties. Proc Natl Acad Sci USA 1988;85:3738–3742.

10 Yoshimura T, Robinson EA, Tanaka S, Appella E, Kuratsu J, Leonard EJ: Purification and amino acid analysis of two human glioma-derived monocyte chemoattractants. J Exp Med 1989:169: 1449–1459.

11 Matsushima K, Larsen CG, DuBois GC, Oppenheim JJ: Purification and characterization of a novel monocyte chemotactic and activating factor produced by a human myelomonocytic cell line. J Exp Med 1989;169:1485–1490.

12 Zachariae CO, Anderson AO, Thompson HL, Appella E, Mantovani A, Oppenheim JJ, Matsushima K: Properties of monocyte chemotactic and activating factor purified from a human fibrosarcoma cell line. J Exp Med 1990;171:2177–2182.

13 Van Damme J, Decock B, Lenaerts JP, Conings R, Bertini R, Mantovani A, Billiau A: Identification by sequence analysis of chemotactic factors for monocytes produced by normal and transformed cells stimulated with virus, double-stranded RNA or cytokine. Eur J Immunol 1989;19: 2367–2373.

14 Graves DT, Jiang YL, Williamson MJ, Valente AJ: Identification of monocyte chemotactic activity produced by malignant cells. Science 1989;245:1490–1493.

15 Furutani Y, Nomura H, Notake M, Oyamada Y, Fukuy T, Yamada M, Larsen CG, Oppenheim JJ, Matsushima K: Cloning and sequencing of the cDNA for human monocyte chemotactic and activating factor. Biochem Biophys Res Commun 1989;159:248–255.

16 Yoshimura T, Yuhki N, Moore SK, Appella E, Lerman MI, Leonard EJ: Human monocyte chemoattractant protein-1. Full-length cDNA cloning, expression in mitogen-stimulation blood mononuclear leukocytes, and sequence similarity to mouse competence gene JE. FEBS Lett 1989;244:487–493.

17 Bottazzi B, Colotta F, Sica A, Nobili N, Mantovani A: A chemoattractant expressed in human sarcoma cells (tumor-derived chemotactic factor) is identical to monocyte chemoattractant protein-1/monocyte chemotactic and activating factor. Int J Cancer 1990;45:795–797.

18 Baggiolini M, Dewald B, Moser B: Human chemokines: An update. Annu Rev Immunol 1997;15: 675–705.

19 Hedrick JA, Zlotnik A: Chemokines and lymphocyte biology. Curr Opin Immunol 1996;8:343–347.

20 Rollins BJ: Chemokines. Blood 1997;90:909–928.

21 Bonecchi R, Bianchi G, Bordignon PP, D'Ambrosio D, Lang R, Borsatti A, Sozzani S, Allavena P, Gray PA, Mantovani A, Sinigaglia F: Differential expression of chemokine receptors and chemotactic responsiveness of type 1 T helper cells (Th1s) and Th2s. J Exp Med 1998;187:129–134.

22 Sallusto F, Mackay CR, Lanzavecchia A: Selective expression of the eotaxin receptor CCR3 by human T helper 2 cells. Science 1997;277:2005–2007.

23 Loetscher P, Uguccioni M, Bordoli L, Baggiolini M, Moser B, Chizzolini C, Dayer JM: CCR5 is characteristic of Th1 lymphocytes. Nature 1998;391:344–345.

24 Sica A, Saccani A, Borsatti A, Power CA, Wells TNC, Luini W, Polentarutti N, Sozzani S, Mantovani A: Bacterial lipopolysaccharide rapidly inhibits expression of C-C chemokine receptors in human monocytes. J Exp Med 1997;185:969–974.

25 Sozzani S, Ghezzi S, Iannolo G, Luini W, Borsatti A, Polentarutti N, Sica A, Locati M, Mackay C, Wells TNC, Biswas P, Vicenzi E, Poli G, Mantovani A: Interleukin-10 increases CCR5 expression and HIV infection in human monocytes. J Exp Med 1998;187:439–444.

26 Ben-Baruch A, Michiel DF, Oppenheim JJ: Signals and receptors involved in recruitment of inflammatory cells. J Biol Chem 1995;270:11703–11706.

27 Schall TJ: The chemokines; in Thomson A (ed): The Cytokine Handbook, ed 2. London, Academic Press, 1994, pp 419–460.

28 Sozzani S, Locati M, Allavena P, Van Damme J, Mantovani A: Chemokines: A superfamily of chemotactic cytokines. Int J Clin Lab Res 1996;26:69–82.

29 Kelner GS, Kennedy J, Bacon KB, Kleyensteuber S, Largaespada DA, Jenkins NA, Copeland NG, Bazan JF, Moore KW, Schall TJ, Zlotnik A: Lymphotactin: A cytokine that represents a new class of chemokine. Science 1994;266:1395–1399.

30 Bazan JF, Bacon KB, Hardiman G, Wang W, Soo K, Rossi D, Greaves DR, Zlotnik A, Schall TJ: A new class of membrane-bound chemokine with a CX3C motif. Nature 1997;385:640–644.

31 Pan Y, Lloyd C, Zhou H, Dolich S, Deeds J, Gonzalo JA, Vath J, Gosselin M, Ma JY, Dussault B, Woolf E, Alperin G, Culpepper J, Gutierrezramos JC, Gearing D: Neurotactin, a membrane-anchored chemokine upregulated in brain inflammation. Nature 1997;387:611–617.

32 Bianchi G, Sozzani S, Zlotnik A, Mantovani A, Allavena P: Migratory response of human NK cells to lymphotactin. Eur J Immunol 1996;26:3238–3241.

33 Baggiolini M, Dewald B, Moser B: Interleukin-8 and related chemotactic cytokines – CXC and CC chemokines. Adv Immunol 1994;55:99–179.

34 Mantovani A, Bussolino F, Introna M: Cytokine regulation of endothelial cell function: From molecular level to the bed side. Immunol Today 1997;18:231–239.

Prof. Alberto Mantovani, Istituto di Ricerche Farmacologiche 'Mario Negri',
Via Eritrea 62, I–20157 Milano (Italy)
Tel. +39 02 390 141, Fax +39 02 3546 277, E-Mail MANTOVANI@IRFMN.MNEGRI.IT

Mantovani A (ed): Chemokines.
Chem Immunol. Basel, Karger, 1999, vol 72, pp 7–29

Monocyte Chemoattractant Protein-1

Long Gu, Susan C. Tseng, Barrett J. Rollins

Department of Adult Oncology, Dana-Farber Cancer Institute,
Harvard Medical School, Boston, Mass., USA

The migration of monocytes into tissues is a highly regulated process that characterizes such diverse situations as the physiological establishment of resident macrophage populations and the pathophysiological accumulation of macrophages at the sites of infection by intracellular pathogens. A common theme uniting all monocyte/macrophage-related conditions is their chronicity. These inflammatory settings take a long time to develop, e.g. atherosclerosis, or persist for an extended period, e.g. granuloma formation. This is in marked contrast to the acute suppurative inflammatory conditions whose hallmark is polymorphonuclear leukocyte infiltration. This has always suggested the possibility that specific signals were available to attract specific leukocyte subsets. For example, in the early 1900s, Russell [1] postulated that cancers secreted a chemotactic factor to account for the peritumoral accumulation of the 'quiescent wandering cells of Maximow,' later shown to be monocytes. The discovery of chemokines fulfilled this prediction.

We now know that many CC chemokines attract monocytes in vitro, and their expression in vivo in association with monocyte accumulation suggests that their in vitro properties are physiologically relevant. However, the only CC chemokine for which formal proof of in vivo relevance currently exists is MCP-1, or monocyte chemoattractant protein-1. MCP-1 specifically attracts monocytes and memory T lymphocytes in vitro, and a variety of transgenic animal models indicates that it has similar properties in vivo. Other animal models have confirmed MCP-1's pathophysiological role in inflammatory diseases characterized by monocyte infiltration. This chapter will summarize the current state of our knowledge about MCP-1.

Purification and Cloning of MCP-1

The identification and characterization of MCP-1 took place in the mid-to-late 1980s during a period of time that witnessed the confluence of two formerly disparate areas of research. On one side were molecular biologists who had demonstrated that cellular activation and proliferation in response to growth factors or cytokines depends on the transcription of otherwise silent genes. Isolating those genes used the technique of differential expression cloning which was employed by many laboratories in diverse cellular systems. In the case of MCP-1, the Stiles laboratory [2] performed a differential screen of a cDNA library prepared from mouse 3T3 fibroblasts that had been treated with platelet-derived growth factor (PDGF). This, of course, was an attempt to capture gene sequences involved in the proliferative response to PDGF. Among the identified clones was *JE*, whose sequence was derived from an mRNA that was induced nearly 300-fold within hours of PDGF treatment.

As in all differential screening experiments, there is no guarantee of isolating genes relevant to the physiological response under investigation. In the case of PDGF-treated fibroblasts, the hope was to isolate mediators of the growth response such as the PDGF-inducible proto-oncogene c-*myc*. However, when the predicted amino acid sequences of the proteins encoded by murine and human *JE* were determined, no insights into cell proliferation were forthcoming [3, 4]. Unlike intracellular mediators of the growth response, the JE protein was secreted, and its predicted amino acid sequence looked similar to sequences of several cytokines, including interferon-α and -β.

At the same time that *JE* was being characterized, several groups were narrowing the search for monocyte-specific chemoattractant factors whose activity could be demonstrated by in vitro chemotaxis assays. Beginning with medium conditioned by baboon arterial smooth muscle cells, Valente's group [5] purified to homogeneity a protein with this activity that they called smooth muscle cell-derived chemotactic factor. At nearly the same time, both Leonard's group [6] and Oppenheim's group [8] purified the human version of this protein from glioblastoma or myelomonocytic leukemia cell lines, respectively. The former group called it Monocyte Chemoattractant Protein-1, while the latter called it Monocyte Chemotactic and Activating Factor.

Some of these groups had been involved in the earlier isolation of IL-8, a neutrophil-specific chemoattractant whose cDNA had also been cloned anonymously in a differential screen [8, 9]. The unexpected result of sequencing MCP-1 was the discovery that its sequence was closely related to that of IL-8, as well as Platelet Factor 4. This, of course, was the discovery of the chemokine family [10, 11]. Even more unexpected, however, was the discovery that the amino acid sequence of MCP-1 was identical to the predicted amino acid sequence of human JE. Thus MCP-1 is a PDGF-inducible gene in fibroblasts, and rather than being part of the proliferative program induced by PDGF, MCP-1 is part of the host defense program initiated when platelets release their contents during wounding. In retrospect, it made sense for PDGF to induce the expression of a factor that would attract mononuclear cell scavengers to the site of tissue injury.

Expression and Activities

High levels of MCP-1 expression were first documented in a variety of mesodermally derived cell types, such as fibroblasts, smooth muscle cells, endothelial cells, and monocytes/macrophages. Induced expression was achieved by a diverse array of activators including growth factors, cytokines, double-stranded RNA, and lipopolysaccharide (LPS) [12]. However, many subsequent studies have demonstrated MCP-1 expression in epithelial cells [13, 14]. As with many other chemokines, it may not be unreasonable to assume that all nucleated cells may be capable of expressing MCP-1 given the appropriate stimulus and circumstances. This may be part of an SOS-like phenomenon built into all cells of higher vertebrates that results in monocyte recruitment in response to physiological insult.

In vitro, MCP-1 attracts monocytes, CD45RO$^+$ T lymphocytes, and NK cells with an EC_{50} of approximately 0.5 n*M* [6, 7, 15, 16]. Surrogates of activation have been measured in vitro, and MCP-1 induces a calcium flux in monocytes with a similar EC_{50}, while induction of the respiratory burst requires approximately 100-fold higher concentrations [17]. Surprisingly, very little has been done to demonstrate MCP-1's ability to enhance phagocytosis or antigen presentation, but MCP-1 does enhance the proliferative response of naive T lymphocytes to anti-CD3 or the response of reactive T-cell clones to autologous antigen presenting cells in the presence of cognate antigen [18]. A similar enhancement of B7-1-induced costimulation was also observed.

MCP-1 induces expression of CD11b, CD11c, IL-1 and IL-6 in monocytes, providing further evidence for the establishment, at least in part, of an activation program [18a]. This fits the suggested role of chemokines in the multistep model of leukocyte emigration, namely stimulating the transition from rolling on the endothelial cell surface to firm adhesion. In flow chambers using monocytes as a target, MCP-1 caused rapid activation then deactivation of VLA-4-mediated adhesion to VCAM-1 or the 40-kD fibronectin fragment [19]. This was followed by prolonged firm adhesion of VLA-5 to the 120-kD fibronectin fragment, suggesting a model of monocyte diapedesis in which VLA-4-mediated endothelial transcytosis is followed by prolonged interaction of VLA-5 with extracellular matrix during subsequent migration. However, in the case of T lymphocytes, which also migrate in response to MCP-1 in vitro, MCP-1 had no effect on arresting their traverse through flow chambers at early times after stimulus (<5 min) [20].

Similar evidence for activation comes from the observation that addition of MCP-1 to purified monocytes in vitro enhanced their ability to inhibit DNA synthesis in several malignant human cell lines [7]. The EC_{50} for this effect was 0.3 n*M*, but it was clearly cytostatic rather than cytocidal. In contrast, combining MCP-1 with LPS stimulated the cytocidal activity of elicited peritoneal macrophages against syngeneic tumor cells in vitro [21, 22].

Thus the weight of evidence indicdates that MCP-1 can activate as well as attract monocytes. However, given the relatively benign appearance of monocytes attracted in vivo in response to transgenically produced MCP-1 (see below), the degree of activation may be somewhat limited. In other words, a variety of monocyte activation states are likely to exist, and while MCP-1 activates monocytes to a degree sufficient for integrin upregulation, it may not, for example, stimulate them to differentiate into macrophages.

MCP-1's Receptor and Signal Transduction

Like all chemokines, MCP-1 binds and signals through a 7-transmembrane spanning G protein-coupled receptor, CCR2 [23]. Unlike most other chemokines, however, this appears to be the sole receptor through which MCP-1 signals. (MCP-1 binds a structurally similar receptor called D6 or, tentatively, CCR9, but it has not yet been demonstrated that this interaction initiates signal transduction.) In contrast, CCR2 binds several other ligands with high affinity including MCP-2, -3, -4, and, in the mouse, MCP-5. CCR2 exists in two forms which are the products of alternatively spliced mRNAs. CCR2A and CCR2B differ only in their C-terminal, intracellular domains and therefore have essentially identical binding characteristics with respect to MCP-1. CCR2B is expressed more abundantly than CCR2A, and its C-terminal tail bears more homology to other 7-TMS receptor tails than does this region of CCR2A. Most biochemical characterizations have been performed on CCR2B.

Monocyte chemotaxis in response to MCP-1 is inhibited by pertussis toxin, indicating that $G_{\alpha i}$ coupling to CCR2 is essential for eliciting this phenomenon [24]. Additional inhibitor studies suggest that downstream targets from $G_{\alpha i}$ include serine/threonine kinases such as PKC [24]. The increase in intracellular calcium induced by MCP-1 is due to influx from extracellular sources and this, too, is inhibited by pertussis toxin and serine/threonine kinase inhibitors [24, 25]. Many of these results in monocytes have been recapitulated in *Xenopus laevis* oocytes and HEK-293 cells engineered to express CCR2B [26].

While these results firmly place $G_{\alpha i}$ in the signal transduction pathway employed by CCR2B, pertussis toxin blocks MCP-1-mediated calcium fluxes and adenylyl cyclase inhibition only by 80% at maximal doses in transfected HEK-293 cells [26]. This suggests that other G proteins and downstream mediators may also be coupled to CCR2B, and there are data consistent with this notion. For example, wortmannin inhibits MCP-1-mediated chemotaxis with an IC_{50} of 2.6 n*M* which is similar to its IC_{50} for inhibiting P13K. While this may implicate P13K in the chemotactic response to MCP-1, wortmannin can also inhibit PLA_2, the activity of which is required for chemotaxis [27]. Additional data, however, also demonstrate that MCP-1 activates MAPK [28, 29] and that MAPK activation is required for chemotaxis [29]. One group investigated a noncloned MCP-1 receptor and found that MAPK activation by MCP-1 was prevented by pertussis toxin [28]. However, a second group examined native monocytes and cloned CCR2B expressed in Chinese hamster ovary cells. They found that MAPK activation by MCP-1 in these systems was insensitive to pertussis toxin, but was PKC-dependent and PTK-independent [29]. This pattern is characteristic of $G_{\alpha q}$ or $G_{\alpha o}$ coupling [30, 31]. Thus it is likely that various subpopulations of CCR2B in a single cell can couple to different G proteins, and that activation of all of the coupled pathways may be required to elicit the complex cellular response of chemotaxis.

Structure/Activity Relationships

Human MCP-1 is a 76 amino acid CC chemokine with an N-terminal pyroglutamic acid. Its sequence places it within the subfamily of CC chemokines that includes MCP-2, -3, -4, -5 and eotaxin, and its gene maps to the crowded CC chemokine locus at 17q11.2-12 [32, 33]. Although MCP-1 has a single canonical N-linked glycosylation site, the native protein appears to have no N-linked sugars. Instead, there is a small amount of O-glycosylation involving one or both of the threonines near the C-terminus that results in the appearance of two isoforms of slightly different apparent molecular weight on SDS-PAGE [34, 37]. These have been called MCP-1α and MCP-1β, the former being the glycosylated version [6]. Based on the potency of bacterially produced MCP-1, glycosylation is clearly not necessary for in vitro chemoattractant activity.

Considering the similarity among chemokines in their primary structure, it is not surprising that they share a considerable amount of secondary and tertiary structural similarities. Like other chemokines, the basic structure of

MCP-1 C-terminal to the paried cysteines is an extended loop that leads into three anti-parallel β-pleated sheets in a Greek key formation, followed by a C-terminal α-helix overlying the flat plane of the Greek key. In the structure inferred from NMR analysis, the region of MCP-1 N-terminal to the paired cysteines is disordered [35]. However, in the crystal structure, amino acids 2–6 form a short, but well-ordered 3_{10} helix [36].

As with all chemokines examined to date, MCP-1 forms oligomers (primarily dimers) under conditions required for structural analysis. The dimeric structure in solution and in one type of crystal shows a dimer interface along a short β sheet near the N-terminus (amino acids 9–11) resulting in a cylindrical molecule quite different in shape from the compact CXC dimers which form through interactions between the first long β-pleated sheet in the Greek key. However, MCP-1 crystals also show tetramers as well as an alternative dimer structure that is very similar to CXC dimers. These striking differences in quaternary structure within the same crystals is apparently unique in the structural literature [36]. Unfortunately, the physiological significance of these alternative structures is completely unclear.

Mutagenesis of MCP-1 has provided some insight into regions and specific amino acids that are required for activity. Most striking and consistent among groups is the observation that truncation of the N-terminal domain severely impairs activity [37, 38]. For example, a variant lacking amino acids 2–8 i.e. having an N-terminal pyroglutamate, lacked activity [37, 39]. In addition, individual truncation variants missing amino acids 1 through 11 were inactive, except for the 5–76 variant [38]. Modifications at the N-terminus such as acetylation to prevent pyroglutamation, adding alanine to the −1 position, or inserting an epitope tag between amino acids 1 and 2 also disrupt activity. (However, in another report, an extra methionine at the N-terminus apparently did not affect MCP-1's activity [40].) In contrast, introduction of amino acids with various aliphatic side chains at position 1 had little effect suggesting that the α carbon backbone is the critical determinant rather than the specific amino acid that occupies this locus.

Individual amino acid changes have helped to map important determinants, and these are summarized in figure 1. Consistent with the truncation data, alteration of some amino acids in the N-terminal domain affect MCP-1 activity. This is, of course, analogous to the critical determinant present in the N-terminal domains of ELR-containing CXC chemokines, although no similarly specific amino acid motif has been documented. Other important areas include parts of the βN sheet (T10), the long loop before the β1 sheet, and several amino acids in the β1 and β2 sheets. For the most part, these are residues whose side chains point in the same direction from the sheets (e.g. Y28 and R30). The proline insertion between S34 and K35 was designed to

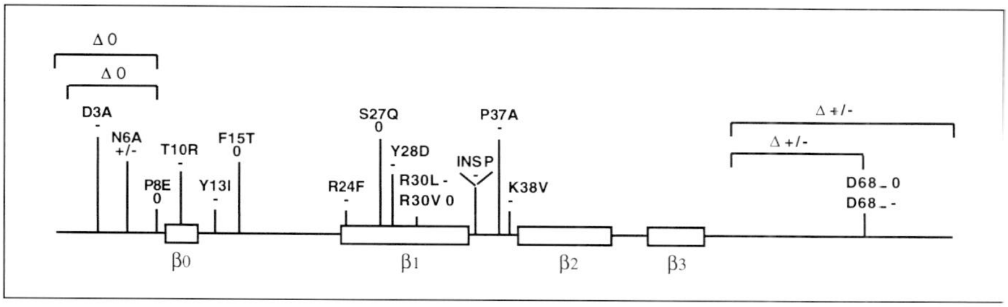

Fig. 1. Effects of amino acid substitutions, deletions, and insertions on MCP-1 monocyte chemoattractant activity. Amino acid substitutions are shown in their appropriate positions, as are various deletions (indicated Δ), and a proline insertion between positions 34 and 35. The scale corresponds to processed human MCP-1, i.e. N-terminal residue number 1 is glutamine. The four β-pleated sheets of MCP-1 are indicated. 0 = No effect; +/− = moderate decrease in activity; − = loss of activity. Data are summarized from various references discussed in the text.

mimic a topographically similar region in IL-8 [41]. While this resulted in a loss of activity, there were no data to rule out the possibility that this maneuver may have caused global alterations in secondary or tertiary structure.

At the C-terminus, partial or complete truncation of the α-helical region resulted in diminution of chemoattractant activity, but not its complete loss [37]. In one report, alteration of D68 to leucine caused a quantitative reduction similar to that observed for truncation [37], but in another report, it had little effect [41]. These observations suggest that the α-helix may not be involved in direct interactions with MCP-1's receptor, and may instead have a function analogous to this region in IL-8 which is involved in binding to glycosaminoglycans [42].

Murine MCP-1

Murine MCP-1, the product of what was originally called the *JE* gene, differs in many respects from human MCP-1. Most strikingly, its primary amino acid sequence extends 49 residues farther in the C-terminal direction and the protein is much more heavily glycosylated [43]. Examined by polyacrylamide gel electrophoresis, murine MCP-1 is a microheterogeneous protein of 25–30 kD. Digestion with neuraminidase collapses the microheterogeneity into a homogeneously distributed band, and subsequent digestion with O-glycanase reduces the size of the protein to 12 kD, which is the expected size of murine MCP-1's core protein. These observations indicate that approximately 50% of murine MCP-1's apparent molecular weight is due to carbohydrate which takes the form of a variable number of terminal sialic acids added to a constant number of O-linked oligosaccharides per peptide chain.

The amino acid sequence of the C-terminal domain of murine MCP-1 is rich in serines and threonines, suggesting that this might be the site of O-linked carbohydrate modification. The absence of this domain in human MCP-1 would also be consistent with its less extensive glycosylation. In fact, expression in COS cells of a truncated version of murine MCP-1 lacking the C-terminal domain produced a protein without detectable carbohydrate, confirming the localization of O-linked glycosylation to this region of the protein [43].

The N-terminal domain of murine MCP-1, i.e. exclusive of the 49 amino acid C-terminal extension, shares 62% amino acid identity with human MCP-1. Furthermore, this N-terminal domain has 100% of the in vitro monocyte chemoattractant activity of the full-length protein, and its specific activity is identical to that of human MCP-1. Thus murine MCP-1 is comprised of two functional domains, namely an N-terminal domain that is responsible for monocyte chemoattractant activity (at least as measured in vitro) and a C-terminal domain that is extensively glycosylated. The function of the C-terminal domain is unknown, but it clearly does not interfere either with in vitro function or with affinity for binding to CCR2. It is tempting to speculate that it functions in a manner similar to the carbohydrate-substituted domain of fractalkine and may be involved in anchoring MCP-1 to sites on endothelial cells or in the extracellular matrix.

Of course, one of the main reasons for characterizing murine MCP-1 in detail is to enable the development of murine models of chemokine function. However, the relevance of these models to human physiology and disease depends on the degree of certainty that the murine gene being manipulated is the true homolog of a given human gene. This is a particularly troublesome problem when dealing with a family of closely related proteins such as chemokines. How can one be sure that a murine chemokine is really a homolog of a human chemokine when they all share so many structural features? In the case of MCP-1, while it is true that the human gene was cloned using murine MCP-1 as a homology probe, the fact remains that the C-terminal domains of the two proteins are quite divergent. The situation has been further clouded by the description of MCP-5, a murine CC chemokine that lacks the C-terminal extension of murine MCP-1 and shares, overall, 66.3% nucleotide and 64.5% amino acid similarity with human MCP-1 [44, 45]. (Considered as a whole, i.e. not just the N-terminal domain, murine MCP-1 shares only 52.7% nucleotide and 45.1% amino acid similarity with human MCP-1.) Despite this mathematical similarity, several observations argue against MCP-5 being the 'true' murine homolog of human MCP-1. First, Southern blot analysis of human DNA using a murine MCP-1 cDNA probe recognizes only human MCP-1 fragments, while a murine MCP-5 cDNA probe hybridizes to non-

MCP-1 fragments [44]. Second, murine MCP-1 is a more potent agonist for murine CCR2 than murine MCP-5 [45]. Third, expression patterns of murine MCP-1 in vivo, e.g. in response to nerve transection or in glomerulonephritis, are similar to human MCP-1 while those of murine MCP-5 are not [R.M. Ransohoff and V.R. Kelley, pers. commun.].

How can the physiological data pointing to murine MCP-1 as human MCP-1's homolog be reconciled with the sequence homology data? The answer lies in the extraordinarily prolific evolution of chemokines. Most genes encoding CC chemokines cluster on the long arm of human chromosome 17 (syntenic with mouse chromosome 11). This clustering plus the high degree of structural similarity among the genes suggests that they arose by duplication and divergence. However, there is an additional subtlety based on structure/activity analyses which indicate that the major specificity and functional domains of chemokines lie in amino acids encoded by exons 1 and 2. In fact, intron/exon boundaries among the CC chemokines are highly conserved and this raises the possibility that chemokines might have evolved through duplication and divergence of exons rather than whole genes.

Reexamined in this light, it becomes clear that exons 1 and 2 of human MCP-1 are more closely related phylogenetically to murine MCP-1 than to MCP-5 (fig. 2). The first two exons of murine MCP-1 share 63.6% nucleotide land 70.7% amino acid similarity with human MCP-1, compared to 55.7 and 65.9%, respectively, for MCP-5. Furthermore, a database search using exon 3 of murine MCP-1 identified regions of 90% similarity in the third exons of the CC chemokines eotaxin and PARC (also known as DC-CK-1 and MIP-4). Exon 3 of murine MCP-5 identifies the third exons of MCP-1, MCP-3, MCP-4, and IP-10. This suggests that in addition to evolution within exons, some shuffling of exons may have occurred.

This analysis indicates that, taking the specificity and functionality domains of these chemokines into account, murine MCP-1 is the closest identified relative of human MCP-1. The conservation of exon 1 likely extends to upstream regulatory regions and explains the similarities in expression patterns between these two chemokines. Thus, while assigning homologs among chemokines is still a hazardous enterprise, it appears that the insights gained from mice genetically modified for murine MCP-1, described in detail below, may be applied to human disease with some assurance.

Lessons from Transgenic Mice

For several years after its isolation, it was not clear that MCP-1's in vitro activities of attracting monocytes and other mononuclear cells would

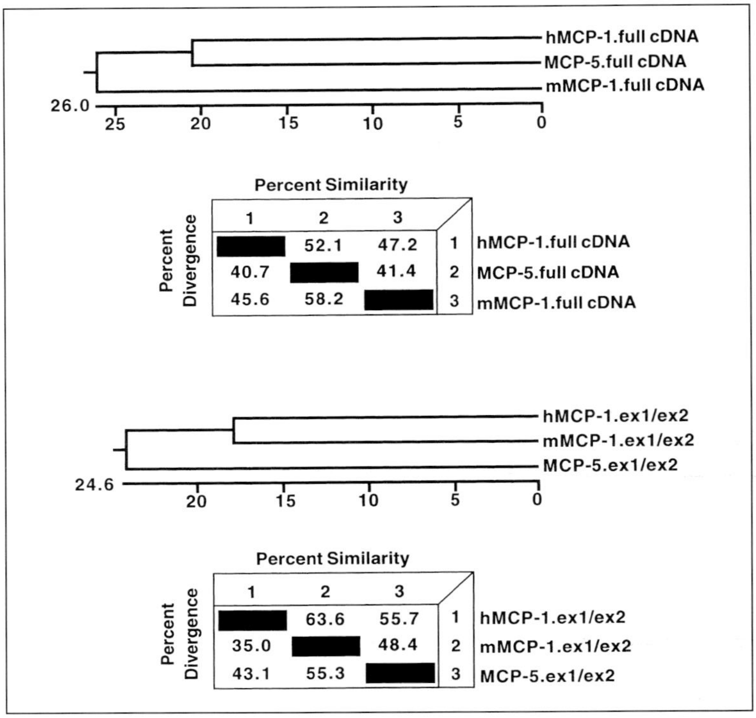

Fig. 2. Phylogenetic trees (phenograms) for human MCP-1, murine MCP-1, and murine MCP-5 using the Clustal method (sequence distances are indicated). Also shown are percentage similarities between sequence pairs (calculated directly) and percentage divergence (calculated with reference to phylogenetic trees). *Upper*, using full cDNA sequences, murine MCP-5 is more closely related to human MCP-1 than murine MCP-1 is. *Lower*, using sequences of exons 1 and 2, murine MCP-1 is more closely related to human MCP-1 than murine MCP-5 is.

accurately predict its in vivo properties. While some investigators reported that purified MCP-1 could elicit a monocytic infiltrate after injection in rodent skin [46, 47], others could not document this [43]. One reason for the meager response to exogenously administered MCP-1 might have been its rapid degradation. Therefore, many groups turned to transgenic technology to provide a continuous source of endogenous MCP-1 in an organ-specific manner. Unfortunately, the path to determining MCP-1's in vivo activities was not completely straightforward.

The first transgenic model to be constructed used sequences from the long terminal repeat of the mouse mammary tumor virus (MMTV) to drive expression of murine MCP-1 [48]. Despite achieving high levels of demonstrably functional MCP-1 expression in a variety of organs, no mononuclear cell infiltrates were ever observed. Ultimately, it became clear that these mice had high plasma levels of MCP-1, perhaps secreted by monocytes themselves, that would be capable of desensitizing MCP-1 receptors on circulating monocytes, thereby rendering them insensitive to locally produced MCP-1. Alternatively, plasma MCP-1 may have simply canceled out the chemoattractant concentration gradient emanating from organs that expressed the transgene.

However, these mice did have an interesting phenotype in their increased susceptibility to lethal infection by intracellular parasites such as *Listeri monocytogenes* and *Mycobacterium tuberculosis.* The LD_{50} for *Listeria* was 10-fold lower and the number of mycobacteria isolated from target organs was 10-fold higher in transgenic mice than in wild-type mice. Although the mechanism has not been elucidated, two possibilities present themselves. On the one hand, this may simply be a consequence of the postulated monocyte desensitization due to high plasma levels of MCP-1. On the other hand, MCP-1 might either stimulate or be part of the effector arm of a Th2 response at the expense of Th1. In fact, data in support of a connection between MCP-1 and Th2 responses have recently been generated and are discussed more fully in the section on knockout mice.

Given the absence of infiltrates in the MMTV model, several groups took the approach of using promoters that would allow transgene expression to occur at lower levels in a more anatomically localized pattern. One of the first groups to do this generated two models in which murine MCP-1 expression was placed under the control of the lck or myelin basic protein (MBP) promoters [49]. In the former case, lck directed expression to the thymus and resulted in a monocytic infiltrate of sufficient subtlety to require flow cytometric examination of transgenic thymi for its detection. However, a more robust monocytic infiltrate was induced by MBP-driven MCP-1. This resulted in perivascular cuffing that occurred in concert with the temporally regulated pattern of MBP expression. The intensity of the infiltrate and the depth to which monocytes invaded in brain parenchyma could be substantially enhanced by systemic treatment with LPS. End-organ dysfunction was not observed in either model suggesting that the recruited monocytes were not activated by the expression of MCP-1 alone.

In another model, murine MCP-1 expression was driven by keratin-14 promoter which directs expression primarily to basal epidermal cells [50]. In the unchallenged state, these mice demonstrated alterations in their dermis consisting of an increased number of cells that were class II MHC^+, $CD45^+$ and $CD11c^+$. These cells had a stellate morphology which, along with their staining pattern, suggested that they were Langerhans-like dermal dendritic cells, although they lacked characteristic Birbeck granules. Nonetheless, their presence is consistent with some observations that MCP-1 can attract dendritic cells in vitro [51].

When challenged in models of cutaneous contact hypersensitivity, these keratin-14-MCP-1 transgenic mice mounted exaggerated inflammatory responses compared to their wild-type littermates. Either or both of two mechanisms could be envisaged to account for this phenotype. First, the increased number of dendritic cells could result in a more efficiently processed afferent arm of the hypersensitivity response. Second, the constitutive expression of MCP-1 by basal keratinocytes could enhance the efferrent arm of the response by recruiting increased numbers of monocytes or T lymphocytes. The relevance of neither mechanism has been established.

A different model used the promoter for surfactant protein C to control the expression of human MCP-1 [52]. This resulted in MCP-1 expression in the lung, but instead of promoting monocyte infiltration into lung parenchyma, this transgene produced increased numbers of monocytes transiting into the alveolar spaces as determined by their presence in bronchoalveolar lavage fluid. As in the MBP-MCP-1 transgenic mouse, the number of mononuclear cells in the lavage could be enhanced by systemic treatment with LPS. Furthermore, embolization of yeast cell wall glucan to the lung resulted in granuloma formation which was more vigorous in the transgenic mice than their wild-type counterparts. One important aspect of this transgenic mouse is its apparent demonstration that murine monocytes can respond in vivo to human MCP-1.

In another model, murine MCP-1 expression driven by the rat insulin promoter (RIP) resulted in expression restricted to the β cells of pancreatic islets [53]. These mice developed a monocytic infiltrate that appeared at birth and persisted throughout the lifetimes of the animals. Despite its presence, the animals never became diabetic and there was no evidence for any local tissue destruction. Thus, as in the other models discussed so far, MCP-1's function in vivo can be restricted to the attraction of monocytes without their activation.

The RIP-MCP-1 mice were also used to investigate questions raised by the MMTV-MCP-1 mice described at the beginning of this section. RIP-MCP-1 transgenic mice were mated to MMTV-MCP-1 transgenic mice. Progeny that inherited only the RIP-MCP-1 transgene expressed 20 ng of MCP-1 per milligram of pancreas protein and showed the monocytic infiltrates characteristic of their RIP-MCP-1 transgenic parent. Progeny that inherited both the RIP-MCP-1 and MMTV-MCP-1 transgenes also expressed 20 ng MCP-1 per milligram of pancreas protein. However, they did not have evidence for a monocytic insulitis. Thus, high levels of circulating MCP-1 can prevent monocytes from infiltrating into organs in which low levels of MCP-1 are expressed. This phenomenon is similar to the ability of intravascular IL-8 to prevent intradermal infiltration of neutrophils in response to locally injected IL-8 [54]. In general, these observations indicate that a chemokine's ability to recruit a leukocyte from the vasculature into a parenchymal site depends on expression of the chemokine occurring at low levels in localized areas.

It should be noted that a recent transgenic model has directed high levels of murine MCP-1 expression to the heart by using the promoter for the α-cardiac myosin heavy chain [55]. This targeting resulted in a monocytic myocarditis. However, unlike all of the other MCP-1 transgenic models, this infiltrate produced serious pathology in the form of cardiac hypertrophy and dilatation, resulting in severe left ventricular dysfunction. Thus something in this model worked synergistically with MCP-1 to cause monocyte activation and tissue damage, although the precise nature of this signal is unknown.

Effects of MCP-1 on Tumor Growth

Although leukocyte infiltration in human cancers has been appreciated since the time of Virchow [56], its role in tumor physiology remains uncertain. In the early part of this century, work on transplantable tumors in animals demonstrated that the inflammatory infiltrate associated with some tumors originated from the host rather than the donor [1, 57]. This led to the concept that tumor cells elaborate chemoattractants that are responsible for eliciting the inflammatory reaction as well as capillary ingrowth [1, 58].

Monocytes comprise a large proportion of the host's inflammatory infiltrate in solid tumors. However, monocytes may play either of two roles in this setting [see 59]. Through their effector functions, either as an arm of innate immunity or directed by T lymphocytes, they may be involved in the host's attempt to reject the tumor. At the same time, monocytes and macrophages are also potent sources of growth factors and it is equally possible that their presence actually enhances tumor growth [60]. There is experimental and observational evidence to support both of these mechanisms. In some murine models [61] as well as human tumors [62, 63], the proportion of macrophages in the tumor correlated with the absence of metastases or with a more favorable clinical outcome. However, others have observed an inverse correlation between macrophage infiltration and survival in breast cancer [64].

Regardless of the precise role played by tumor-associated macrophages, these observations suggest the hypothesis that tumor cells secrete monocyte chemoattractants. In the early 1980s, Mantovani and colleagues [65] showed that tumor cells cultured in vitro secreted monocyte chemoattractant activity that correlated directly with the extent of monocyte/macrophage infiltration elicited by tumors that were formed by the same cells in vivo. Human ovarian cancer explants showed a similar correlation [66]. It later became clear that MCP-1 was primarily responsible for this tumor cell-derived monocyte chemoattractant activity [67, 68].

Experimental models have documented MCP-1's ability to inhibit tumor growth. In vitro, MCP-1 appeared to have a cytostatic effect on several human tumor cell lines, although the mechanism has not been elucidated [7]. In vivo, Chinese hamster ovary (CHO) cells engineered to express high levels of MCP-1 were unable to form tumors in nude mice despite their unchanged proliferative rate in vitro [69]. In this case, two lines of evidence suggested that this was due to secreted MCP-1's ability to attract monocytes and macrophages into the tumor mass. First, monocyte-rich infiltrates were observed in the tumor inoculation sites within 24 h of injection. Second, the effect was non-cell autonomous since MCP-1-expressing CHO cells could also suppress tumor formation by coinjected wild-type CHO cells or HeLa cells.

Several other studies support the notion that MCP-1 can direct monocyte antitumor effects in immunocompetent as well as athymic animals. For example, individual clones of Rous sarcoma virus-induced sarcomas have been analyzed and found to express varying amounts of MCP-1 [70]. Clones with high level MCP-1 expression formed tumors in syngeneic animals with an increased proportion of macrophage infiltration compared to low level expressors, and these tumors appeared later and grew more slowly. In another study, B16 melanoma cells were engineered to express MCP-1 [71]. High level expressors again showed macrophage infiltration and slower growth rates. Interestingly, however, the MCP-1 expressors actually had a higher rate of tumor-forming efficiency at low inocula, even though the growth rates of the tumors that formed were slower than those of nonexpressing cells. This may be evidence for the growth-promoting effects of macrophages at early stages of tumors formation [60] which is superseded later by antitumor effects. However, when CT26 colon carcinoma cells were injected intravenously so that they would metastasize to the lungs, MCP-1 expressors formed fewer metastases [22]. This occurred despite the fact that expressors and nonexpressors homed to the lungs in similar numbers. In this model, therefore, MCP-1 expression was not advantageous even for an 'inoculum' of one cell.

Correlations have also been reported between levels of MCP-1 expression, macrophage infiltration, and diminished tumor growth in rat models [72] and in human tumors. For example, MCP-1 expression was quantified by in situ hybridization of 20 human ovarian carcinomas, and the number of epithelial cells expressing MCP-1 correlated with the numbers of $CD68^+$ and $CD8^+$ cells in the tumor infiltrate [73].

Most of the animal models described in the foregoing paragraphs depend on local effects of MCP-1. For example, injection of MCP-1-expressing cells in one anatomic site has no effect on tumor formation by nonexpressing cells injected synchronously at a distant site [69]. This suggests that MCP-1 exerts its effects in these models in a nonspecific manner by recruiting monocytes that engage in local antitumor activity. However, given MCP-1's ability to attract T lymphocytes, it might be imagined that in the proper circumstances, MCP-1 could also contribute to the formation of systemic antitumor immunity. This has been demonstrated by immunizing rats with γ-irradiated 9L glioma cells engineered to express high levels of MCP-1 [74]. Upon subsequent challenge with wild-type 9L cells, immunized rats were resistant to tumor growth indicating that immunization with MCP-1-expressing cells afforded systemic protection from syngeneic tumor growth. It remains to be seen whether MCP-1 can be effective in preventing the growth of other less immunogenic tumor cells.

It must be mentioned that a paradox underlies any discussion of MCP-1's antitumor activities. Despite correlations between MCP-1 expression and diminished tumor growth in human cancers, and despite direct demonstrations in animal models of its tumor-suppressive effects, the fact remains that a large proportion of human tumors express MCP-1 and clearly grow with impunity. One possible explanation may be found in the phenotype of MMTV-MCP-1 transgenic mice, described above, in which high levels of MCP-1 expression prevented monocytes from migrating properly and engaging their effector functions. It may be that some tumor cells secrete MCP-1 in order to accomplish the same sort of disarming of monocyte antitumor activity. Although this concept is unproved, it may also explain the rich descriptive literature that connects tumor burden with monocyte dysfunction in cancer patients [75–79]. Alternatively, systemic MCP-1 may stimulate Th2 polarization which could enhance tumor growth indirectly by suppressing Th1-associated cell-mediated immunity.

Lessons from 'Knockout' Mice

In the 1990s, the central question for the chemokine field was whether the functional redundancy of chemokines in vitro was recapitulated in vivo. In other words, a large number of CC chemokines are able to attract monocytes in vitro and, what is more, at least five CC chemokines bind to CCR2 with high affinity. Given this scenario, could a single chemokine such as MCP-1 possibly play an essential role in normal physiology or disease?

Evidence for unique functions of MCP-1 came first from antibody neutralization experiments. In models of pulmonary granuloma formation, pulmonary hypersensitivity responses, and glomerulonephritis, antibody treatment significantly ameliorated manifestations of disease [80–86]. More recently, genetic proof for this concept has come from MCP-1-deficient animals created by targeted gene disruption [87]. These animals express no detectable MCP-1, but do express other CC chemokines whose genes map to the same locus on mouse chromosome 11, including MCP-3 and MCP-5, two other ligands for CCR2.

Despite the absence of MCP-1, mice develop normally, have normal hematologic profiles, and have normal numbers of resident tissue macrophages, suggesting that MCP-1 does not have an obvious role to play in development. However, these mice do show serious abnormalities in several inflammatory and immunological models. For example, in response to intraperitoneal instillation of thioglycollate broth, MCP-1-deficient mice recruit essentially no macrophages but the same number of neutrophils and eosinophils as wild-type mice. Similarly, in models of delayed-type hypersensitivity, the lesions in *MCP-1*$^{-/-}$ mice have normal amounts of local edema (which is probably mediated by neutrophils) but greatly reduced numbers of monocytes and macrophages. Thus MCP-1 apparently plays a nonredundant role in these models of macrophage recruitment in vivo. These phenotypes also appear in *CCR2*$^{-/-}$ mice described elsewhere in this volume as well as reported by others, suggesting that MCP-1 and CCR2 comprise a 'closed' ligand/receptor loop in these settings [88–90].

In immunological settings, it has been observed that naive T lymphocytes from T-cell receptor transgenic mice will polarize toward a Th2 phenotype when stimulated with antigen and MCP-1 in vitro [91]. Some evidence for MCP-1's connection to Th2 responses in vivo came from observations on MMTV-MCP-1 transgenic mice which showed increased susceptibility to intracellular pathogens. One hypothesis to explain this phenotype was that high levels of systemic MCP-1 could be stimulating a Th2 response at the expense of Th1 which would be required for the host to be resistant to such pathogens. Stronger evidence came from a model of pulmonary granuloma formation in response to eggs of *Schistosoma mansoni* embolized to the pulmonary vasculature. When this procedure is performed in mice sensitized to Schistosome egg antigen, the granulomatous response has a Th2 character and is partially inhibited by anti-MCP-1 antibodies [92]. Almost identical quantitative inhibition is observed in genetically MCP-1-deficient mice [87].

In a more direct examination of MCP-1's effects on the immune response, *MCP-1*$^{-/-}$ mice in a pure C57Bl/6 background were immunized with trinitrophenyl-derivatized ovalbumin [Gu et al., in prep.]. Cells from draining lymph nodes were then stimulated in vitro with ovalbumin and patterns of cytokine secretion were observed. Levels of IFN-γ and IL-12 were the same as those in wild-type mice indicating an intact Th1 response. However, levels of IL-5 and IL-10 were nearly undetectable in cultures from *MCP-1*$^{-/-}$ mice, consistent with a severe Th2 defect. It has not yet been determined whether this reflects

MCP-1's direct influence on T-helper cell polarization or a requirement for MCP-1-mediated trafficking of naive T cells to appropriate microenvironments where their polarization is effected by other cytokines. Also unresolved is the apparent contradiction between this Th2 defect in *MCP-1*$^{-/-}$ mice and the reported Th1 defect in *CCR2*$^{-/-}$ mice [88]. This may reflect the ability of some of the other CCR2 ligands to induce Th1 responses while MCP-1 is required for developing a Th2 response.

Some of these concepts about MCP-1's unique role in macrophage recruitment have been put to the test in a disease model of atherosclerosis. The justification for examining MCP-1's role in this disease comes from a decade of observations connecting MCP-1 to atherogenesis. For example, endothelial cells, arterial smooth muscle cells, and fibroblasts have all been shown to express MCP-1 in vitro in response to relevant stimuli including minimally modified low-density lipoprotein (LDL) [93–96]. Furthermore, MCP-1 expression occurs in vivo in animal models of atherogenic conditions such as hypercholesterolemia, hypertension, and balloon angioplasty [95, 97, 98]. Finally, MCP-1 has been found in human plaques [99].

To test MCP-1's role in atherogenesis, the disrupted *MCP-1* alleles were placed in an LDL receptor-deficient background, and doubly deficient mice were fed a defined high cholesterol diet [100]. In the absence of MCP-1, total plasma cholesterol levels and lipoprotein profiles were exactly the same as those in animals with wild-type *MCP-1* alleles. However, the MCP-1-deficient mice had 80% less lesion formation in their aortas, and this difference persisted for up to 25 weeks of hypercholesterolemia. Furthermore, they had a significant decrease in the number of macrophages in their aortic walls. This suggests a model of atherosclerosis in which arterial damage due to hypercholesterolemia induces local MCP-1 expression which is required for recruitment of macrophages that take up residence in the arterial wall. These macrophages ingest lipid and become the foam cells of the atherosclerotic plaque. Notably, again, MCP-1's role in this pathophysiological picture appears to be unique and other CC chemokines cannot act as substitutes.

The mouse is a relatively poor model for human atherosclerosis. However, the central role of MCP-1 and CCR2 in atherogenesis has now been observed in two additional and distinct murine models of atherosclerosis. The disrupted *MCP-1* alleles have been crossed into an apolipoprotein B background, and a similar reduction in lesion formation has been observed [Gosling et al., submitted]. Finally, disrupted *CCR2* alleles have been placed in an apolipoprotein E-deficient background [101]. Although lesion reduction is neither so substantial nor prolonged as in the other models, amelioration of disease is still significant. Thus similar results in several murine models suggest that MCP-1 and CCR2 are likely to play important roles in human atherosclerosis.

Conclusions

There have been two competing forces in the chemokine world during the past 10 years. On one hand, genetic and biochemical approaches have conspired to reveal the existence of nearly 60 chemokines and, probably, 30 receptors. On the other hand, the need to understand what chemokines do and how they do it has led some investigators to concentrate on tiny subpopulations of the chemokine family. Most of the information contained in this chapter derives from the latter approach. Through the use of detailed structural studies, we are beginning to glimpse mechanisms that underlie MCP-1's interaction with its receptor. Genetic manipulation of the mouse has revealed that MCP-1's in vitro properties tend to predict what it will do in vivo and, in contrast, gene disruption has shown that in vitro redundancy does not predict the unique roles played by MCP-1 and CCR2 in physiology and disease.

The next set of challenges will involve understanding the rest of the members of this diverse family and determining how they fit with each other into a network of signals that influence leukocyte physiology. Many of the approaches discussed in this chapter can serve as paradigms for the investigation of other chemokines.

References

1 Russell BRG: The nature of resistance to the inoculation of cancer. Third Sci Rep ICRF 1908;3: 341–358.

2 Cochran BH, Reffel AC, Stiles CD: Molecular cloning of gene sequences regulated by platelet-derived growth factor. Cell 1983;33:939–947.

3 Rollins BJ, Stier P, Ernst TE, Wong GG: The human homologue of the *JE* gene encodes a monocyte secretory protein. Mol Cell Biol 1989;9:4687–4695.

4 Rollins BJ, Morrison ED, Stiles CD: Cloning and expression of *JE*, a gene inducible by platelet-derived growth factor and whose product has cytokine-like properties. Proc Natl Acad Sci USA 1988;85:3738–3742.

5 Valente AJ, Graves DT, Vialle-Valentin CE, Delgado R, Schwartz CJ: Purification of a monocyte chemotactic factor secreted by nonhuman primate vascular cells in culture. Biochemistry 1988;27: 4162–4168.

6 Yoshimura T, Robinson EA, Tanaka S, Appella E, Kuratsu JI, Leonard EJ: Purification and amino acid analysis of two human glioma-derived monocyte chemoattractants. J Exp Med 1989;169:1449–1459.

7 Matsushima K, Larsen CG, DuBois GC, Oppenheim JJ: Purification and characterization of a novel monocyte chemotactic and activating factor produced by a human myelomonocytic cell line. J Exp Med 1989;169:1485–1490.

8 Yoshimura T, Matsushima K, Tanaka S, Robinson EA, Appella E, Oppenheim JJ, Leonard EJ: Purification of a human monocyte-derived neutrophil chemotactic factor that has peptide sequence similarity to other host defense cytokines. Proc Natl Acad Sci USA 1987;84:8233–9237.

9 Schmid J, Weissmann C: Induction of mRNA for a serine protease and a β-thromboglobulin-like protein in mitogen-stimulated human leukocytes. J Immunol 1987;139:250–256.

10 Baggiolini M, Dewald B, Moser B: Interleukin-8 and related chemotactic cytokines – CXC and CC chemokines. Adv Immunol 1994;55:97–179.

11 Rollins BJ: Chemokines. Blood 1997;90:909–928.
12 Rollins BJ: Monocyte chemoattractant protein 1: A potential regulator of monocyte recruitment in inflammatory disease. Mol Med Today 1996;2:198–204.
13 Standiford TJ, Kunkel SL, Basha MA, Chensue SW, Lynch JPI, Toews GB, Westwick J, Strieter RM: Interleukin-8 gene expression by a pulmonary epithelial cell line. A model for cytokine networks in the lung. J Clin Invest 1990;86:1945–1953.
14 Barker JNWN, Jones ML, Swenson CL, Sarma V, Mitra RS, Ward PA, Johnson KJ, Fantone JC, Dixit VM, Nickoloff BJ: Monocyte chemotaxis and activating factor production by keratinocytes in response to IFN-γ. J Immunol 1991;146:1192–1197.
15 Carr MW, Roth SJ, Luther E, Rose SS, Springer TA: Monocyte chemoattractant protein 1 acts as a T-lymphocyte chemoattractant. Proc Natl Acad Sci USA 1994;91:3652–3656.
16 Taub DD, Sayers TJ, Carter CR, Ortaldo JR: α and β chemokines induce NK cell migration and enhance NK-mediated cytolysis. J Immunol 1995;155:3877–3888.
17 Rollins BJ, Walz A, Baggiolini M: Recombinant human MCP-1/JE induces chemotaxis, calcium flux, and the respiratory burst in human monocytes. Blood 1991;78:1112–1116.
18 Taub DD, Turkovski-Carrales SM, Key ML, Longo DL, Murphy WJ: Chemokines and T lymphocyte activation. I. β Chemokines costimulate human T lymphocyte activation in vitro. J Immunol 1996;156:2095–2103.
18a Jiang Y, Beller DI, Frendl G, Graves DT: Monocyte chemoattractant protein-1 regulates adhesion molecule expression and cytokine production in human monocytes. J Immunol 1992;148:2423–2428.
19 Weber C, Alon R, Moser B, Springer TA: Sequential regulation of $\alpha4\beta1$ and $\alpha5\beta1$ integrin avidity by CC chemokines in monocytes: Implications for transendothelial chemotaxis. J Cell Biol 1996;134:1063–1073.
20 Campbell JJ, Hedrick J, Zlotnik A, Siani MA, Thompson DA, Butcher EC: Chemokines and the arrest of lymphocytes rolling under flow conditions. Science 1998;279:381–384.
21 Singh RK, Berry K, Matsushima K, Yasumoto K, Fidler IJ: Synergism between human monocyte chemotactic and activating factor and bacterial products for activation of tumoricidal properties in murine macrophages. J Immunol 1993;151:2786–2793.
22 Huang S, Singh RK, Xie K, Gutman M, Berry KK, Bucana CD, Fidler IJ, Bar-Eli M: Expression of the JE/MCP-1 gene suppresses metastatic potential in murine colon carcinoma cells. Cancer Immunol Immunother 1994;39:231–238.
23 Charo IF, Myers SJ, Herman A, Franci C, Connolly AJ, Coughlin SR: Molecular cloning and functional expression of two monocyte chemoattractant protein 1 receptors reveals alternative splicing of the carboxyl-terminal tails. Proc Natl Acad Sci USA 1994;91:2752–2756
24 Sozzani S, Luini W, Molino M, Jilek P, Bottazzi B, Cerletti C, Matsushima K, Mantovani A: The signal transduction pathway involved in the migration induced by a monocyte chemotactic cytokine. J Immunol 1991;147:2215–2221.
25 Sozzani S, Molino M, Locati M, Luini W, Cerletti C, Vecchi A, Mantovani A: Receptor-activated calcium influx in human monocytes exposed to monocyte chemotactic protein-1 and related cytokines. J Immunol 1993;150:1544–1553.
26 Myers SJ, Wong LM, Charo IF: Signal transduction and ligand specificity of the human monocyte chemoattractant protein-1 receptor in transfected embryonic kidney cells. J Biol Chem 1995;270:5786–5792.
27 Locati M, Lamorte G, Luini W, Introna M, Bernasconi S, Mantovani A, Sozzani S: Inhibition of monocyte chemotaxis to C-C chemokines by antisense oligonucleotide for cytosolic phospholipase A_2. J Biol Chem 1996;271:6010–6016.
28 Dubois PM, Palmer D, Webb ML, Ledbetter JA, Shapiro RA: Early signal transduction by the receptor to the chemokine monocyte chemoattractant protein-1 in a murine T cell hybrid. J Immunol 1996;156:1356–1361.
29 Yen H, Penfold S, Zhang Y, Rollins BJ: MCP-1-mediated chemotaxis requires activation of non-overlapping signal transduction pathways. J Leukoc Biol 1997;61:529–532.
30 Hawes BE, van Biesen T, Koch WJ, Luttrell LM, Lefkowitz RJ: Distinct pathways of Gi- and Gq-mediated mitogen-activated protein kinase activation. J Biol Chem 1995;270:17148–17153.

31 Van Biesen T, Hawes BE, Raymond JR, Luttrell LM, Koch WJ, Lefkowitz RJ: G_o-protein α-subunits activate mitogen-activated protein kinase via a novel protein kinase C-dependent mechanism. J Biol Chem 1996;271:1266–1269.

32 Rollins BJ, Morton CC, Ledbetter DH, Eddy RL, Shows TB: Assignment of the human small inducible cytokine A2 gene, SCYA2 (encoding JE or MCP-1) to 17q11.2-12: Evolutionary relatedness of cytokines clustered at the same locus. Genomics 1991;10:489–492.

33 Mehrabian M, Sparkes RS, Mohandas T, Fogelman AM, Lusis AJ: Localization of monocyte chemotactic protein-1 gene (SCYA2) to human chromosome 17q11.2-q21.1. Genomics 1991;9:200–203.

34 Jiang Y, Valente AJ, Williamson MJ, Zhang L, Graves DT: Post-translational modification of a monocyte-specific chemoattractant synthesized by glioma, osteosarcoma, and vascular smooth muscle cells. J Biol Chem 1990;265:18318–18321.

35 Hendel TM, Domaille PJ: Heteronuclear (1H, 13C, 15N) NMR assignments and solution structure of the monocyte chemoattractant protein-1 (MCP-1) dimer. Biochemistry 1996;35:6569–6584.

36 Lubkowski J, Bujacz G, Boque L, Domaille PJ, Handel TM, Wlodawer A: The structure of MCP-1 in two crystal forms provides a rare example of variable quaternary interactions. Nat Struct Biol 1997; 4:64–69.

37 Zhang YJ, Rutledge BJ, Rollins BJ: Structure/activity analysis of human monocyte chemoattractant protein-1 (MCP-1) by mutagenesis: Identification of a mutated protein that inhibits MCP-1-mediated monocyte chemotaxis. J Biol Chem 1994;269:15918–15924.

38 Gong JH, Clark-Lewis I: Antagonists of monocyte chemoattractant protein 1 identified by modification of functionally critical NH_2-terminal residues. J Exp Med 1995;181:631–640.

39 Zhang Y, Rollins BJ: A dominant negative inhibitor indicates that monocyte chemoattractant protein 1 functions as a dimer. Mol Cell Biol 1995;15:4851–4855.

40 Beall CJ, Mahajan S, Kolattukudy PE: Conversion of monocyte chemoattractant protein-1 into a neutrophil attractant by substitution of two amino acids. J Biol Chem 1992;267:3455–3459.

41 Beall CJ, Mahajan S, Kuhn DE, Kolattukudy PE: Site-directed mutagenesis of monocyte chemoattractant protein-1 identifies two regions of the polypeptide essential for biological activity. Biochem J 1996;313:633–640.

42 Webb LMC, Ehrengruber MU, Clark-Lewis I, Baggiolini M, Rot A: Binding to heparan sulfate or heparin enhances neutrophil responses to interleukin-8. Proc Natl Acad Sci USA 1993;90:7158–7162.

43 Ernst CA, Zhang YJ, Hancock PR, Rutledge BJ, Corless CL, Rollins BJ: Biochemical and biological characterization of murine MCP-1: Identification of two functional domains. J Immunol 1994;152: 3541–3549.

44 Jia GQ, Gonzalo JA, Lloyd C, Kremer L, Lu L, Martinez AC, Wershil BK, Guttierez-Ramos JC: Distinct expression and function of the novel mouse chemokine monocyte chemotactic protein-5 in lung allergic inflammation. J Exp Med 1996;184:1939–1951.

45 Sarafi MN, Garcia-Zepeda EA, MacLean JA, Charo IF, Luster AD: Murine monocyte chemoattractant protein (MCP)-5: A novel CC chemokine that is a structural and functional homologue of human MCP-1. J Exp Med 1997;185:99–109.

46 Zachariae COC, Anderson AO, Thompson HL, Appella E, Mantovani A, Oppenheim JJ, Matsushima K: Properties of monocyte chemotactic and activating factor purified from a human fibrosarcoma cell line. J Exp Med 1990;171:2177–2182.

47 Van Damme J, Proost P, Lenaerts JP, Opdenakker G: Structural and functional identification of two human, tumor-derived monocyte chemotactic proteins (MCP-2 and MCP-3) belonging to the chemokine family. J Exp Med 1992;176:59–65.

48 Rutledge BJ, Rayburn H, Rosenberg R, North RJ, Gladue RP, Corless CL, Rollins BJ: High level monocyte chemoattractant protein-1 expression in transgenic mice increases their susceptibility to intracellular pathogens. J Immunol 1995;155:4838–4843.

49 Fuentes ME, Durham SK, Swerdel MR, Lewin AC, Barton DS, Megill JR, Bravo R, Lira SA: Controlled recruitment of monocytes/macrophages to specific organs through transgenic expression of MCP-1. J Immunol 1995;155:5769–5776.

50 Nakamura K, Williams IR, Kupper TS: Keratinocyte-derived monocyte chemoattractant protein 1 (MCP-1): Analysis in a transgenic model demonstrates MCP-1 can recruit dendritic and Langerhans' cells to skin. J Invest Dermatol 1995;105:635–643.

51 Xu LL, Warren MK, Rose WL, Gong W, Wang JM: Human recombinant monocyte chemotactic protein and other C-C chemokines bind and induce directional migration of dendritic cells in vitro. J Leuk Biol 1996;60:365–371.
52 Gunn MD, Nelken NA, Liao X, Williams LT: Monocyte chemoattractant protein-1 is sufficient for the chemotaxis of monocytes and lymphocytes in transgenic mice but requires an additional stimulus for inflammatory activation. J Immunol 1997;158:376–382.
53 Grewal IS, Rutledge BJ, Fiorillo JA, Gu L, Gladue RP, Flavell RA, Rollins BJ: Transgenic monocyte chemoattractant protein-1 (MCP-1) in pancreatic islets produces monocyte-rich insulitis without diabetes: Abrogation by a second transgene expressing systemic MCP-1. J Immunol 1997;159:401–408.
54 Hechtman DH, Cybulsky MI, Fuchs HJ, Baker JB, Gimbrone MA: Intravascular IL-8: Inhibitor of polymorphonuclear leukocyte accumulation at sites of acute inflammation. J Immunol 1991;147: 883–892.
55 Kolattukudy PE, Quach T, Bergese S, Breckenridge S, Hensley J, Altschuld R, Gordillo G, Klenotic S, Orosz C, Parker-Thornburg J: Myocarditis induced by targeted expression of the MCP-1 gene in murine cardiac muscle. Am J Pathol 1998;152:101–111.
56 Virchow R: Die krankhaften Geschwülste. Dreissig Vorlesungen, gehalten während des Wintersemesters 1862–1863 an der Universität zu Berlin. Vorlesungen über Pathologie. Berlin, Verlag von August Hirschwald, 1863.
57 Bashford EF, Murray JA, Cramer W: The growth of cancer under natural and experimental conditions. Sci Rep Invest. ICRF, 1905.
58 Ehrlich P: Experimentelle Studien an Maustumoren. Z Krebsforsch 1907;5:59–81.
59 Mantovani A, Bottazzi B, Colotta F, Sozzani S, Ruco L: The origin and function of tumor-associated macrophages. Immunol Today 1992;13:265–270.
60 Prehn RT: The immune reaction as a stimulator of tumor growth. Science 1972 176:170–171.
61 Eccles SA, Alexander P: Macrophage content of tumors in relation to metastatic spread and host immune reaction. Nature 1974;250:667–669.
62 Black MM, Opler SR, Speer FD: Survival in breast cancer cases in relation to the structure of the primary tumor and regional lymph nodes. Surg Gynecol Obstet 1955;100:543–551.
63 Takahashi K: Squamous cell carcinoma of the esophagus. Stromal inflammatory cell infiltration as a prognostic factor. Cancer 1961;14:921–933.
64 Leek RD, Lewis CE, Whitehouse R, Greenall M, Clarke J, Harris AL: Association of macrophage infiltration with angiogenesis and prognosis in invasive breast carcinoma. Cancer Res 1996;56 4625–4629.
65 Bottazzi B, Polentarutti N, Acero R, Balsari A, Boraschi D, Ghezzi P, Salmona M, Mantovani A Regulation of the macrophage content of neoplasms by chemoattractant. Science 1983 220:210–212
66 Bottazzi B, Ghezzi P, Taraboletti G, Salmona M, Colombo N, Bonazzi C, Mangioni C, Mantovani A: Tumor-derived chemotactic factor(s) from human ovarian carcinoma: Evidence for a role in the regulation of macrophage content of neoplastic tissues. Int J Cancer 1985;36:167–173.
67 Graves DT, Jiang YL, Williamson MJ, Valente AJ: Identification of monocyte chemotactic activity produced by malignant cells. Science 1989;245:1490–1493.
68 Bottazzi B, Colotta F, Sica A, Nobili N, Mantovani A: A chemoattractant expressed in human sarcoma cells (tumor-derived chemotactic factor) is identical to monocyte chemoattractant protein-1/monocyte chemotactic and activating factor. Int J Cancer 1990;45:795–797.
69 Rollins BJ, Sunday ME: Suppression of tumor formation in vivo by expression of the *JE* gene in malignant cells. Mol Cell Biol 1991;11:3125–3131.
70 Walter S, Bottazzi B, Govoni D, Colotta F, Mantovani A: Macrophage infiltration and growth of sarcoma clones expressing different amounts of monocyte chemotactic protein/JE. Int J Cancer 1991;49:431–435.
71 Bottazzi B, Walter S, Govoni D, Colotta F, Mantovani A: Monocyte chemotactic cytokine gene transfer modulates macrophage infiltration, growth, and susceptibility to IL-2 therapy of a murine melanoma. J Immunol 1992;148:1280–1285.
72 Yamashira S, Takeya M, Nishi T, Kuratsu J, Yoshimura T, Ushio Y, Takahashi K: Tumor-derived monocyte chemoattractant protein-1 induces intratumoral infiltration of monocyte-derived macrophage subpopulation in transplanted rat tumors. Am J Pathol 1994;145:856–867.

73 Negus RP, Stamp GW, Hadley J, Balkwill FR: Quantitative assessment of the leukocyte infiltrate in ovarian cancer and its relationship to the expression of C-C chemokines. Am J Pathol 1997;150: 1723–1734.

74 Manome Y, Wen PY, Hershowitz A, Tanaka T, Rollins BJ, Kufe DW, Fine HA: Monocyte chemoattractant protein-1 gene transduction: An effective tumor vaccine strategy for non-intracranial tumors. Cancer Immunol Immunother 1995;41:227–235.

75 Dizon QS, Southam CM: Abnormal cellular response to skin abrasion in cancer patients. Cancer 1963;16:1288–1292.

76 Goldsmith HS, Levin AG, Southam CM: A study of cellular responses in cancer patients by qualitative and quantitative Rebuck tests. Surg Forum 1965;16:102–104.

77 Boetcher DA, Leonard EJ: Abnormal monocyte chemotactic response in cancer patients. J Natl Cancer Inst 1974;52:1091–1099.

78 Snyderman R, Pike MC, Meadows L, Hemstreet G, Wells S: Depression of monocyte chemotaxis by neoplasia. Clin Res 1975;34:297A.

79 Normann SJ, Sorkin E: Inhibition of macrophage chemotaxis by neoplastic and other rapidly proliferating cells in vitro. Cancer Res 1977;37:705–711.

80 Jones ML, Mulligan MS, Flory CM, Ward PA, Warren JS: Potential role of monocyte chemoattractant protein 1/JE in monocyte/macrophage-dependent IgA immune complex alveolitis in the rat. J Immunol 1992;149:2147–2154.

81 Flory CM, Jones ML, Warren JS: Pulmonary granuloma formation in the rat is partially dependent on monocyte chemoattractant protein 1. Lab Invest 1993;69:396–404.

82 Fujinaka H, Yamamoto T, Takeya M, Feng L, Kawasaki K, yaoita E, Kondo D, Wilson CB, Uchiyama M, Kihara I: Suppression of anti-glomerular basement membrane nephritis by administration of anti-monocyte chemoattractant protein-1 antibody in WKY rats. J Am Soc Nephrol 1997;8:1174–1178.

83 Lloyd CM, Minto AW, Dorf ME, Proudfoot A, Wells TN, Salant DJ, Gutierrez-Ramos JC: RANTES and monocyte chemoattractant protein-1 (MCP-1) play an important role in the inflammatory phase of crescentic nephritis, but only MCP-1 is involved in crescent formation and interstitial fibrosis. J Exp Med 1997;185:1371–1380.

84 Tang WW, Qi M, Warren JS: Monocyte chemoattractant protein 1 mediates glomerular macrophage infiltration in anti-GBM Ab GN. Kidney Int 1996;50:665–671.

85 Wada T, Yokoyama H, Furuichi K, Kobayashi KI, Harada K, Naruto M, Su SB, Akiyama M, Mukaida N, Matsushima K: Intervention of crescentic glomerulonephritis by antibodies to monocyte chemotactic and activating factor (MCAF/MCP-1). FASEB J 1996;10:1418–1425.

86 Wenzel U, Schneider A, Valente AJ, Abboud HE, Thaiss F, Helmchen UM, Stahl RA: Monocyte chemoattractant protein-1 mediates monocyte/macrophage influx in anti-thymocyte antibody-induced glomerulonephritis. Kidney Int 1997;51:770–776.

87 Lu B, Rutledge BJ, Gu L, Fiorillo J, Lukacs NW, Kunkel SL, North R, Gerard C, Rollins BJ: Abnormalities in monocyte recruitment and cytokine expression in monocyte chemoattractant protein 1-deficient mice. J Exp Med 1998;187:601–608.

88 Boring L, Gosling J, Chensue SW, Kunkel SL, Farese RVJ, Broxmeyer HE, Charo IF: Impaired monocyte migration and reduced type 1 (Th1) cytokine responses in C-C chemokine receptor 2 knockout mice. J Clin Invest 1997;100:2552–2561.

89 Kurihara T, Warr G, Loy J, Bravo R: Defects in macrophage recruitment and host defense in mice lacking the CCR2 chemokine receptor. J Exp Med 1997;186:1757–1762.

90 Kuziel WA, Morgan SJ, Dawson TC, Griffin S, Smithies O, Ley K, Maeda N: Severe reduction in leukocyte adhesion and monocyte extravasation in mice deficient in CC chemokine receptor 2. Proc Natl Acad Sci USA 1997;94:12053–12058.

91 Karpus WJ, Lukacs NW, Kennedy KJ, Smith WS, Hurst SD, Barrett TA: Differential CC chemokine-induced enhancement of T-helper cell cytokine production. J Immunol 1997;158:4129–4136.

92 Chensue SW, Warmington KS, Lukacs NW, Lincoln PM, Burdick MD, Strieter RM, Kunkel SL: Monocyte chemotactic protein expression during schistosome egg granuloma formation. Sequence of production, localization, contribution, and regulation. Am J Pathol 1995;146:130–138.

93 Rollins BJ, Pober JS: Interleukin-4 induces the synthesis and secretion of MCP-1/JE by human endothelial cells. Am J Pathol 1991;138:1315–1319.

94 Strieter RM, Wiggins R, Phan SH, Wharram BL, Showell HJ, Remick DG, Chensue SW, Kunkel SL: Monocyte chemotactic protein gene expression by cytokine-treated human fibroblasts and endothelial cells. Biochem Biophys Res Commun 1989;162:694–700.
95 Taubman MB, Rollins BJ, Poon M, Marmur J, Green RS, Berk BC, Nadal-Ginard B: *JE* mRNA accumulates rapidly in aortic injury and in PDGF-stimulated vascular smooth muscle cells. Circ Res 1992;70:314–325.
96 Cushing SD, Berliner JA, Valente AJ, Territo MC, Navab M, Parhami F, Gerrity R, Schwartz CJ, Fogelman AM: Minimally modified low density lipoprotein induces monocyte chemotactic protein 1 in human endothelial cells and smooth muscle cells. Proc Natl Acad Sci USA 1990;87:5134–5138.
97 Yu X, Dluz S, Graves DT, Zhang L, Antoniades HN, Hollander W, Prusty S, Valente AJ, Schwartz CJ, Sonenshein GE: Elevated expression of monocyte chemoattractant protein 1 by vascular smooth muscle cells in hypercholesterolemic primates. Proc Natl Acad Sci USA 1992;89:6953–6957.
98 Capers Q IV, Alexander RW, Lou P, De Leon H, Wilcox JN, Ishizaka N, Howard AB, Taylor WR: Monocyte chemoattractant protein-1 expression in aortic tissues of hypertensive rats. Hypertension 1997;30:1397–1402.
99 Nelken NA, Coughlin SR, Gordon D, Wilcox JN: Monocyte chemoattractant protein-1 in human atheromatous plaques. J Clin Invest 1991;88:1121–1127.
100 Gu L, Okada Y, Clinton SK, Gerard C, Sukhova GK, Libby P, Rollins BJ: Absence of monocyte chemoattractant protein-1 reduces atherosclerosis in low density lipoprotein receptor-deficient mice. Mol Cell 1998;2:275–281.
101 Boring L, Gosling J, Cleary M, Charo IF: Decreased lesion formation in $CCR2^{-/-}$ mice reveals a role for chemokines in the initiation of atherosclerosis. Nature 1998;394:894–897.

B. J. Rollins, Dana-Farber Cancer Institute, Department of Medical Oncology,
Bldg. D930, 44 Binney Street, Boston, MA 02115 (USA)
Tel. +1 617 632 3896, Fax +1 617 632 5417, E-Mail Barrett_Rollins@macmailgw.dfci.harvard.edu

Mantovani A (ed): Chemokines.
Chem Immunol. Basel, Karger, 1999, vol 72, pp 30–41

CCR2: From Cloning to the Creation of Knockout Mice

Israel F. Charo

Gladstone Institute of Cardiovascular Disease, San Francisco, Calif., and
Cardiovascular Research Institute, Department of Medicine,
University of California, San Francisco, Calif., USA

In this chapter, the author reviews the current state of knowledge concerning the structural and signaling properties of CCR2. Evidence for important roles for this receptor in human disease based on recent in vivo studies in knockout mice will also be discussed.

Identification and Molecular Cloning of the Receptor

CCR2 is the receptor for MCP-1 as well as for several other members of the 'MCP' family of CC chemokines. By way of brief introduction, MCP-1 was first identified as a monocyte chemotactic factor in medium conditioned by baboon smooth muscle cells and human glioma cells [for a recent review, see 1a]. Amino acid sequencing revealed that it was identical to the predicted sequence of human *JE*, previously cloned as a platelet-derived, growth factor-inducible gene. MCP-1 is a potent agonist for monocytes and memory-type T cells and induces histamine release from basophils. It does not attract or activate eosinophils or neutrophils.

To begin to understand the mechanisms whereby MCP-1 activates mononuclear cells, we initiated an effort to clone the MCP-1 receptor. The receptor for MCP-1, and indeed all of the cloned receptors for chemokines, are members of the superfamily of G-protein-coupled receptors. Our efforts resulted in the cloning of two forms of this receptor, originally designated MCP-1RA and MCP-1RB, which when expressed in *Xenopus* oocytes mediated release of calcium in response to MCP-1 [1]. The presence of mRNA for these receptors

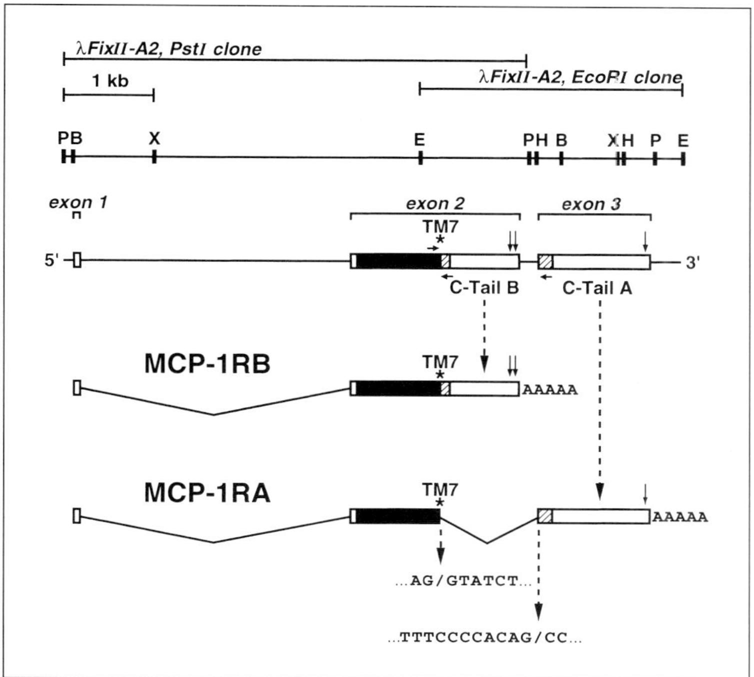

Fig. 1. Organization of the MCP-1 receptor (CCR2) gene.

correlated with the ability of leukocytes to signal in response to MCP-1. More recent studies have confirmed that CCR2 is specific for members of the 'MCP' chemokines: MCP-1, MCP-3, MCP-4, and MCP-5 [2–4].

Comparison of the deduced amino acid sequence of the MCP-1 receptor with other 7-transmembrane proteins revealed that it was most closely related to the MIP1α/RANTES receptor (CCR1) with 51% amino acid identity, but had converged considerably in the amino-terminal domain. A striking identity between CCR2 and CCR1 was also noted in second intracellular loop (the sequence DRYLAIVHAV), in a region known to participate in G-protein binding [5]. The amino acid sequences of CCR2A and CCR2B differed only in their putative carboxyl tails, which suggested that they might be splice variants of a single gene. Further work confirmed this hypothesis and revealed that both isoforms of the receptor were encoded in three exons spanning approximately 7 kb of genomic sequence (fig. 1) [6]. Whereas exon 1 encodes part of the 5′ untranslated region (UTR) of both receptor isoforms, exon 2 encodes the entire open reading frame and the 3′ UTR of CCR2B. Exon 3, on the other hand, codes for only the carboxyl tail and the 3′ UTR of CCR2A. Therefore, both isoforms share a common 5′ end composed of exon 1 and the 5′ half of exon 2, but differ in their carboxyl tails and 3′ UTRs. In the CCR2 gene, if exon 2 polyadenylation signals are recognized, then cleavage and polyadenylation would be expected to produce CCR2B transcripts. However, if these signals are not recognized, mRNA synthesis would continue through exon 3, thereby providing the 3′ acceptor site necessary for the splicing and synthesis of CCR2A mRNA. In this case, full-length pre-mRNA encoding both carboxyl-tail and 3′ UTR isoforms would be synthesized, and any expression of the CCR2 isoform would be predominantly regulated by the degree of splicing of these pre-mRNAs.

We examined the relative expression of CCR2A and CCR2B in monocytic cell lines and freshly isolated human monocyte/macrophages. CCR2B was readily detected in monocytic cell lines, as well as in freshly isolated human monocytes, whereas CCR2A was less abundant. To examine CCR2 expression in macrophages, human monocytes were maintained in culture for up to 7 days, during which time they differentiated into cells that morphologically resembled macrophages. Both CCR2A and CCR2B mRNA levels fell as the monocytes differentiated into macrophages.

We also noted significant differences in the cell-surface expression of CCR2A and CCR2B. In a number of different transfected cell types, including HEK-293 cells, fibroblasts, COS-7 cells, T cells, and basophilic cells, CCR2A was expressed at lower levels than CCR2B at the cell surface. When these cells were permeabilized, CCR2A was retained in the cytoplasm. Studies in which the carboxyl-terminal tails of CCR2A and CCR2B were exchanged confirmed that the amino acid sequences that signal cytoplasmic retention were contained within the carboxyl tail. Thus, the major form of CCR2 present on both primary and cultured cells examined to date is CCR2B. The physiological role of CCR2A remains unclear at this time.

Signaling and G-Protein Coupling

We investigated the signal transduction pathways activated by MCP-1 in a number of cell lines stably transfected with CCR2. In HEK-293 cells, MCP-1 induced a robust and dose-dependent increase in intracellular calcium (fig. 2); this increase was substantially but not completely blocked by pretreating the cells with pertussis toxin [7]. To identify pertussis toxin-resistant G proteins that coupled to CCR2, we performed cotransfection experiments in COS-7 and HEK-293 cells. The C-C chemokine receptors, but not the IL-8 or C5a receptor, coupled to Gαq [8]. Significantly, virtually all of the coupling could

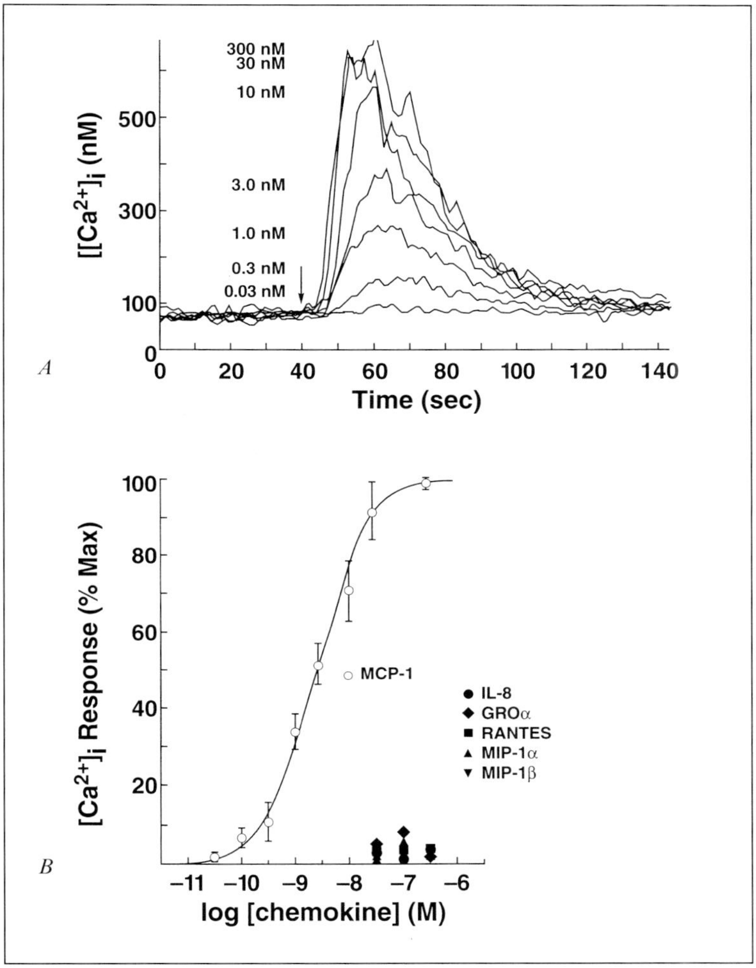

Fig. 2. A, B CCR2-mediated calcium mobilization.

be attributed to the third intracellular loop of the receptor [8]. The MCP-1 receptors, but not CCR1, coupled to Gα16 in COS-7 cells, but none of the C-C chemokine receptors coupled to Gα16 in HEK-293 cells. These results indicated important differences in coupling between the C-X-C and C-C chemokine receptors and further suggested that the spectrum of G proteins to which a chemokine receptor coupled was likely to be highly dependent on cell type.

Chemotaxis

Chemotaxis is the prototypic function of the chemokines, but the signal transduction pathways utilized to initiate directed cell migration are not well understood. Moreover, accurate tracking of changing chemokine gradients may require rapid modulation of signaling at the level of the receptor. To investigate these issues, we asked whether receptor deactivation is required for chemotaxis. Our earlier work had established that the carboxyl terminus of CCR2B plays an important role in both receptor deactivation and internalization [9], but it was unclear whether or not this domain of the receptor is important for chemotaxis. To answer this question, we created and analyzed a series of CCR2 mutants with carboxyl-tail truncations. We found that the 12 amino acids between CCR2-328 and CCR2-316 were critically involved in signal transduction, agonist-dependent internalization, and chemotaxis. Surprisingly, rapid deactivation of the receptor, either by agonist-induced phosphorylation of carboxyl-domain serine and threonine residues or by receptor internalization, was not required for chemotaxis [10]. This result was particularly interesting and, at face value, suggests that chemotaxis is not modulated at the level of the receptor. It should be emphasized, however, that a unidirectional chemotaxis assay was used for these experiments. Receptor deactivation may play a role in the directed migration of leukocytes in vivo, in which changes in cell direction are frequent.

To identify the G proteins critical for chemotaxis, we stably expressed CCR2 and prototypic Gαi- and Gαq-coupled receptors in 300-19 cells, an immortalized pre-B cell line [11]. Activation of Gαi, but not Gαq- or Gαs-coupled receptors, led to chemotaxis. Moreover, the large intracellular calcium flux typically seen in response to activation of serpentine receptors was not sufficient to cause chemotaxis. In addition, production of G protein βγ dimers, rather than activated Gαi, was required for chemotaxis. Gαi-coupled receptors not found on leukocytes or traditionally associated with the directed migration of cells, such as the κ opioid receptor, also mediated chemotaxis when expressed in a hematopoietic cell line. Our results support the hypothesis that activation of Gαi-coupled receptors and the subsequent release of Gβγ dimers are required to initiate signal transduction leading to directed cell migration. Athough the κ receptor mediated chemotaxis, it was clearly less efficient than the chemokine receptors. That is, the chemotactic index for 300-19 cells expressing the κ receptor was significantly lower than that of cells expressing CCR2. A reasonable interpretation of these data is that chemotaxis requires the generation of G protein βγ dimers and that cytoplasmic domains of the receptor help to optimize directed migration, perhaps by acting as a scaffold for the assembly of other signaling molecules.

CCR2 as an HIV-1 Coreceptor

The role of chemokines in disease has recently been greatly expanded by the discovery that chemokine receptors act as coreceptors for HIV-1 entry into cells. Work by many different laboratories has identified CCR5 and CXCR4 as the major coreceptors for macrophage-tropic and T-cell-tropic viruses, respectively. Although it is not one of the major coreceptors, CCR2B acts in vitro as a coreceptor for certain strains of HIV-1, particularly dual-tropic strains such as the virus 89.6 [12].

Recently, a genetic variant of CCR2 was found to correlate with disease progression in AIDS [13]. Smith et al. [13] reported a mutation that changes valine to isoleucine at amino acid 64 of CCR2 (CCR2-64I) and found that HIV-1-infected subjects carrying the CCR2-64I allele progressed to AIDS 2–4 years later than subjects homozygous for the wild-type allele. The CCR2-64I allele was found to occur invariably on a CCR5 wild-type allele.

The mechanism for the delayed progression is not clear. Lee et al. [14] examined the CCR264I mutation in some detail and found that this very conservative change in the first transmembrane domain does not affect CCR2 expression or signaling. Kostrikis et al. [15] confirmed the delayed disease progression in subjects with the CCR2-64I allele and found that this allele was associated with a point mutation in the CCR5 promoter, suggesting that the CCR264I mutation may be exerting its protective effect through expression of CCR5. However, Lee et al. [14] found similar levels of CCR5 in blood mononuclear cells from subjects heterozygous for the CCR2-64I allele or homozygous for the wild-type allele. The reason why the CCR2-64I allele delays AIDS progression is thus not clear at this time.

Creation of a CCR2 Knockout Mouse

To determine the role of MCP-1 and related family members in vivo, we used homologous recombination in embryonic stem cells to create mice with a targeted disruption of CCR2 [16]. The mice were viable, developed normally, and showed no overt morphological or behavioral defects. Examination of the hematopoietic system revealed no reduction in the number of myeloid progenitor cells or defects in the development of lymphocyte subsets. Although the mice exhibited no obvious phenotype in the unstressed state, exposure to both antigenic and nonantigenic challenges revealed significant defects in monocyte/macrophage recruitment and immunological responses, most notably a profound impairment in IFN-γ production. We concluded from these preliminary studies that activation of CCR2 by MCP-1 and related chemokines is critically involved in macrophage accumulation at sites of inflammation, as well as in modulating the immune response and cyokine production.

Using an antigen-dependent model of lung inflammation, we found that CCR2 played a role in both granuloma induction and modulation of the immune response. In *CCR2–/–* mice, lung granulomas induced by purified protein derivative (PPD) were significantly smaller 4 days after challenge, and this reduction was preceded by a selective decrease in the macrophage component of the granuloma on day 2. This result provided further evidence that CCR2 participates in the recruitment of monocyte/macrophages to regions of inflammation. PPD bead challenge also resulted in a marked monocytosis in wild-type mice but not in the *CCR2–/–* mice. These data suggested that antigen-induced monocyte recruitment into the circulation, like nonantigenic recruitment into the peritoneum, is highly dependent on activation of CCR2.

Lung granulomas induced by *Mycobacterium bovis* PPD are characterized by a Th1 (IL-2, IFN-γ) cytokine response [17, 18]. In the absence of CCR2, IFN-γ production decreased dramatically after PPD challenge. At least two lines of evidence demonstrate that CCR2 is necessary for robust IFN-γ production in PPD-challenged mice. First, examination of cytokine profiles of draining lymph node cells revealed no increase in IFN-γ production in *CCR2–/–* mice, but showed a large, time-dependent increase in this cytokine in wild-type mice. Second, purified T cells from PPD-sensitized *CCR2–/–* mice had a marked reduction in PPD-induced IFN-γ production and a less marked reduction in IL-2. This defect was not corrected by inclusion of wild-type APCs. Thus, the genotype of the T cells, rather than the APCs, is critical in mediating upregulation of IFN-γ. These data show that *CCR2–/–* mice have defects in macrophage recruitment and in the development of a Th1-type response.

Two other groups have independently created and reported on CCR2 knockout mice. Kuziel et al. [19] and Kurihara et al. [20] also noted decreases in macrophage accumulation in the peritoneum after injection of thioglycollate. In addition, Kuziel et al. [19] found a decrease in granulomas in the liver parenchyma after intravenous injection of yeast β-glucan, and Kurihara et al. [30] found that CCR2-deficient mice were unable to clear infection by the bacteria *Listeria monocytogenes.* Taken together with the studies cited above, these data provide strong evidence for an important and nonredundant role for MCP-1 in host defense and cytokine production.

CCR2 in Atherosclerosis

The arterial fatty streak is composed of lipid-laden macrophages (foam cells) and is the precursor of more complex and dangerous lesions. Morpho-

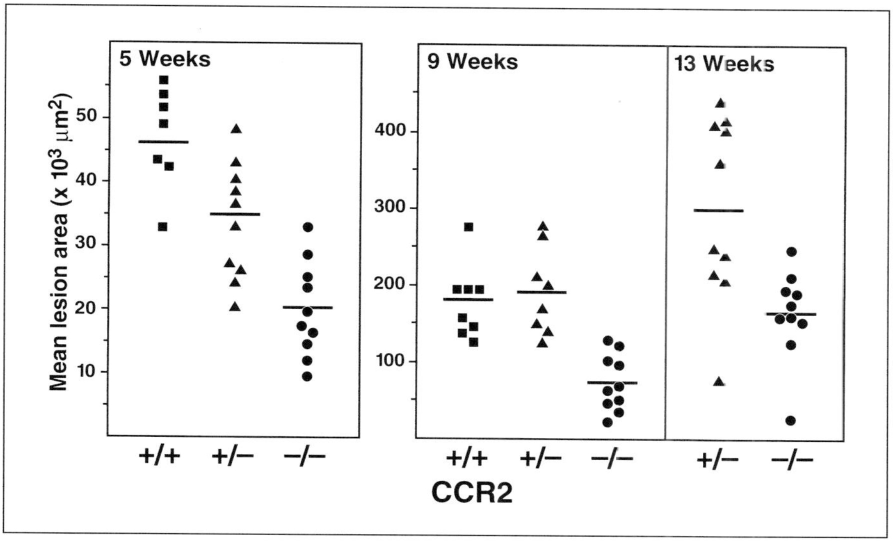

Fig. 3. Reduced atherosclerotic lesion size in *CCR2–/–* mice.

logical studies in swine and nonhuman primates have suggested that circulating monocytes are the precursors of foam cells, but the molecular signals that initiate monocyte recruitment to the vessel wall are not well understood. To determine if MCP-1 or related CCR2 agonists are important in macrophage recruitment and foam cell formation in vivo, we utilized the *CCR2–/–* mice, which, as noted above, have profound defects in macrophage recruitment in response to inflammatory stimuli. Because mice do not develop robust atherosclerosis, we crossed the *CCR2–/–* mice with mice deficient in apolipoprotein E (apoE) to place the CCR2 mutation onto an atherogenic background. ApoE-null mice have high plasma cholesterol levels and develop progressive atherosclerotic lesions that mimic human disease [21, 22]. Lesion progression and severity are further enhanced by feeding these mice a diet rich in cholesterol and saturated fat (Western diet). The double-knockout (*apoE–/–CCR2–/–*) mice were born at the expected mendelian ratios, developed normally, and were disease-free while maintained in a pathogen-free environment.

To examine early fatty-streak lesions for the presence of macrophages, we stained aortic root sections with MOMA2, a macrophage-specific antibody. Macrophages were abundant in *CCR2+/+apoE–/–* mice fed the high-fat diet for as little as 5 weeks and were the most abundant cell population in the lesion. In contrast, markedly fewer macrophages were present in sections from the same level in *CCR2–/–* mice [23]. These data indicated that activation of

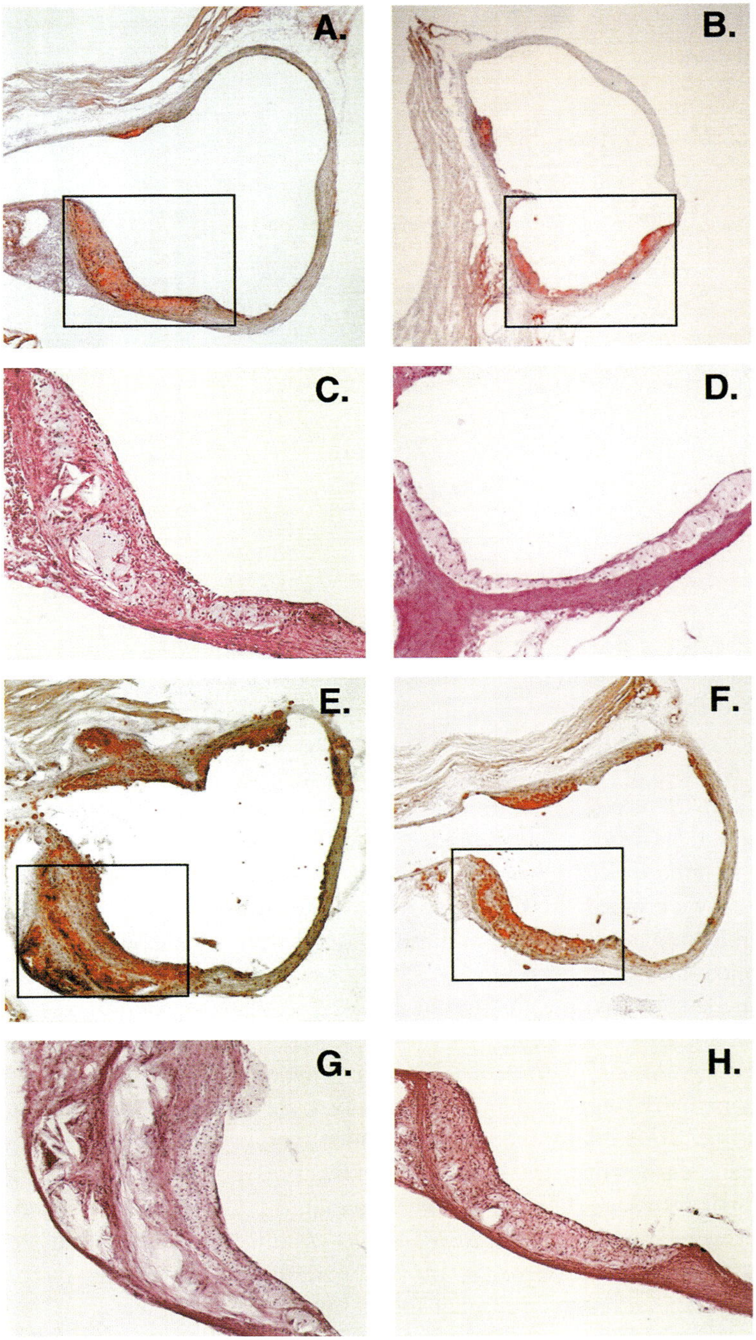
A.
B.
C.
D.
E.
F.
G.
H.

CCR2 is important in monocyte/macrophage recruitment to the vessel wall. We next asked whether the reduced macrophage content would diminish or delay the formation of fatty streaks, the earliest recognizable sign of atherosclerosis. To address this question, we studied mice fed on the Western diet for up to 13 weeks. Atherosclerotic lesion size was quantitated by staining serial sections through the aortic root with Oil Red O. At each of three time points, the *CCR2–/–* mice had significantly smaller lesions than the *CCR2+/+* or *CCR2+/–* mice (fig. 3). Analysis of sections through the proximal aorta revealed that whereas lesions size was greatest between the valve leaflets and coronary arteries in the *CCR2+/+* mice, lesion area was uniformly low at all points in the *CCR2–/–* mice. Analysis of the lipoprotein and lipid profiles of these animals confirmed that the absence of CCR2 had no effect on total cholesterol lelvels, plasma triglycerides, or the distribution of lipoprotein particles in the plasma.

Representative sections from mice fed on the Western diet for 9 and 13 weeks are shown in figure 4. At 9 weeks, *CCR2+/+* mice frequently had developing lesions (fig. 4A). Staining with hematoxylin and eosin revealed an abundance of foam cell macrophages, the beginning of fibrous caps, and evidence of cholesterol clefts (fig. 4B). In contrast, the *CCR2–/–* mice had smaller lesions composed almost exclusively of foam cells (fig. 4C, D). At 13 weeks, *CCR2+/+* mice had large, raised multifocal lesions that were intensely Oil Red O positive, with evidence of possible necrosis (fig. 4E, F). The *CCR2–/–* mice had smaller and generally less complex lesions (fig. G, H). These data suggest that the decreased recruitment of macrophages at 5 weeks results in delayed lesion development at the later time points.

Next, we examined lesion development along the entire aorta. Whole-mount, *en face* preparations were stained with Sudan IV, and lesion area was quantitated by digital morphometry. In mice on the Western diet for 5 or 9 weeks, < 1% of the entire aorta was covered with lesions, and no significant differences between the CCR2 genotypes were observed (data not shown). At 13 weeks, however, lesions covered 5.1% of the aorta in the *CCR2+/–* mice but only 2.9% in the *CCR–/–* mice. Thus, *CCR2–/–* mice had approximately a 50% reduction in total aortic lesion area. Very similar results were reported by Gu et al. [24], who crossed MCP-1 knockout mice with low-density lipoprotein receptor knockout mice. Thus, absence of either MCP-1 or its receptor, CCR2, dramatically reduces atheroma formation in mice genetically modified to develop atherosclerosis.

Fig. 4. Lesion histology in *CCR2–/–* versus *CCR2+/+* mice. Aortic cross sections from *CCR2+/+* (*A, C, E, G*) or *CCR2–/–* (*B, D, F, H*) mice were stained with hematoxylin and eosin (*C, D, G, H*) or Oil Red O (*A, B, E, F*).

Concluding Remarks

The past several years have witnessed rapid advances in our understanding of the biology of monocyte recruitment to sites of inflammation and injury. MCP-1 has been identified as an extremely potent monocyte chemoattractant, and its receptor, CCR2, has been cloned and characterized in some detail. The availability of mice genetically altered to be deficient in specific chemokines or chemokine receptors has provided us with very powerful tools to probe the biology of this family of cytokines. With regard to CCR2, the available data support an important role for MCP-1 in the development of early atherosclerotic lesions and in T-cell polarization. Studies are currently in progress to further define the role of MCP-1/CCR2 in these important settings.

References

1a Rollins BJ: Chemokines. Blood 1997;90:909–928.

1 Charo IF, Myers SJ, Herman A, Franci C, Connolly AJ, Coughlin SR: Molecular cloning and functional expression of two monocyte chemoattractant protein 1 receptors reveals alternative splicing of the carboxyl-terminal tails. Proc Natl Acad Sci USA 1994;91:2752–2756.

2 Franci C, Wong LM, Van Damme J, Proost P, Charo IF: Monocyte chemoattractant protein-3, but not monocyte chemoattractant protein-2, is a functional ligand of the human monocyte chemoattractant protein-1 receptor. J Immunol 1995;154:6511–6517.

3 Sarafi MN, Garcia-Zepeda EA, MacLean JA, Charo IF, Luster AD: Murine monocyte chemoattractant protein (MCP)-5: A novel CC chemokine that is a structural and functional homologue of human MCP-1. J Exp Med 1997;185:99–109.

4 Berkhout TA, Sarau HM, Moores K, White JR, Elshourbagy N, Appelbaum E, Reape RJ, Brawner M, Makwana J, Foley JJ, Schmidt DB, Imburgia C, McNulty D, Matthews J, O'Donnell K, O'Shannessy D, Scott M, Groot PHE, Macphee C: Cloning, in vitro expression, and functional characterization of a novel human CC chemokine of the monocyte chemotactic protein (MCP) family (MCP-4) that binds and signals through the CC chemokine receptor 2B. J Biol Chem 1997;272:16404–16413.

5 Namba T, Sugimoto Y, Negishi M, Irie A, Ushikubi F, Kakizuka A, Ito S, Ichikawa A, Narumiya S: Alternative splicing of C-terminal tail of prostaglandin E receptor subtype EP3 determines G-protein specificity. Nature 1993;365:166–170.

6 Wong LM, Myers SJ, Tsou CL, Gosling J, Arai H, Charo IF: Organization and differential expression of the human monocyte chemoattractant protein 1 receptor gene. Evidence for the role of the carboxyl-terminal tail in receptor trafficking. J Biol Chem 1997;272:1038–1045.

7 Myers SJ, Wong LM, Charo IF: Signal transduction and ligand specificity of the human monocyte chemoaatractant protein-1 receptor in transfected embryonic kidney cells. J Biol Chem 1995;270: 5786–5792.

8 Arai H, Charo IF: Differential regulation of G-protein-mediated signaling by chemokine receptors. J Biol Chem 1996;271:21814–21819.

9 Franci C, Gosling J, Tsou CL, Coughlin SR, Charo IF: Phosphorylation by a G protein-coupled kinase inhibits signaling and promotes internalization of the monocyte chemoattractant protein-1 receptor. Critical role of carboxyl-tail serines/threonines in receptor function. J Immunol 1996;157:5606–5612.

10 Arai H, Monteclaro FS, Tsou CL, Franci C, Charo IF: Dissociation of chemotaxis from agonist-induced receptor internalization in a lymphocyte cell line transfected with CCR2B. Evidence that directed migration does not require rapid modulation of signaling at the receptor level. J Biol Chem 1997;272:25037–25042.

11 Arai H, Tsou CL, Charo IF: Chemotaxis in a lymphocyte cell line transfected with C-C chemokine receptor 2B: Evidence that directed migration is mediated by βγ dimers released by activation of $G_{\alpha i}$-coupled receptors. Proc Natl Acad Sci USA 1997;94:14495–14499.
12 Doranz BJ, Rucker J, Yi Y, Smyth RJ, Samson M, Peiper SC, Parmentier M, Collman RG, Doms RW: A dual-tropic primary HIV-1 isolate that uses fusin and the β-chemokine receptors CKR-5, CKR-3, and CKR-2b as fusion cofactors. Cell 1996;85:1149–1158.
13 Smith MW, Dean M, Carrington M, Winkler C, Huttley GA, Lomb DA, Goedert JJ, O'Brien TR, Jacobson LP, Kaslow R, Buchbinder S, Vittinghoff E, Vlahov D, Hoots K, Hilgartner MW, Hemophilia Growth and Development Study (HGDS), Multicenter AIDS Cohort Study (MACS), Multicenter Hemophilia Cohort Study (MHCS), San Francisco City Cohort (SFCC) AS, O'Brien SJ: Contrasting genetic influence of *CCR2* and *CCR5* variants on HIV-1 infection and disease progression. Science 1997;15:959–965.
14 Lee B, Doranz BJ, Rana S, Yi Y, Mellado M, Frade JM, Martinez-A C, O'Brien SJ, Dean M, Collman RG, Doms RW: Influence of the CCR2-V64I polymorphism on human immunodeficiency virus type 1 coreceptor activity and on chemokine receptor function of CCR2b, CCR3, CCR5, and CXCR4. J Virol 1998;72:7450–7458.
15 Kostrikis LG, Huang Y, Moore JP, Wolinsky SM, Zhang L, Guo Y, Deutsch L, Phair J, Neumann AU, Ho DD: A chemokine receptor CCR2 allele delays HIV-1 disease progression and is asociated with a CCR5 promoter mutation. Nat Med 1998;4:350–353.
16 Boring L, Gosling J, Chensue SW, Kunkel SL, Farese RV Jr, Broxmeyer HE, Charo IF: Impaired monocyte migration and reduced type 1 (Th1) cytokine responses in C-C chemokine receptor 2 knockout mice. J Clin Invest 1997;100:2552–2561.
17 Chensue SW, Warmington K, Ruth J, Lincoln P, Kuo MC, Kunkel SL: Cytokine responses during mycobacterial and schistosomal antigen-induced pulmonary granuloma formation. Production of Th1 and Th2 cytokines and relative contribution of tumor necrosis factor. Am J Pathol 1994;145: 1105–1113.
18 Chensus SW, Warmington KS, Ruth JH, Lincoln P, Kunkel SL: Cytokine function during mycobacterial and schistosomal antigen-induced pulmonary granuloma formation. Local and regional participation of IFN-γ, IL-10, and TNF. J Immunol 1995;154:5969–5976.
19 Kuziel WA, Morgan SJ, Dawson TC, Griffin S, Smithies O, Ley K, Maeda N: Severe reduction in leukocyte adhesion and monocyte extravasation in mice deficient in CC chemokine receptor 2. Proc Natl Acad Sci USA 1997;94:12053–12058.
20 Kurihara T, Warr G, Loy J, Bravo R: Defects in macrophage recruitment and host defense in mice lacking the CCR2 chemokine receptor. J Exp Med 1997;186:1757–1762.
21 Zhang SH, Reddick RL, Piedrahita JA, Maeda N: Spontaneous hypercholesterolemia and arterial lesions in mice lacking apolipoprotein E. Science 1992;258:468–471.
22 Nakashima Y, Plump AS, Raines EW, Breslow JL, Ross R: ApoE-deficient mice develop lesions of all phases of atherosclerosis throughout the arterial tree. Arterioscler Thromb 1994;14:133–140.
23 Boring L, Gosling J, Cleary M, Charo IF: Decreased lesion formation in $CCR2^{-/-}$ mice reveals a role for chemokines in the initiation of atherosclerosis. Nature 1998;394:894–897.
24 Gu L, Okada Y, Clinton SK, Gerard C, Sukhova GK, Libby P, Rollins BJ: Absence of monocyte chemoattractant protein-1 reduces atherosclerosis in low density lipoprotein receptor-deficient mice. Mol Cell 1998;2:275–281.

Israel F. Charo, MD, PhD, Gladstone Institute of Cardiovascular Disease,
PO Box 419100, San Francisco, CA 94141-9100 (USA)
Tel. +1 415 826 7500, Fax +1 415 285 5632, E-Mail icharo@gladstone.ucsf.edu

Mantovani A (ed): Chemokines.
Chem Immunol. Basel, Karger, 1999, vol 72, pp 42–56

The Role of CD26/DPP IV in Chemokine Processing

Jo Van Damme[a], *Sofie Struyf*[a], *Anja Wuyts*[a], *Els Van Coillie*[a], *Patricia Menten*[a], *Dominique Schols*[b], *Silvano Sozzani*[c], *Ingrid De Meester*[d], *Paul Proost*[a]

Laboratories of
[a] Molecular Immunology and
[b] Experimental Chemotherapy, Rega Institute for Medical Research, University of Leuven, Belgium;
[c] Department of Immunology and Cell Biology, Istituto di Ricerche Farmacologiche 'Mario Negri', Milan, Italy, and
[d] Department of Clinical Biochemistry, University of Antwerp, Wilrijk, Belgium

Dipeptidyl-peptidase IV (DPP IV) identified as the activation antigen CD26 [1, 2] is expressed on the membrane of memory T lymphocytes, as well as on endothelial and epithelial cells. CD26/DPP IV is a pluripotent molecule which interferes with many immune functions both in vitro and in vivo. T-lymphocyte activation and signaling by CD26/DPP IV is not solely attributed to its proteolytic effect. In addition to its membrane-associated form, CD26/DPP IV is also present as a soluble exopeptidase in seminal fluid, urine and plasma. Indeed, this glycoprotein exerts peptidase activity through its extracellular domain. CD26/DPP IV has a unique aminopeptidase activity since it cleaves dipeptides from the NH_2-terminus of proteins having a Pro or Ala residue at the penultimate position. The presence of a Pro in the NH_2-terminal region protects proteins from proteolytic degradation by aminopeptidases [3]. Although several cytokines including interleukins (e.g. IL-1β, IL-2, IL-5, IL-6 and IL-10) and colony-stimulating factors (G-CSF, GM-CSF) are potential substrates, they are not processed by CD26/DPP IV [4]. The finding that the NH_2-terminal residues of these cytokines cannot be removed by CD26/DPP IV and that short natural substrates such as substance P are effectively processed, indicates that the size or the structural conformation of proteins is important [4]. This review describes the effects of CD26/DPP IV on a large group of small proinflammatory cytokines, i.e. the chemokines. For each individual chemoattractant the different biological consequences of processing by CD26/DPP IV are evaluated in comparison with the intact molecule. These examples clearly show that chemokines are important natural substrates for CD26/DPP IV and illustrate the impact of this serine protease in immunological processes.

Chemokines of both the CXC and CC subfamilies have been reported to naturally occur as posttranslationally modified isoforms. For example, two predominant isoforms of the neutrophil chemoattractant IL-8 have been described, which differ by an extension of five residues in the NH_2-terminal region [5]. Additional NH_2-terminally processed forms of natural IL-8 have been identified and a number of proteases, except CD26/DPP IV, are reported to be responsible for these truncations [6]. It was demonstrated that shortening the NH_2-terminal region of other neutrophil-specific CXC chemokines in front of the conserved ELR motif, increases the biological potency of these chemoattractants. A striking example is human neutrophil activating protein-2 (NAP-2) which is generated by proteolytic cleavage from its precursor platelet basic protein through a number of intermediates such as connective tissue activating peptide III and β-thromboglobulin [5, 7]. Remarkably, only NAP-2 (and not its precursors) has potent chemotactic activity for neutrophils. In contrast, four NH_2-terminally truncated forms of the human ELR-CXC chemokine granulocyte chemotactic protein-2 (GCP-2) have been purified from connective tissue cells, but no difference in chemotactic potency was observed [8]. For CC chemokines the picture is rather different. For example, deletion of a single NH_2-terminal residue from monocyte chemotactic protein-1 (MCP-1) results in a drastic reduction of its chemotactic potency [9]. In contrast, posttranslational removal of residues from the COOH-terminus implies less pronounced consequences for its biological activity. Indeed, natural human MCP-1 missing 7 COOH-terminal residues was found to be equally active as intact MCP-1 [10]. Finally, posttranslational modification of cytokines and chemokines by glycosylation has a moderate effect on their potency [11]. For example, naturally glycosylated 30 kDa mouse MCP-1 was found to be only 3-fold less chemotactic than 7 kDa unglycosylated MCP-1 [12].

Experimental Procedures

Production and Purification of Chemokines

Chemotactic activity in the conditioned media from freshly isolated peripheral blood mononuclear cells or MG-63 osteosarcoma cells was first concentrated and partially purified by adsorption to controlled pore glass or silicic acid. After dialysis, concentrated proteins were loaded on a heparin-Sepharose column and eluted in a linear NaCl gradient. Alternatively, chemotactic activity was isolated by antibody affinity chromatography and eluted at pH 2.0. Fractions containing the chemotactic activity were prepared for Mono S cation exchange FPLC (Pharmacia, Uppsala, Sweden) by dialysis against 50 m*M* formiate pH 4.0. A linear NaCl gradient was used to elute proteins. Finally, the natural chemokines were purified to homogeneity by reversed-phase (RP-) HPLC. Samples were injected on a C-8 Aquapore RP-300 column (220×2.1 mm; Perkin Elmer, Foster City, Calif., USA), equilibrated with 0.1% trifluoroacetic acid (TFA) in water and the proteins were eluted with an acetonitrile gradient. Alternatively, intact MCP-2, MCP-3 and GCP-2 were synthesized by Fmoc chemistry, folded into biologically active proteins and purified by C-8 RP-HPLC.

Purification of CD26/DPP IV and Cleavage of Chemokines

Human membrane-bound CD26/DPP IV was obtained from prostasomes (prostate-derived organelles which occur freely in seminal plasma) and soluble CD26/DPP IV, starting at amino acid Gly-31, was isolated from total seminal plasma. The enzyme was purified to homogeneity by anion exchange chromatography and affinity chromatography on immobilized adenosine deaminase. The enzymatic activity was determined using the fluorogenic substrate Gly-Pro-4-methoxy-2-naphthylamide. A 100–1,000 *M* excess of chemokine was incubated overnight at 37 °C with CD26/DPP IV in 100 m*M* Tris/HCl pH 7.7. Control chemokine incubations were performed without the addition of CD26/DPP IV. Chemokines were separated from CD26/DPP IV by SDS-PAGE on a Tris/Tricine gel system. Proteins were electroblotted on PVDF (polyvinylidene fluoride) membranes (Problott; Perkin Elmer) and stained with Coomassie brilliant blue R250. After destaining, membranes were rinsed at least 5 times with ultrapure water (Milli Q; Millipore, Bedford, Mass., USA). To obtain sufficient amounts of pure truncated chemokines for biological assays, recombinant or synthetic chemokines (PeproTech, Rocky Hill, N.J., USA or R&D Systems Europe, Abingdon, UK) were treated with CD26/DPP IV and the cleavage product was acidified with 0.1% TFA. Tween 20 (0.01%) was added to prevent the chemokines from sticking to the tubes. Chemokines were separated from CD26/DPP IV in an acetonitrile gradient on a C-8 Aquapore RP-300 column (1×50 mm) (Perkin Elmer). Fractions containing proteins were analyzed by SDS-PAGE and silver stained. CD26/DPP IV-treated chemokines, purified by RP-HPLC or excised from PVDF blots, were NH_2-terminally sequenced by Edman degradation on a pulsed liquid phase 477A/120A protein sequencer (Perkin Elmer) using *N*-methylpiperidine as a coupling base.

Isolation of Leukocytes

Neutrophilic granulocytes and mononuclear cells were isolated from heparinized peripheral blood from a single donor. Briefly, erythrocytes were removed by sedimentation for 30 min at 37 °C in hydroxyethyl-starch solution (Plasmasteril; Fresenius AG, Bad Homburg, Germany). Mononuclear cells and granulocytes were separated by gradient centrifugation for 30 min at 400 g on Ficoll-sodium metrizoate (Lymphoprep; Life Technologies, Paisley, UK). Remaining erythrocytes in the granulocyte pellet were removed by lysis in bidistilled water for 30 s. Neutrophilic granulocytes were used in the microchamber assay at a concentration of 10^6 cells/ml in Hanks' balanced salt solution (HBSS; Life Technologies) supplemented with 1 mg/ml human serum albumin (HSA).

To isolate eosinophils from the granulocyte pellet, the cells were incubated for 30 min at 4 °C with paramagnetic microbeads conjugated with mAb against CD16 (Miltenyi Biotec GmbH, Bergisch Gladbach, Germany). The cell suspension was passed over a column placed in a strong magnetic field (VarioMACS; Miltenyi Biotec GmbH). The cells that passed through the column were for more than 90% eosinophils. Eosinophils were used in the microchamber assay at a concentration of 10^6 cells/ml.

Monocytes and lymphocytes were isolated from the mononuclear cell fraction by incubation of the cell suspension with paramagnetic microbeads conjugated with mAb against CD14 and CD3 (both Miltenyi Biotec GmbH), respectively, for 15 min at 4 °C. Cells were passed over a column in a magnetic field. Labeled cells were retained on the column and were eluted with buffer after the column was removed from the magnetic field. Monocytes and lymphocytes (>90% purity) were used in the microchamber assay at a concentration of 2×10^6 cells/ml and 10×10^6 cells/ml, respectively. The presence of paramagnetic beads did not influence the chemotaxis of the cells.

Chemotaxis Assay

Chemotaxis assays were performed in a 48-well microchamber (Neuro Probe Inc., Cabin John, Md., USA). The lower compartment, containing test sample or control, was separated from the upper compartment, containing cells, by a 5-µm pore size polycarbonate filter (Nuclepore, Pleasanton, Calif., USA; polyvinylpyrrolidone (PVP)-free for neutrophils and eosinophils; PVP-treated for monocytes and coated with fibronectin for lymphocytes). The incubation times were 45, 60, 120 min and 4 h for neutrophils, eosinophils, monocytes and lymphocytes, respectively. The chemotactic activity was expressed as a chemotactic index, being the number of cells migrated to the sample divided by the number of cells migrated to the negative control.

Detection of Intracellular Ca^{2+} Concentrations

Purified leukocytes or THP-1 cells (10^7 cells/ml) were incubated in Eagle's Minimum Essential Medium (EMEM; Life Technologies) + 0.5% FCS with the fluorescent indicator fura-2 (fura-2/AM 2.5 μ*M*; Molecular Probes Europe BV, Leiden, The Netherlands) and 0.01% Pluronic F-127 (Sigma, St. Louis, Mo., USA). After 30 min at 37 °C, the cells were washed twice and resuspended at 10^6 cells/ml in HBSS with 1 m*M* Ca^{2+} and 0.1% FCS (buffered with 10 m*M* Hepes/NaOH at pH 7.4). The cells were equilibrated at 37 °C for 10 min before fura-2 fluorescence was measured in an LS50B luminescence spectrophotometer (Perkin Elmer). Upon excitation at 340 and 380 nm, fluorescence was detected at 510 nm. The $[Ca^{2+}]_i$ was calculated using the Grynkiewicz equation. In order to determine R_{max}, the cells were lysed with 50 μ*M* digitonin. Subsequently, the pH was adjusted to 8.5 with 20 m*M* Tris and R_{min} was obtained by addition of 10 m*M* EGTA to the lysed cells. The K_d used was 224 n*M*.

For desensitization experiments, leukocytes or THP-1 cells were first stimulated with buffer or chemokine at different concentrations. As a second stimulus, chemokines were used at a concentration inducing a significant increase in the $[Ca^{2+}]_i$ after prestimulation with buffer. The second stimulus was applied 2 min after addition of the first stimulus. The percentage inhibition of the $[Ca^{2+}]_i$ increase in response to the second stimulus was calculated comparing the signal after prestimulation with chemokine with the signal after addition of buffer.

Receptor Binding Assay

CCR-transfected HEK293 cells (kindly provided by Dr. J.M. Wang, NCI-NIH, Frederick, Md., USA) were incubated with ^{125}I-RANTES for 2 h in the presence or in the absence of varying concentrations of intact RANTES or RANTES(3-68). Cells were washed 3 times with phosphate-buffered saline (PBS) supplemented with 2% bovine serum albumin (BSA) and the radioactivity present on the CCR-transfected cells was counted in a γ counter. Nonspecific binding was subtracted from the total binding to obtain specific binding.

Inhibition of HIV-1 Infection

The macrophage-tropic (M-tropic) HIV-1 strain BaL and the T-cell-tropic (T-tropic) HIV-1 strain NL4.3 were obtained through the MRC AIDS reagent project (Herts, UK) and from the National Institute of Allergy and Infectious Disease, AIDS reagent program (Bethesda, Md., USA), respectively. Peripheral blood mononuclear cells (PBMC) from healthy donors were isolated by density gradient centrifugation and stimulated with PHA at 1 μg/ml (Sigma) for 3 days at 37 °C. The activated cells (PHA-stimulated blasts) were washed 3 times with PBS, and infected with virus. After 1 h, nonadsorbed virus was removed

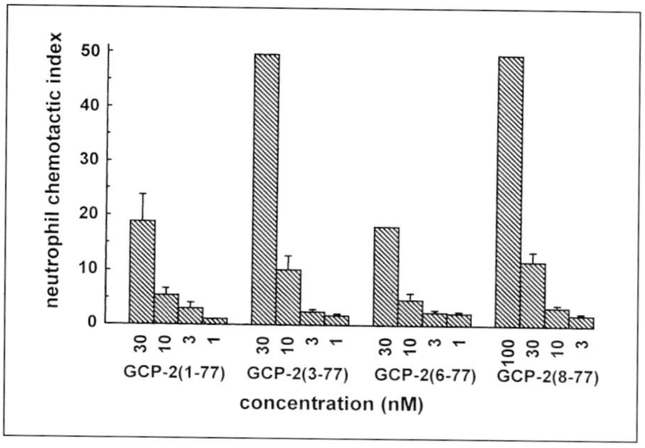

Fig. 1. Chemotactic activity of natural truncated GCP-2 forms. Natural GCP-2, produced by cytokine-induced MG-63 osteosarcoma cells, was isolated by subsequent purification on heparin-Sepharose, cation exchange and RP-HPLC columns (cf. Experimental Procedures). Pure GCP-2 forms were tested for neutrophil chemotaxis using the microchamber assay. Cell migration is represented as chemotactic indexes.

by washing 3 times with PBS and HIV-1-infected or mock-infected PHA-stimulated blasts were cultured in the presence of 25 U/ml of IL-2 and varying concentrations of intact or truncated chemokine. Cell supernatant was collected at day 10 and HIV-1 core antigen in the supernatant was determined by a commercial p-24 Ag ELISA kit (du Pont, Wilmington, Del., USA).

Results and Discussion

CD26/DPP IV Cleaves Human GCP-2 without Affecting Its Granulocyte Chemotactic Activity

Human, bovine and mouse GCP-2 isolated from in vitro cultured cell lines show significant NH_2-terminal heterogeneity [8, 13]. The distinct natural isoforms of human and bovine GCP-2 have been separated from each other by RP-HPLC [8]. One of the human GCP-2 isoforms, i.e. GCP-2(3-77), is truncated beyond Pro at the penultimate position, indicating the possible involvement of CD26/DPP IV. To investigate this protease-chemokine interaction, intact synthetic GCP-2 was incubated overnight at 37 °C with CD26/DPP IV purified from seminal plasma. Cleavage of the chemokine into GCP-2(3-77) was confirmed by NH_2-terminal sequence analysis. Since the neutrophil chemotactic potency of GCP-2(3-77) as well as of further processed forms, e.g. GCP-2(8-77) was found to be similar to that of intact GCP-2 (fig. 1), the

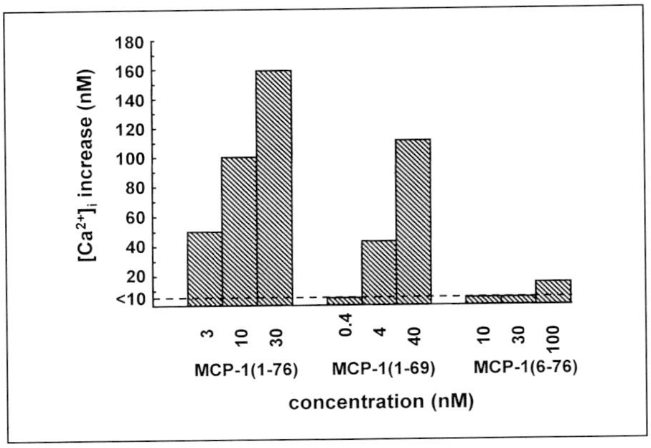

Fig. 2. NH_2-terminal, but not COOH-terminal processing reduces the receptor signaling capacity of human MCP-1. Posttranslationally processed forms of human MCP-1 were produced by stimulated PBMC and purified to homogeneity (cf. fig. 1). Measurements of intracellular calcium concentrations ($[Ca^{2+}]_i$) were performed on THP-1 cells as described in the section Experimental Procedures.

physiological significance of GCP-2 processing by CD26/DPP IV is still illusive. Forms of bovine GCP-2, which are NH_2-terminally processed in front of their conserved ELR motif, also remained biologically intact [8]. Mouse GCP-2 is also a potential substrate for CD26/DPP IV but NH_2-terminal truncation does affect its neutrophil chemotactic potency [13]. However, in the mouse system, the effect of CD26/DPP IV on chemokines remains to be investigated.

Monocyte Chemotactic Proteins (MCPs) are Protected from CD26/DPP IV Cleavage by a Pyroglutamate

Human MCP-1, -2, -3 and -4 all possess a Pro at the penultimate position. Although NH_2-terminally truncated forms of MCP-1 and MCP-2 have been isolated from stimulated peripheral blood leukocytes [10], no MCP(3-76) forms (missing the two NH_2-terminal residues corresponding to CD26/DPP IV cleavage) were recovered from these cells. Naturally processed MCP-1(5-76), MCP-1(6-76) and MCP-2(6-76) have a drastically reduced monocyte chemotactic potency [10] and retain only a weak ability to induce signal transduction as measured by diminished increases in the intracellular calcium concentration (fig. 2). In contrast, COOH-terminally processed MCP-1(1-69) and MCP-2(1-74) have no significant change in specific biological activity compared to the intact chemokines [10]. Similarly, posttranslational modification by glycosylation has only a minor effect on the activity of human MCP-1 [10]. Since it has been demonstrated that deletion or modification of the

NH_2-terminal residue of MCP-1 and MCP-3 is detrimental for their biological activity [9, 14], the NH_2-terminus of these CC chemokines must be essential for receptor binding and signaling.

With regard to MCP truncation by CD26/DPP IV, the existing literature is apparently conflicting [15, 16]. Recombinant MCP-2 with an NH_2-terminal Gln-Pro dipeptide was efficiently cleaved by CD26/DPP IV, whereas synthetical MCP-2 with an NH_2-terminal pyroglutamate (like natural MCP-2) remained intact after CD26/DPP IV treatment. This indicates that NH_2-terminal cyclization provides a structural protection against this specific proteolytic degradation. Indeed, chemical conversion of the Gln residue into a pyroglutamate protects MCP-2 from CD26/DPP IV cleavage [17]. Such cyclization is essential for chemotactic activity, but not for signal transduction (calcium mobilization). Removal of Gln_1-Pro_2 from MCP-2 by CD26/DPP IV also reduces the calcium-mobilizing capacity of the chemokine, showing that not the cyclization, but the presence of the two NH_2-terminal residues is essential for signal transduction [17]. NH_2-terminal extension of recombinant MCP-3 and MCP-4 also resulted in a significant (MCP-4) to complete (MCP-3) loss of biological activity [14, 18]. Thus, MCP-2, and probably also the other MCPs, are examples of chemokine substrates that are protected from CD26/DPP IV degradation by a pyroglutamate. This situation is exactly the opposite to that for GCP-2, which is effectively processed by CD26/DPP IV but is biologically not affected.

CD26/DPP IV Converts RANTES into a Potent Inhibitor of Chemotaxis and HIV-1 Infection

When the CC chemokine RANTES was purified from cytokine-induced fibroblasts or osteosarcoma cells, no intact chemokine, but truncated RANTES(3-68) missing two NH_2-terminal residues was recovered, whereas conditioned medium from mononuclear cells contained a mixture of intact and truncated RANTES [19]. In contrast to MCPs, RANTES is effectively cleaved by CD26/DPP IV into RANTES(3-68) with far-reaching consequences for its biological function [15, 16]. Indeed, RANTES(3-68) shows impaired binding (fig. 3) to and signaling [19] through its receptors CCR1 and CCR3, whereas the opposite occurs for CCR5. As a consequence, the chemotactic effect of RANTES(3-68) on monocytes and eosinophils is significantly reduced, but its antiviral activity against M-tropic HIV-1 strains using CCR5 is clearly enhanced [16, 19]. The increased anti-HIV-1 activity of RANTES(3-68) observed on PBMC is even more pronounced on CD4/CCR5 transfected cells [20]. Furthermore, RANTES(3-68) serves as a potent inhibitor of monocyte migration induced by intact RANTES as well as by other CC chemokines [16, 19]. Thus, CD26/DPP IV may downregulate the inflammatory response induced by RANTES by reducing its chemotactic potency and by generating

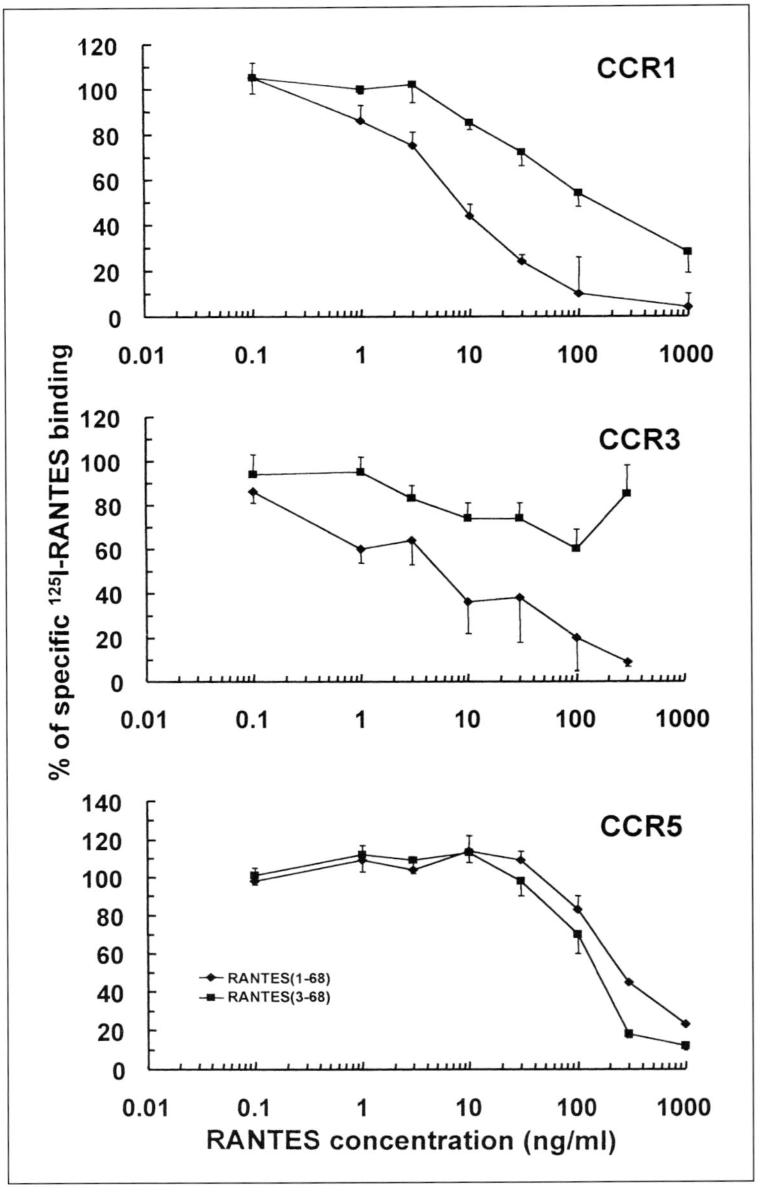

Fig. 3. Cleavage of RANTES by CD26/DPP IV results in reduced binding to CCR1 and CCR3 but enhanced recognition of CCR5. The percentage of specific ^{125}I-RANTES binding in the presence of different concentrations of cold RANTES(1-68) or RANTES(3-68) to CCR1-, CCR3- and CCR5-transfected HEK293 cells is shown.

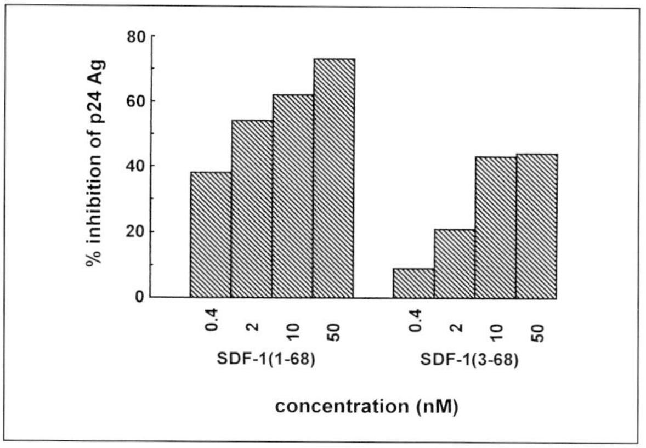

Fig. 4. Reduced anti-HIV-1 activity of SDF-1 after NH_2-terminal cleavage by CD26/DPP IV. PBMC were protected from infection with the HIV-1 strain NL4.3 by different concentrations of intact SDF-1(1-68) and CD26/DPP IV-truncated SDF-1(3-68). The viral replication was quantified by viral p24 antigen (p24 Ag) ELISA. Results are expressed as the percentage inhibition of p24 Ag production.

at the same time a natural competitor of intact RANTES for receptor binding. Undeliberately, impairment of RANTES activity by CD26/DPP IV cleavage results in increased antiviral activity. This demonstrates that physiologically generated RANTES(3-68) may exert both anti-inflammatory and anti-HIV-1 activities in vivo.

Truncation of SDF-1 by CD26/DPP IV Results in Reduction of Both Its Chemotactic and Antiviral Activity

Stromal cell-derived factor-1 (SDF-1) is a CXC chemokine which exerts antiviral activity by blocking its receptor CXCR4, which is used for entry by T-tropic HIV-1 strains. SDF-1, also a substrate for CD26/DPP IV, is efficiently cleaved into SDF-1(3-68), lacking the two NH_2-terminal residues. In contrast to RANTES, such processing results in a diminished potency to prevent HIV-1 infection of PBMC [21, 22] (fig. 4). The reduced antiviral effect of SDF-1(3-68) coincides with the loss of both chemotactic activity for lymphocytes and signaling through CXCR4 [21, 22]. However, SDF-1(3-68) still weakly binds to CXCR4 (10-fold reduction in receptor affinity) whereas further deletion of an additional Val residue results in a 100-fold weaker receptor binding [23]. Weak receptor binding of SDF-1(3-68) to CXCR4 is confirmed by its capacity to desensitize the calcium response induced by intact SDF-1 [21]. By comparing the effect of CD26/DPP IV on SDF-1 and RANTES, it must be concluded that although for both chemokines a similar reduction in chemotactic potential occurs, CD26/DPP IV truncation has complete opposing effects on their antiviral activity. This may be due to the fact that SDF-1 exerts its antiviral chemotactic activity through a single receptor (CXCR4), whereas RANTES chemoattracts through CCR1, CCR3 and CCR5, but inhibits HIV-1 mainly through CCR5.

Unexpected Alternative Cleavage of MDC by CD26/DPP IV

Macrophage-derived chemokine (MDC) is a recently discovered chemoattractant for dendritic cells, NK cells, monocytes and activated lymphocytes [24, 25]. Truncated MDC(3-69) was previously identified from lymphocyte-conditioned medium based on its anti-HIV-1 activity against both M- and T-tropic virus strains [26]. Since the primary structure of MDC has a Pro residue at the penultimate position, it was expected to be processed by CD26/DPP IV. Similar to the previously discussed chemokines GCP-2, RANTES and SDF-1, intact MDC is quickly converted (within hours) into MDC(3-69). However, it is further cleaved (within 24 h) to MDC(5-69) by enzymatic removal of the subsequent Tyr_3-Gly_4 dipeptide [27]. This unexpected additional truncation by CD26/DPP IV proves that the substrate specificity of this peptidase is less restricted than anticipated. Confirmation of this second cleavage was obtained using the NH_2-terminal peptides MDC(1-9) and MDC(3-9) which both yielded MDC(5-9) after CD26/DPP IV treatment [27].

MDC(3-69) and MDC(5-69) both show impaired signaling through CCR4, the only identified MDC receptor [27, 28]. Furthermore, in CCR4-transfected cells, MDC(3-69) and MDC(5-69) fail to desensitize intracellular calcium mobilization induced by MDC or TARC, another ligand for CCR4 [28]. T lymphocytic (HUT-78 and SUP-T1) cells are only marginally attracted by the truncated MDC forms compared to intact MDC. A similar reduction in chemotactic potency is noticed on monocyte-derived dendritic cells. However, MDC(3-69) and MDC(5-69) remain equally potent as intact MDC to chemoattract peripheral blood monocytes and to desensitize MDC-induced monocyte chemotaxis [27, 28].

Testing of MDC(1-69) and MDC(3-69) for antiviral activity showed that both intact and CD26/DPP IV-truncated MDC can partially prevent infection of PBMC with either M-tropic (Bal) or T-tropic (NL4.3) HIV-1 strains [28]. This anti-HIV-1 activity is probably not mediated through binding of MDC to CXCR4 or CCR5 nor to the orphan receptors BOB/GPR15 and Bonzo/STRL33. Since the antiviral effect of MDC(3-69) is even more pronounced than that of intact MDC and because MDC(3-69) and MDC(5-69) retain their monocyte chemotactic activity without signaling through CCR4, an additional MDC receptor must be involved [28].

Table 1. NH_2-terminal processing of chemokines by CD26/DPP IV

	Chemokine	CD26/DPP IV treatment	NH_2-terminal sequence	CD26/DPP IV truncation	Receptor signaling	Chemotaxis	Anti-HIV-1 effect
CXC	GCP-2	–	**G P** V S A V L T E L R C T C		CXCR1,2	+	–
		+	V S A V L T E L R C T C	Yes	CXCR1,2	+	–
	SDF-1	–	**K P** V S L S Y R C P C		CXCR4	+	+
		+	V S L S Y R C P C	Yes	–	–	–
CC	MIP-1α	–	A S L A A D T P T A C C		CCR1,5	+	+
		+	A S L A A D T P T A C C	No	CCR1,5	+	+
	MCP-1	–	**Q P** D A I N A P V T C C		CCR2	+	–
		+	**Q P** D A I N A P V T C C	No	CCR2	+	–
	MCP-3	–	**Q P** V G I N T S T T C C		CCR1,2,3	+	±
		+	**Q P** V G I N T S T T C C	No	CCR1,2,3	+	±
	RANTES	–	**S P** Y S S D T T P C C		CCR1,3,5	+	+
		+	Y S S D T T P C C	Yes	CCR5	–	+ +
	Eotaxin	–	**G P** A S V P T T C C		CCR3	+	+
		+	A S V P T T C C	Yes	–	–	+
	MDC	–	**G P** Y G A N M E D S V C C		CCR4	+	±
		+	Y G A N M E D S V C C	Yes	–	±	±
		+	A N M E D S V C C	Yes	–	±	±

Taken together, the results on MDC illustrate that this chemokine is processed by CD26/DPP IV in an unusual way, resulting in the removal of four NH_2-terminal residues. This truncation has far-reaching but selective consequences for the chemotactic activity of MDC on its various target cells.

Conclusions: Consequences of the Chemokine – CD26/DPP IV Interaction in Pathology

In previous sections it has been documented that the outcome, both biologically and biochemically, of chemokine processing by CD26/DPP IV is variable. Within the group of putative CD26/DPP IV substrates, some chemokines (MCPs) are protected from proteolytic degradation. Other chemokines (GCP-2) are cleaved, but their biological activity remains unaffected. For most chemokines (RANTES, SDF-1, MDC) truncation by CD26/DPP IV is accompanied by reduced receptor binding and signaling and by impaired chemotactic responses (table 1). For all these chemokines a Pro and not Ala residue at the penultimate position is involved. As an exception, MDC is processed beyond this cleavage site. In order to verify whether chemokine processing by CD26/DPP IV occurs according to a predictable pattern, more molecules need to be investigated. In such an attempt the CC chemokine eotaxin, a selective eosinophil chemoattractant operating through CCR3, was also found to be cleaved by CD26/DPP IV. As a consequence, eotaxin(3-74) fails to chemoattract eosinophils and to induce calcium responses in CCR3 transfectants. However, eotaxin(3-74) still binds to CCR3 and inhibits the chemotactic response towards intact eotaxin [29]. With respect to the consequences of posttranslational processing by CD26/DPP IV, eotaxin(3-74) behaves almost like SDF-1, a CXC chemokine activating also a single receptor.

Although the effect of CD26/DPP IV on a substantial number of chemokines has been investigated by now, the remaining putative CD26/DPP IV substrates (e.g. γIP-10, Mig, I-TAC, MIP-1β) must be studied before firm conclusions can be drawn. Even then, the biochemical and biological in vivo outcome of a single chemokine-CD26/DPP IV interaction remains unpredictable. Furthermore, the combined effect of multiple chemokines being processed by CD26/DPP IV cannot be estimated. In addition, multiple immunological properties can be attributed to CD26/DPP IV, since it interacts with CD45 (a protein tyrosine phosphatase) and with adenosine deaminase [1, 2]. For CC chemokines, the reduction of chemotactic potency due to processing by CD26/DPP IV may weaken the inflammatory response. In contrast to CC chemokines, posttranslational processing of CXC chemokines (e.g. IL-8, NAP-2) by other proteases results in enhanced proinflammatory activities. Further experimental evidence must allow to estimate the net balance of proteolytic cleavage of chemokines by proteases during disease. At this moment, no immunoassays, that discriminate between intact and truncated chemokines, are available to measure their relative appearance during pathological disorders characterized by leukocyte infiltration. Finally, the conflicting literature on the role of CD26/DPP IV in HIV-1 infection [30] may be partially explained by the opposing consequences of chemokine (such as SDF-1 and RANTES) processing by CD26/DPP IV for their antiviral activity.

Acknowledgments

The authors thank Sandra Claes, René Conings, Erik Fonteyn, Jean-Pierre Lenaerts and Willy Put for technical assistance. This work was supported by the Fund for Scientific Research of Flanders (FWO-Vlaanderen), the Concerted Research Actions (GOA) of the Regional Government of Flanders, the InterUniversity Attraction Pole (IUAP) initiative of the Belgian Federal Government and the Biomed Program of the European Community. S.S. P.M., I.D.M. and P.P. hold fellowships of the FWO-Vlaanderen and E.V.C. holds a specialization fellowship of the Flemish Institute for the Enhancement of Scientific and Technological Research in Industry 'IWT'.

References

1 Von Bonin A, Hühn J, Fleischer B: Dipeptidyl-peptidase IV/CD26 on T cells: Analysis of an alternative T-cell activation pathway. Immunol Rev 1998;161:43–53.

2 Morimoto C, Schlossman SF: The structure and function of CD26 in the T-cell immune response. Immunol Rev 1998;161:55–70.

3 Vanhoof G, Goossens F, De Meester I, Hendriks D, Scharpé S: Proline motifs in peptides and their biological processing. FASEB J 1995;9:736–744.

4 De Meester I, Korom S, Van Damme J, Scharpé S: CD26, let it cut or cut it down. Immunol. Today 1999, in press.

5 Van Damme J, Van Beeumen J, Conings R, Decock B, Billiau A: Purification of granulocyte chemotactic peptide/interleukin-8 reveals N-terminal sequence heterogeneity similar to that of β-thromboglobulin. Eur J Biochem 1989;181:337–344.

6 Wuyts A, Proost P, Van Damme J: Interleukin-8 and other CXC chemokines; in Thomson A (ed): The Cytokine Handbook. London, Academic Press, 1998, chap 10, pp 271–311.

7 Walz A, Baggiolini M: Generation of the neutrophil-activating peptide NAP-2 from platelet basic protein or connective tissue-activating peptide III through monocyte proteases. J Exp Med 1990;171:449–454.

8 Proost P, Wuyts A, Conings R, Lenaerts JP, Billiau A, Opdenakker G, Van Damme J: Human and bovine granulocyte chemotactic protein-2: Complete amino acid sequence and functional characterization as chemokines. Biochemistry 1993;32:10170–10177.

9 Gong JH, Clark-Lewis I: Antagonists of monocyte chemoattractant protein 1 identified by modification of functionally critical NH_2-terminal residues. J Exp Med 1995;181:631–640.

10 Proost P, Struyf S, Couvreur M, Lenaerts JP, Conings R, Menten P, Verhaert P, Wuyts A, Van Damme J: Posttranslational modifications affect the activity of the human monocyte chemotactic proteins MCP-1 and MCP-2: Identification of MCP-2(6-76) as a natural chemokine inhibitor. J Immunol 1998;160:4034–4041.

11 Opdenakker G, Rudd PM, Wormald M, Dwek RA, Van Damme J: Cells regulate the activities of cytokines by glycosylation. FASEB J 1995;9:453–457.

12 Liu ZG, Haelens A, Wuyts A, Struyf S, Pang XW, Proost P, Chen WF, Van Damme J: Isolation of a lymphocyte chemotactic factor produced by the murine thymic epithelial cell line MTEC1: Identification as a 30 kDa glycosylated form of MCP-1. Eur Cytokine Netw 1996;7:381–388.

13 Wuyts A, Haelens A, Proost P, Lenaerts JP, Conings R, Opdenakker G, Van Damme J: Identification of mouse granulocyte chemotactic protein-2 from fibroblasts and epithelial cells. Functional comparison with natural KC and macrophage inflammatory protein-2. J Immunol 1996;157:1736–1743.

14 Masure S, Paemen L, Proost P, Van Damme J, Opdenakker G: Expression of a human mutant monocyte chemotactic protein-3 (MCP-3) in *Pichia pastoris* and characterization as an MCP-3 receptor antagonist. J Interferon Cytokine Res 1995;15:955–963.

15 Proost P, De Meester I, Schols D, Struyf S, Lambeir AM, Wuyts A, Opdenakker G, De Clercq E, Scharpé S, Van Damme J: Amino-terminal truncation of chemokines by CD26/dipeptidyl-peptidase IV. J Biol Chem 1998;273:7222–7227.

16 Oravecz T, Pall M, Roderiquez G, Gorrell MD, Ditto M, Nguyen NY, Boykens R, Unsworth E, Norcross MA: Regulation of the receptor specificity and function of the chemokine RANTES (regulated on activation, normal T cell expressed and secreted) by dipeptidyl peptidase IV (CD26)-mediated cleavage. J Exp Med 1997;186:1865–1872.

17 Van Coillie E, Proost P, Van Aelst I, Struyf S, Polfliet M, De Meester I, Harvey DJ, Van Damme J, Opdenakker G: Functional comparison of two human monocyte chemotactic protein-2 isoforms. Role of the amino-terminal pyroglutamic acid and processing by CD26/dipeptidyl peptidase IV. Biochemistry 1998;37:12672–12680.

18 Uguccioni M, Loetscher P, Forssmann U, Dewald B, Li H, Hensche Lima S, Li Y, Kreider E, Garotta G, Thelen M, Baggiolini M: Monocyte chemotactic protein 4 (MCP-4), a novel structural and functional analogue of MCP-3 and eotaxin. J Exp Med 1996;183:2379–2384.

19 Struyf S, De Meester I, Scharpé S, Lenaerts J-P, Menten P, Wang JM, Proost P, Van Damme J: Natural truncation of RANTES abolishes signaling through the CC chemokine receptors CCR1 and CCR3, impairs its chemotactic potency and generates a CC chemokine inhibitor. Eur J Immunol 1998;28:1262–1271.

20 Schols D, Proost P, Struyf S, Wuyts A, De Meester I, Scharpé S, Van Damme J, De Clercq E: CD26-processed RANTES(3-68), but not intact RANTES, has potent anti-HIV-1 activity. Antivir Res 1998;39:175–187.

21 Proost P, Struyf S, Schols D, Durinx C, Wuyts A, Lenaerts JP, De Clercq E, De Meester I, Van Damme J: Processing by CD26/dipeptidyl-peptidase IV reduces the chemotactic and anti-HIV-1 activity of stromal cell-derived factor-1α. FEBS Lett 1998;432:73–76.

22 Ohtsuki T, Hosono O, Kobayashi H, Munakata Y, Souta A, Shioda T, Morimoto C: Negative regulation of the anti-human immunodeficiency virus and chemotactic activity of human stromal cell-derived factor 1α by CD26/dipeptidyl peptidase IV. FEBS Lett 1998;431:236–240.

23 Crump MP, Gong JH, Loetscher P, Rajarathnam K, Amara A, Arenzana-Seisdedos F, Virelizier JL, Baggiolini M, Sykes BD, Clark-Lewis I: Solution structure and basis for functional activity of stromal cell-derived factor-1; dissociation of CXCR4 activation from binding and inhibition of HIV-1. EMBO J 1997;16:6996–7007.

24 Godiska R, Chantry D, Raport CJ, Sozzani S, Allavena P, Leviten D, Mantovani A, Gray PW: Human macrophage-derived chemokine (MDC), a novel chemoattractant for monocytes, monocyte-derived dendritic cells, and natural killer cells. J Exp Med 1997;185:1595–1604.

25 Chang MS, McNinch J, Elias C III, Manthey CL, Grosshans D, Meng T, Boone T, Andrew DP: Molecular cloning and functional characterization of a novel CC chemokine, stimulated T cell chemotactic protein (STCP-1) that specifically acts on activated T lymphocytes. J Biol Chem 1997; 272:25229–25237.

26 Pal R, Garzino-Demo A, Markham PD, Burns J, Brown M, Gallo RC, DeVico AL: Inhibition of HIV-1 infection by the β-chemokine MDC. Science 1997;278:695–698.

27 Proost P, Struyf S, Van Damme J, Opdenakker G, Sozzani S, Allavena P, Mantovani A, Augustijns K, Bal G, Haemers A, Lambeir AM, Scharpe S, De Meester I: Truncation of macrophage-derived chemokine by CD26/dipeptidyl-peptidase IV beyond its predicted cleavage site affects chemotactic activity and CC chemokine receptor 4 interaction. J Biol Chem 1999;274:3988–3993.

28 Struyf S, Proost P, Sozzani S, Mantovani A, Wuyts A, De Clercq E, Schols D, Van Damme J: Cutting edge: Enhanced anti-HIV-1 activity and altered chemotactic potency of NH_2-terminally processed macrophage-derived chemokine imply an additional MDC receptor. J Immunol 1998; 161:2672–1676.

29 Struyf S, Proost P, Schols D, De Clercq E, Opdenakker G, Lenaerts JP, Detheux M, Parmentier M, De Meester I, Scharpe S, Van Damme J: CD26/dipeptidyl-peptidase IV down-regulates the eosinophil chemotactic potency, but not the anti-HIV activity of human eotaxin by affecting its interaction with CC chemokine receptor 3. J Immunol 1999;162:4903–4909.

30 Callebaut C, Jacotot E, Blanco J, Krust B, Hovanessian AG: Increased rate of HIV-1 entry and its cytopathic effect in $CD4^+/CXCR4^+$ T cells expressing relatively high levels of CD26. Exp Cell Res 1998;241:352–362.

Dr. J. Van Damme, Laboratory of Molecular Immunology, Rega Institute for Medical Research, University of Leuven, Minderbroedersstraat 10, B–3000 Leuven (Belgium)
Tel. +32 16 337348, Fax +32 16 337340, E-Mail jozef.vandamme@rega.kuleuven.ac.be

Mantovani A (ed): Chemokines.
Chem Immunol. Basel, Karger, 1999, vol 72, pp 57–68

Chemokines and Chemokine Receptors in T-Cell Development

Joseph A. Hedrick[a], *Albert Zlotnik*[b]

[a] Schering-Plough Research Institute, Kenilworth, N.J. and
[b] DNAX Research Institute, Palo Alto, Calif., USA

The process of thymic differentiation is extremely complicated and involves a variety of checkpoints and selection processes [1]. An additional complication is that this process, while similar overall between mouse and man, is not identical when comparing the temporal regulation of various markers. For a review in the human system, see Blom et al. [2]. In order to simplify our discussion we will generally employ four intrathymic stages of differentiation in this review. The most immature thymocytes will be described as triple negative (TN) for CD3–CD4–CD8–, the next stage will be double negative (DN) for CD3+CD4–CD8–, followed by double positive (DP) for CD3+ CD4+CD8+ (the stage at which selection occurs and which represents >80% of all thymocytes), and finally single positive (SP) referring to either CD3+ CD4+CD8– or CD3–CD4–CD8+ as indicated. The latter include mature thymocytes which are ready to emigrate from the thymus. These stages and markers are common between mouse and man.

In the earliest TN stages, developing thymocytes are subject to as yet unknown signals that induce them to commit to the T-cell lineage and to start rearranging T-cell receptor (TCR) genes [3, 4]. A further decision is to select either the γδ or the αβ T-cell lineages [4]. Thymocytes that have passed these steps and that successfully rearrange the β chain of the TCR undergo a step called 'β selection' where the rearranged TCR β chain is recognized with a surrogate TCR α chain specifically expressed by developing thymocytes. This step represents a 'quality control' step that allows only those thymocytes that successfully rearranged a productive β chain to advance to the DP stage, where they will rearrange the TCR α chain and will express a 'mature' TCR, thus allowing the cell to undergo positive and negative selection mechanisms that define the TCR repertoire prior to becoming SP and exiting the thymus. Seen from the overview angle, the passage of the lymphoid precursors that arrive in the thymus includes the following control points: (1) commitment to the T-cell lineage; (2) selection of the $\gamma\delta$ or $\alpha\beta$ lineage; (3) rearrangement of TCR genes; (4) β selection; (5) positive and negative selection, and (6) selection of CD4 or CD8 lineages, final maturation and exit from the thymus.

The mechanisms regulating each one of these steps remain obscure. What makes them even more interesting is that we can replicate essentially all thymic development in a 'semi-in vivo' model using fetal thymus organ culture (FTOC) [3]. In this model, a mouse fetal thymus is placed on top of a filter which is on top of a piece of surgical foam placed in a Petri dish that contains tissue culture media up to the level of the filter. In this model, the fetal thymocytes grow and differentiate along the differentiation pathway described above. Surprisingly, it is even possible to reconstitute fetal thymi depleted of thymocytes with a few lymphoid precursors (TN thymocytes). The reconstituted organs develop and form a normal thymus. These observations indicate that the thymus is essentially a self-contained organ, and that the interactions between the lymphoid precursors and the thymic stromal cells have all the signals necessary to carry out for thymic development.

In the 1980s there was significant interest in the role that cytokines could play in thymic development. However, the use of monoclonal antibodies in FTOC as well as analysis of mice rendered genetically deficient in a particular cytokine by homologous recombination (knockout mice) revealed that only IL-7 plays a significant role in T-cell development, making it a critical cytokine in the survival of TN thymocytes. This despite the fact that most cytokines can be readily demonstrated to be expressed in the thymus. It therefore became clear that other signals, as yet unrecognized, must exist to regulate thymic development events. It is also known that structurally, the thymus undergoes significant changes during its development, with a distinct boundary appearing between the cortex and medulla appearing at roughly the time when DP thymocytes appear. This observation indicates a very active and specific cellular distribution process, affecting not only the migration of the developing thymocytes but the organization and possibly differentiation of the thymic stroma as well. Yet, virtually nothing is known about the signals regulating this process.

In the 1990s our ability to find genes increased significantly with the availability of EST (expressed sequence tag) databases. One of the molecular families most affected by these developments has been the chemokines, whose number significantly increased between 1994 and 1997. Expression analysis of many of these chemokines and their receptors indicated that many were highly expressed in the thymus. Their known function (regulation of leukocyte migration) suggests a role for chemokines in thymic development as regulators of intrathymic cell migration. Against this backdrop, it is interesting that thymic development and chemokines have not received significant attention as a combined field until recently. This has been mostly due to the fact that few researchers spanned these fields. Given the sharp increase in reports of chemokine expression in the thymus as well as the renewed interest in this family of molecules, we can expect significant advances in this field in the near future. Here, we will review the data available on the expression and possible role of chemokines in the thymus. The aim of this review is to summarize what little we do know and to suggest possible directions for future investigation.

Thymically-Expressed Chemokines and Chemokine Receptors

A wide range of chemokines have now been cloned and characterized. Several among these (or their receptors) have been shown to be expressed in the thymus. We will review the available information.

Although a number of chemokines have been associated with hematopoiesis, the best characterized of these is stromal cell-derived factor (SDF)-1. The first characterized activity of SDF-1 was its ability to stimulate pre-B-cell proliferation. In addition, SDF-1 has been shown to be a chemoattractant for CD34+ hematopoietic progenitor cells [5] as well as for mature T lymphocytes and monocytes [6]. Expression of SDF-1 in the thymus of both mouse and human has been reported and both human and mouse thymocytes have been shown to migrate in response to SDF-1 [7, 8]. The source of SDF-1 in human thymus seems to be thymic stromal elements rather than the thymocytes themselves. Zaitseva et al. [8] using RT-PCR examined expression of SDF-1 in thymically-derived fibroblasts as well as DN, DP, and SP thymocytes. SDF-1 was detected only in fibroblasts and not in any of the thymocyte subsets examined.

While the response of human thymocytes to SDF-1 has been reported only for total thymocytes [8], the response of murine thymocytes to SDF-1 has been more thoroughly dissected. A summary of available data is presented in figure 1. Kim et al. [7] have reported that the response of separated DN, DP, and CD8+ SP thymocytes is roughly equivalent while CD4+ SP thymocytes were somewhat less responsive. Similarly, when unseparated thymocytes were allowed to migrate to SDF-1, the proportion of CD4+ SP thymocytes recovered was reduced compared to the other thymic subsets, supporting the conclusion that these cells are less responsive to SDF-1 than other thymocyte subsets.

The receptor for SDF-1 has been identified as CXCR4. In mouse, CXCR4 expression has been examined only at the level of mRNA. Kim et al. [7]

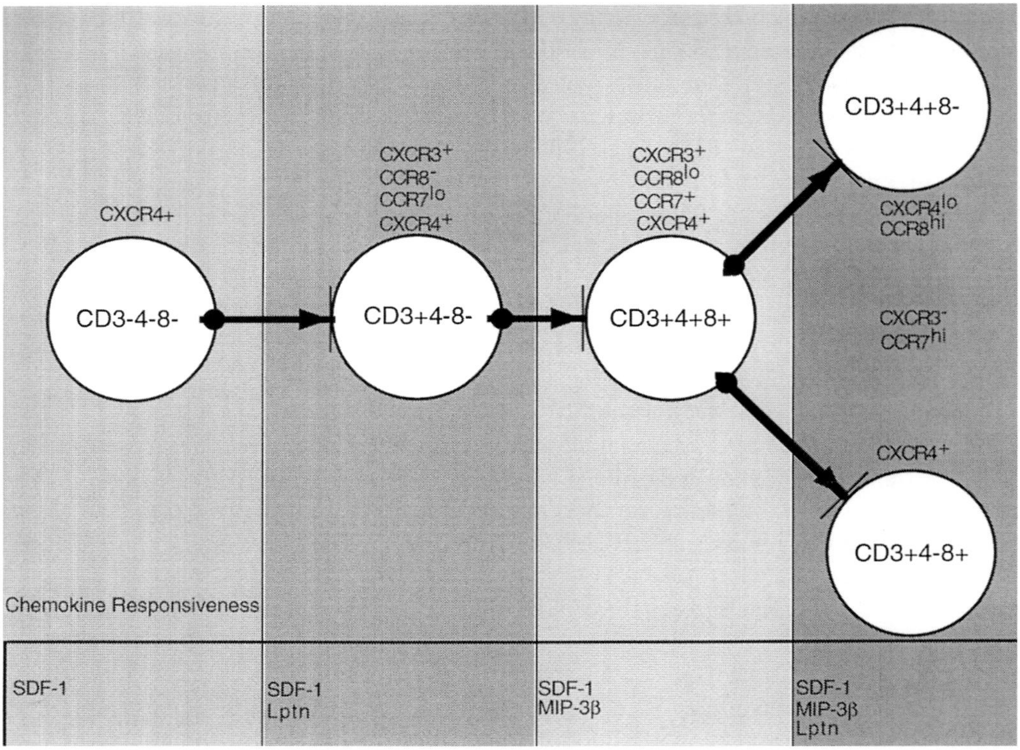

Fig. 1. Summary of chemokine receptor expression and chemokine responsiveness during mouse intrathymic T-cell development.

reported that, by RT-PCR, CXCR4 expression appeared low in DN and increased with maturation with CD8+ SP showing more expression than CD4+ SP thymocytes. These results correlate well with the pattern of SDF-1 responsiveness observed in the same study. The expression of this receptor in human thymic subsets has been examined in greater detail due principally to its role as a coreceptor for HIV-1. Flow cytometric studies from Zaitseva et al. [8] have shown that CXCR4 expression in human thymocytes is generally high and stable throughout early thymic differentiation declining in the most mature thymocytes to very low levels and is then upregulated in the periphery. Kitchen and Zack [9] also reported an inverse relationship between thymocyte maturity and CXCR4 expression. In a separate study using a SCID-hu model of thymopoiesis, Berkowitz et al. [10] reported similar findings although they observed CD4+ SP thymocytes to be negative for CXCR4 expression.

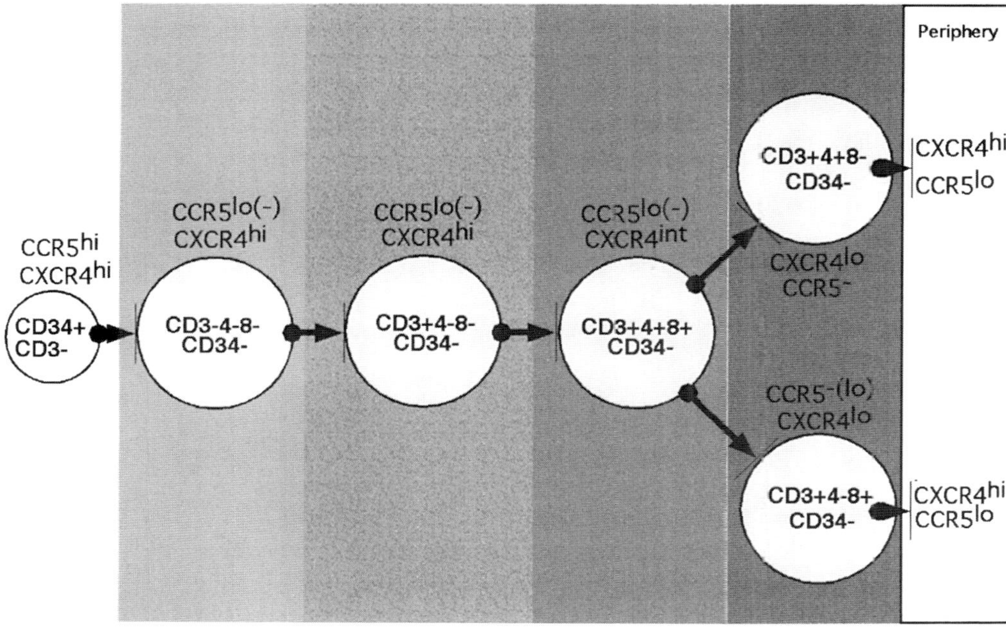

Fig. 2. Summary of chemokine receptor expression during intrathymic human T-cell development.

The exact nature of the cell that migrates from the bone marrow to the thymus is not known and it is not yet clear whether the first thymic progenitor cells are already CXCR4-positive upon entry into the thymus or not. Berkowitz et al. [10] reported that the more mature CD34+CD38+CD10+lin-bone marrow progenitor cells lack CXCR4 expression while Zaitseva et al. [8] reported CD34+CD3– cells isolated directly from thymus were very high for CXCR4 expression suggesting that CXCR4 is already expressed by the first cells to colonize the thymus. Indeed Berkowitz et al. [10] did report that a small subset of TN cells expressed high levels of CXCR4. The expression of CXCR4 has also been examined in the thymus of rhesus macaques and largely confirms expression of CXCR4 in both immature and mature thymocytes [11]. A summary of these data is presented in figure 2.

The recent reports of null mice for both the SDF-1 and the CXCR4 genes would seem to indicate that despite the temporal regulation of SDF-1/CXCR4 expression in thymocytes, this chemokine system plays little role in T-cell development or at least in the emigration of thymic precursors from the bone marrow to the thymus. SDF-1–/– and CXCR4–/– mice each had significant defects in B-cell lymphopoiesis, but thymic subsets and thymic architecture at day 18.5 of embryonic life appear unperturbed. Furthermore, if CXCR4–/– thymocytes were allowed to mature in fetal thymic organ culture, there was no difference in their capability to advance to the SP stage compared with thymocytes derived from a littermate control. While these experiments do not rule out a role for SDF-1/CXCR4 in thymic differentiation, they suggest that this interaction is not absolutely required for normal thymocyte development.

The expression of other CXC chemokines in the thymus has also been examined. In particular the chemokines interferon IFNγ induced protein (IP)-10 and monokine induced by interferon-γ (Mig) have been shown to be expressed in thymus. Interestingly, the cellular source of these chemokines does not appear to be thymocytes themselves, but rather thymic stromal cells [12, 13]. IP-10 expression in murine thymus is constitutive and separation of thymic cells into thymocytes and thymic stroma demonstrates that IP-10 expression segregates with the stromal cells [13, 14]. Although thymocytes do not appear to express IP-10 constitutively they can be induced to express IP-10 if stimulated by PMA and ionomycin or anti-Thy-1 antibody while ConA or PMA alone are ineffective [13].

The expression of murine Mig also appears to be regulated by activation [12]. Surprisingly the source of Mig in these studies was not the thymocytes themselves but rather thymic stromal cells. The expression of Mig in this case may be regulated by IFNγ secreted by activated thymocytes as induction was limited in IFNγ–/– mice [12]. Another CXC chemokine related to Mig and IP-10, interferon-inducible T-cell α chemoattractant (I-TAC), has recently been identified. Like Mig and IP-10, I-TAC is regulated by IFNγ and is expressed in human thymus as well as several other organs [15]. A mouse counterpart for this chemokine has yet to be identified and regulation of this chemokine in the thymic environment has not been investigated.

The receptor for these CXC chemokines, CXCR3, is also expressed in the murine thymus and appears to be both developmentally and activation-state regulated. Expression of CXCR3 in DN thymocytes is high and is reduced upon activation while resting TN thymocytes do not express CXCR3, but do so upon activation in a manner similar to that of mature T cells.

The thymic expression of CCR5, a receptor for macrophage inflammatory protein (MIP)-1α and -1β as well as the regulated upon activation, normal T-cell expressed and secreted (RANTES) chemokine, has also been examined. As with CXCR4, the principle motivation for this examination is related more to the role of CCR5 as an HIV coreceptor than its role as a thymic chemokine receptor. Zaitseva et al. [8] found that CCR5 expression in human thymocytes declined with increasing expression of TCR in a manner similar to that observed for CXCR4. These investigators also reported expression of CCR5 on CD3–CD34+ cells isolated from thymus. They were unable, however, to detect a calcium flux in thymocytes in response to RANTES, MIP-1α, or MIP-1β and could not observe chemotaxis using MIP-1α. These results contrast with those of Dairaghi et al. [16] who reported that human DP and SP thymocytes migrate vigorously in response to MIP-β while DN thymocytes were nonresponsive. In these studies, thymocytes also produced a modest calcium flux in response to MIP-1β.

The results of CCR5 expression analysis on various thymocyte subpopulations also differs among various studies. As discussed above, Zaitseva et al. [8] observed CCR5 expression in thymocytes which declined with maturation. In contrast to these results, Dairaghi et al. [16] reported CCR5 expression only in DP and CD8+ SP thymocytes with DN and CD4+ SP cells being negative. A similar result was also obtained by Berkowitz et al. [10] in the SCID-hu model discussed previously. The explanation for these differences is not entirely clear, but may be related to the reagents used by the various groups to examine CCR5 expression. It has been reported in the literature that various anti-CCR5 antibodies differ in their ability to detect CCR5 in thymocytes [10].

Other chemokines and chemokine receptors are also reported to be expressed in the thymus, however little has been done to investigate the role of these molecules in thymic development. Thymus and activation regulated chemokine (TARC) for example was originally characterized as a chemokine constitutively expressed at high levels in the thymus and not in spleen or circulating T cells [17]. Its specific receptor, CCR4 [18], is likewise expressed constitutively in thymus [19], suggesting the possibility of intrathymic interactions. As has been reported for many other thymic chemokines, the expression of TARC in the thymus seems to originate from stromal elements rather than thymocytes themselves [17]. Another ligand for CCR4, macrophage-derived chemokine (MDC), has also been described [20] and is likewise constitutively expressed in the human thymus as well as lymph node and appendix [20, 21]. As with TARC, the activity of MDC on thymocytes has not been reported.

Another particularly intriguing chemokine receptor expressed in the thymus is CCR8. Originally reported as thymus-expressed receptor (TER)-1, CCR8 is highly expressed in human and mouse thymus, but only weakly or not at all in spleen and lymph node [22–25]. The temporal expression of CCR8 in mouse thymus has also been examined by RT-PCR [26]. Interestingly, CCR8 was not detected in DN thymocytes but was present at low levels in DP thymocytes. This expression increased in CD4+ SP thymocytes but declined in CD8+ SP thymocytes. The property of CCR8 which makes it particularly interesting is the ability of its reported ligand, I-309, to inhibit apoptosis in BW5147 thymoma cells [27]. Although formal proof that this effect is mediated by interaction with CCR8 has not been published, it is worthwhile to note that BW5147 cells express very high levels of CCR8 mRNA [25, 26]. This makes it tempting to speculate that CCR8 is somehow involved in thymic selection. One problem with this hypothesis is that I-309 does not appear to be expressed in thymus. Two alternative ligands, TARC and MIP-1β, have been advanced as ligands for CCR8 [28]. In contrast to I-309, both TARC (discussed above) and MIP-1β are present in thymus. MIP-1β has also been reported to interact with CCR4 [19]. Other investigators, however, have been unable to observe the interaction between CCR8 and TARC or MIP-1β. Similarly the interaction of MIP-1β with CCR4 remains controversial, thus the significance of these findings remains unclear.

The chemokine MIP-3β, also known as EBI-1 ligand chemokine (ELC), is also known to be expressed in thymus as well as in other tissues and its activity on murine thymocytes has recently been examined in greater detail. Kim et al. [7] report that MIP-3β is for SP thymocytes, but not for DP or DN thymocytes. The expression of CCR7, the receptor for MIP-3β, was also determined by RT-PCR and showed increasing expression throughout differentiation beginning with DN thymocytes and ending with highest levels expressed in SP thymocytes [29]. This study also correlated the onset of MIP-3β responsiveness with expression of CD69, typically thought to mark postselection thymocytes.

Lymphotactin is a unique molecule containing only two of four normally conserved cysteines that are the structural signature of a chemokine. Lymphotactin was originally cloned from activated TN cells in an effort to identify sequences unique to that subset of cells. Interestingly, lymphotactin is also chemotactic for DN and SP thymocytes [30], while DP thymocytes are nonresponsive. The receptor for lymphotactin, GPR5 or XCR1 [31], is also expressed in thymus though its expression in specific subsets has not yet been examined.

Probably the most interesting thymically-expressed chemokine described so far is TECK (thymus-expressed chemokine). While performing an EST analysis from RAG-1–/– knockout mouse thymus, we identified a novel chemokine and designated it TECK because it appeared specifically expressed in the thymus [32]. TECK was found to be expressed by class II MHC-positive cells and also positive for the dendritic cell marker N418. These observations suggest that TECK is produced by thymic dendritic cells. Interestingly, these cells have been postulated to derive from a lymphoid precursor as opposed to a myeloid precursor for other dendritic cells. The fact that TECK is expressed by thymic dendritic cells but not, under normal circumstances, by other dendritic cells suggests that TECK may be a marker of lymphoid dendritic cells. It is possible, however, that other thymic stromal cells may also express TECK although thymic stromal cell lines examined did not express TECK. Interestingly, TECK was also detected in the small intestine, a site that has long been suspected to be a site for extrathymic T-cell development. In fact, we cloned human TECK from a human small intestine cDNA library. Both human and mouse TECK share the same expression pattern. TECK attracts monocytes and dendritic cells, and possibly some thymocyte subsets, which remain to be characterized. We have recently observed that antibodies against TECK block T-cell development in FTOC, suggesting an important role for this chemokine in T-cell development. However, it has not been easy to pinpoint the role that this chemokine plays in T-cell development. The FTOC exposed to anti-TECK does not 'stop' at a particular stage of thymocyte development, rather it simply fails to develop after a certain time in culture, making it impossible to recover enough cells for detailed analysis. These observations are more consistent with an essential role for TECK in overall thymic architecture although this does not rule out a specific role at some stage of thymic development. Importantly, TECK has also been detected in the spleens of mice injected with LPS. This indicates that TECK is inducible under inflammatory conditions in extrathymic sites, suggesting that besides homeostatic functions in the thymus, it may also have other functions under inflammatory conditions.

Future Directions

The overlap in chemokine expression and thymic biology is now very compelling and warrants increased attention to this area. Some of the future directions are fairly straightforward. Firstly, it is important to map more precisely the expression of all chemokines and their receptors in both thymic subsets and stromal cell subtypes. This information should point to more specific hypotheses on the role of each chemokine in T-cell development. Secondly, functional experiments (chemotaxis) should be performed using purified thymocyte subsets in order to more precisely identify the responding cells, particularly for those chemokine for which receptors have not yet been identified. Finally, experiments using neutralizing antibodies against either chemokines or chemokine receptors in FTOC should be performed in order to evaluate the role of these molecules in T-cell development. The latter step may in many cases be replaced by the analysis of the thymus of chemokine or chemokine receptor knockout mice which are now being produced in many laboratories. We can predict that some of these mice will show thymic defects.

Conclusions

Despite our expanded knowledge of chemokine function, there has been little advancement of our understanding of chemokine function in thymic biology. We have no clear understanding of several key processes where chemokines are very likely to be involved, for example, how a thymic progenitor cell finds its way from the bone marrow to the thymus. We have to establish whether the role of chemokines in thymic development is restricted to the regulation of intrathymic cell migration or whether they also have direct effects in thymocyte differentiation. Finally, we should explore their possible roles in the discrete steps that have been recognized during intrathymic T-cell development. We should expect rapid progress in these areas in the near future.

Another exciting aspect of this area is that it represents a direct consequence of the progress of genomics and bioinformatics as well as an example of the impact that the human genome project will have in virtually every aspect of biology.

Acknowledgment

DNAX Research Institute is supported by Schering-Plough Corporation.

References

1 Godfrey DI, Zlotnik A: Control points in early T-cell development. Immunol Today 1993;14:547.

2 Blom B, Res P, Spits H: T cell precursors in man and mice. Crit Rev Immunol 1998;18:371–378.

3 Moore T, Zlotnik A: T cell lineage commitment and cytokine responses of thymic progenitors. Blood 1995;86:1850–1860.

4 Capone MC, Gorman DM, Ching EP, Zlotnik A: Identification through bioinformatics of cDNAs encoding human thymic shared Ag-1/stem cell Ag-2. J Immunol 1996;157:969–973.

5 Aiuti A, Webb IJ, Bleul C, Springer T, Gutierrez-Ramos JC: The chemokine SDF-1 is a chemoattractant for human CD34+ hematopoietic progenitor cells and provides a new mechanism to explain the mobilization of CD34+ progenitors to peripheral blood. J Exp Med 1997;185:111–120.

6 Bleul CC, Fuhlbrigge RC, Casasnovas JM, Aiuti A, Springer TA: A highly efficacious lymphocyte chemoattractant, stromal cell-derived factor 1 (SDF-1). J Exp Med 1996;184:1101–1109.

7 Kim CH, Pelus LM, White JR, Broxmeyer HE: Differential chemotactic behavior of developing T cells in response to thymic chemokines. Blood 1998;91:4434–4443.

8 Zaitseva MB, Lee S, Rabin RL, Tiffany HL, Farber JM, Peden KW, Murphy PM, Golding H: CXCR4 and CCR5 on human thymocytes: Biological function and role in HIV-1 infection. J Immunol 1998;161:3103–3113.

9 Kitchen SG, Zack JA: CXCR4 expression during lymphopoiesis: Implications for human immunodeficiency virus type 1 infection of the thymus. J Virol 1997;71:6928–6934.

10 Berkowitz RD, Beckerman KP, Schall TJ, McCune JM: CXCR4 and CCR5 expression delineates targets for HIV-1 disruption of T cell differentiation. J Immunol 1998;161:3702–3710.

11 Zhang L, He T, Talal A, Wang G, Frankel SS, Ho DD: In vivo distribution of the human immunodeficiency virus/simian immunodeficiency virus coreceptors: CXCR4, CCR3, and CCR5. J Virol 1998;72:5035–5045.

12 Lerner A, Clayton LK, Mizoguchi E, Ghendler Y, van Ewijk W, Koyasu S, Bhan AK, Reinherz EL: Cross-linking of T-cell receptors on double-positive thymocytes induces a cytokine-mediated stromal activation process linked to cell death. EMBO J 1996;15:5876–5887.

13 Gattass CR, King LB, Luster AD, Ashwell JD: Constitutive expression of interferon-gamma-inducible protein 10 in lymphoid organs and inducible expression in T cells and thymocytes. J Exp Med 1994;179:1373–1378.

14 Tamaru M, Tominaga Y, Yatsunami K, Narumi S: Cloning of the murine interferon-inducible protein 10 (IP-10) receptor and its specific expression in lymphoid organs. Biochem Biophys Res Commun 1998;251:41–48.

15 Cole KE, Strick CA, Paradis TJ, Ogborne KT, Loetscher M, Gladue RP, Lin W, Boyd JG, Moser B, Wood DE, Sahagan BG, Neote K: Interferon-inducible T cell alpha chemoattractant (I-TAC): A novel non-ELR CXC chemokine with potent activity on activated T cells through selective high affinity binding to CXCR3. J Exp Med 1998;187:2009–2021.

16 Dairaghi DJ, Franz-Bacon K, Callas E, Cupp J, Schall TJ, Tamraz SA, Boehme SA, Taylor N, Bacon KB: Macrophage inflammatory protein-1β induces migration and activation of human thymocytes. Blood 1998;91:2905–2913.

17 Imai T, Yoshida T, Baba M, Nishimura M, Kakizaki M, Yoshie O: Molecular cloning of a novel T-cell-directed CC chemokine expressed in thymus by signal sequence trap using Epstein-Barr virus vector. J Biol Chem 1996;271:21514–21521.

18 Imai T, Baba M, Nishimura M, Kakizaki M, Takagi S, Yoshie O: The T-cell-directed CC chemokine TARC is a highly specific biological ligand for CC chemokine receptor 4. J Biol Chem 1997;272: 15036–15042.

19 Hoogewerf A, Black D, Proudfoot AE, Wells TN, Power CA: Molecular cloning of murine CC CKR-4 and high affinity binding of chemokines to murine and human CC CKR-4. Biochem Biophys Res Commun 1996;218:337–343.

20 Godiska R, Chantry D, Raport CJ, Sozzani S, Allavena P, Leviten D, Mantovani A, Gray PW: Human macrophage-derived chemokine, a novel chemoattractant for monocytes, monocyte-derived dendritic cells, and natural killer cells. J Exp Med 1997;185:1595–1604.

21 Chang M, McNinch J, Elias CR, Manthey CL, Grosshans D, Meng T, Boone T, Andrew DP: Molecular cloning and functional characterization of a novel CC chemokine, stimulated T cell chemotactic protein (STCP-1) that specifically acts on activated T lymphocytes. J Biol Chem 1997; 272:25229–25237.

22 Napolitano M, Zingoni A, Bernardini G, Spinetti G, Nista A, Storlazzi CT, Rocchi M, Santoni A: Molecular cloning of TER1, a chemokine receptor-like gene expressed by lymphoid tissues. J Immunol 1996;157:2759–2763.

23 Zaballos A, Varona R, Gutierrez J, Lind P, Marquez G: Molecular cloning and RNA expression of two new human chemokine receptor-like genes. Biochem Biophys Res Commun 1996;227:846–853; Erratum in Biochem Biophys Res Commun 1997;231:519–520.

24 Tiffany HL, Lautens LL, Gao JL, Pease J, Locati M, Combadiere C, Modi W, Bonner TI, Murphy PM: Identification of CCR8: A human monocyte and thymus receptor for the CC chemokine I-309. J Exp Med 1997;186:165–170.

25 Goya I, Gutiérrez J, Varona R, Kremer L, Zaballos A, Márquez G: Identification of CCR8 as the specific receptor for the human β-chemokine I-309: Cloning and molecular characterization of murine CCR8 as the receptor for TCA-3. J Immunol 1998;160:1975–1981.

26 Zingoni A, Soto H, Hedrick JA, Stoppacciaro A, Storlazzi CT, Sinigaglia F, D'Ambrosio D, O'Garra A, Robinson D, Rocchi M, Santoni A, Zlotnik A, Napolitano M: The chemokine receptor CCR8 is preferentially expressed in Th2 but not Th1 cells. J Immunol 1998;161:547–551.

27 Van Snick J, Houssiau F, Proost P, Van Damme J, Renauld JC: I-309/T cell activation gene-3 chemokine protects murine T cell lymphomas against dexamethasone-induced apoptosis. J Immunol 1996;157:2570–2576.

28 Bernardini G, Hedrick J, Sozzani S, Luini W, Gaia S, Weiss M, Menon S, Zlotnik A, Mantovani A, Santoni A, Napolitano M: Identification of the CC chemokines TARC and macrophage inflammatory protein-1β as novel functional ligands for the CCR8 receptor. Eur J Immunol 1998;28: 582–588.

29 Kim C, Pelus L, White J, Applebaum E, Johanson K, Broxmeyer H: CKβ-11/macrophage inflammatory protein-3β/EBI1-ligand chemokine is an efficacious chemoattractant for T and B cells. J Immunol 1998;160:2418–2424.

30 Kelner GS, Kennedy J, Bacon KB, Kleyensteuber S, Largaespada DA, Jenkins NA, Copeland NG, Bazan JF, Moore KW, Schall TJ, Zlotnik A: Lymphotactin: A cytokine that represents a new class of chemokine. Science 1994;266:1395–1399.

31 Yoshida T, Imai T, Kakizaki M, Nishimura M, Takagi S, Yoshie O: Identification of single C motif-1/lymphotactin receptor XCR1. J Biol Chem 1998;273:16551–16554.

32 Vicari AP, Figueroa DJ, Hedrick JA, Foster JS, Singh KP, Menon S, Copeland NG, Gilbert DJ, Jenkins NA, Bacon KB, Zlotnik A: TECK: A novel CC chemokine specifically expressed by thymic dendritic cells and potentially involved in T cell development. Immunity 1997;7:291–301.

Dr. Albert Zlotnik, DNAX Research Institute of Cellular and Molecular Biology,
901 California Avenue, Palo Alto, CA 94304 (USA)
Tel. +1 650 496 1131, Fax +1 650 496 1200, E-Mail zlotnik@dnax.org

Mantovani A (ed): Chemokines.
Chem Immunol. Basel, Karger, 1999, vol 72, pp 69–85

Chemokines and Chemokine Receptors in the Regulation of Dendritic Cell Trafficking

Paola Allavena[a], *Walter Luini*[a], *Raffaella Bonecchi*[a], *Giovanna D'Amico*[a], *Giancarlo Bianchi*[a], *Daniela Longoni*[c], *Annunciata Vecchi*[a], *Alberto Mantovani*[a, b], *Silvano Sozzani*[a]

[a] Istituto di Ricerche Farmacologiche Mario Negri, Milan;
[b] Department of Biotechnology, Section of General Pathology, University of Brescia, and
[c] Fondazione Tettamanti, Department Clinical Pediatrics, University of Milan, Italy

Dendritic cells (DC) are a heterogeneous system of leukocytes highly specialized in priming of T-cell-dependent immune responses. DC are potent accessory cells and are believed to be indispensable to activate quiescent lymphocytes [1–3]. The hallmark of DC is an extraordinary ability to capture soluble antigens, to process and present antigenic peptides, and to migrate through tissues to reach secondary lymphoid organs, where the stimulation of naive T cells takes place [4]. DC have peculiar trafficking properties: circulating precursors of tissue DC leave the blood compartment and localize at diverse anatomical sites, where they develop into specialized antigen-presenting cells (APC) with distinct morphological features such as Langerhans' cells (LC) in epithelia [1–3]. Upon exposure to immune or inflammatory signals, DC undergo functional maturation and reenter the circulatory system to home to the T-cell areas of lymphoid organs. They do so via two routes, lymphatic vessels to reach lymph nodes and blood to reach the spleen. DC in transit to lymph nodes have long been recognized as veiled cells [1, 2, 4]. This trafficking of DC to lymph nodes is critical to their overall function as APC; in fact, it is established that surgical removal of afferent lymphatic vessels prevents sensitization to skin transplants or to contact allergens [5, 6].

The DC population is highly heterogeneous: a myeloid-derived and a lymphoid-derived DC have been recognized [2, 3]. Nonlymphoid as well as lymphoid tissues contain DC with different names but similar properties. For instance, DC of the skin are the well-known LC and interstitial DC harbor several organs (lung, heart, kidney, etc.). Veiled DC are cells circulating in the lymph after tissue trafficking. Interdigitating cells (IDC) and follicular dendritic cells (FDC) are found within the lymphoid organs but the latter may not be bone marrow-derived. Thymic DC and DC of Peyer's patches have also been recognized [1, 2].

In vivo studies have demonstrated that DC use specific pathways of tissue trafficking. Application of a fluorescent marker to skin induces migration of LC and a day later fluorescent LC are found in the draining lymph nodes [7]. It has also been described that inhaled pathogens induce a very rapid mobilization of DC in the airway epithelium [8, 9]. The systemic treatment with LPS provokes a massive egress of DC from several organs, such as skin, heart, kidney, intestine, and causes DC migration from the marginal zone of the spleen to T-cell areas [10–12]. After intravenous injection of inert particles, cells with DC characteristic are recruited to the hepatic sinusoid and then translocate to the hepatic lymph [13].

A major difficulty in the study of DC is the paucity of cells recovered ex vivo, as they are scattered all over tissues. In the last few years new methods have been described allowing the in vitro differentiation of DC from precursors, either from CD34+ stem cells or monocytes, providing large quantities of cells feasible for in vitro studies [14–17].

Cell migration involves the coordinate activation of two classes of effector molecules – adhesion proteins and their counterreceptors, and chemotactic proteins [18]. In this review we will discuss the current understanding on the molecular basis of DC migration in vitro and in vivo, and how the regulated expression of chemotactic receptors may account for the different distribution of DC at a different stage of maturation.

Response of DC to Chemokines

Chemotactic agonists are key effector molecules in the process of leukocyte recruitment and tissue trafficking. The discovery of a large family of chemotactic cytokine (chemokines) has vigorously contributed to identify the molecular basis of the motility of different leukocyte subpopulations [19–22]. A number of studies have addressed the stimuli that induce chemotaxis of human DC, in vitro. In most experiments, DC were obtained from blood monocytes (mono-DC) cultured in the presence of GM-CSF and IL-4 or IL-13 [23–27]. These in vitro differentiated DC can be considered at an immature stage, as demonstrated by their high endocytic activity and by membrane phenotype expression (CD1a++, MHC II++, CD80+/–, CD86+/–, CD83–) [16, 24, 28]. In a microwell chemotaxis assay human mono-DC migrate in response to classical chemotactic agonists, such as formylated peptides, platelet-activating factor (PAF), C5a and to many CC chemokines including MCP-3, MCP-4, RANTES, MIP-1α, MIP-1β, MIP-5, MIP-3β, and MDC. Unlike monocytes, mono-DC do not respond to MCP-1 and MCP-2, two CC chemokines. All of the CXC chemokines tested were inactive, with the exception of SDF-1. Lymphotactin, the only C chemokine, was also inactive [23–25]. In general, peak active concentration and the percentage of migrating DC in response to chemokines were comparable to those observed with human monocytes. Active chemokines also induced calcium fluxes in DC [24, 27, 29, 30, and unpubl. data].

Experiments using DC originated from CD34+ stem cells (CD34-DC) differentiated with GM-CSF and TNF, confirmed these results [26, 31], but also showed a response to MIP-3α, a chemokine inactive on mono-DC [32, 33]. Interestingly, also murine CD34-DC differentiated with GM-CSF and fLT3L behaved very similarly to human DC [34]. Therefore, DC differentiated in vitro from different species, from different sources, and with a different cocktail of cytokines, have a very similar pattern of chemotactic response. The only major difference between mouse and man was MCP-1. Human mono-DC and CD34-DC express the MCP-1 receptor CCR2 and bind labelled MCP-1, but show little or no response [23, 24]. In contrast, mouse DC show a chemotactic response to MCP-1 [34]. It is of note the report that transgenic mice overexpressing MCP-1 in the basal layer of the epidermis had local accumulation of cells with DC morphology [35].

DC also represent a source of chemokines in vitro and in vivo. Immature DC constitutively produce MDC, MIP-1γ and DCK1/PARC [25, 36, 37]. Furthermore, thymic DC selectively express TECK, a CC chemokine active on thymocytes, macrophages and DC [38]. Mature DC obtained in vitro by stimulation with inflammatory agonists or engagement of CD40, produce a number of chemokines such as MCP-1, IL-8 and MIP-3β [30, 39, 40]. Of note, MIP-3β is also produced by mature DC in the T-cell areas of lymphoid organs, in vivo [29, 41].

In vivo Migration of DC to Chemokines

In order to investigate the in vivo role of chemokines in DC recruitment, we recently transfected tumor cells with MCP-3, a chemokine able to induce DC chemotaxis, in vitro [23, 24, 31]. After MCP-3 gene transfer, P815 mastocytoma cells grew, but subsequently underwent rejection [42] MCP-3-elicited rejection was associated with increased leukocyte infiltration. Analysis of leukocyte subsets infiltrating tumor tissues revealed that macrophages, T cells, eosinophils and neutrophils were increased in MCP-3-transfected tumors. DC (i.e. DEC205+, MHC class II+ and CD11c+ cells) did not substantially increase in the tumor mass, but accumulated in peritumoral tissues and were found in proximity of blood vessels. This peculiar localization has been found also in human carcinoma, and improved patient survival was indeed correlated with peritumoral – and not intratumoral – DC infiltration [43]. The evidence that MCP-3-transfected tumor cells grow normally in nude mice and in immunocompetent mice depleted of CD4+, or CD8+ T lymphocytes, indicates that MCP-3 gene transfer elicits tumor rejection by activating type I T-cell-dependent immunity. It is tempting to speculate that altered trafficking of antigen-presenting cells, which express receptors and respond to MCP-3, together with recruitment of activated T cells, underlies activation of specific immunity by MCP-3-transfected cells. Therefore, gene transfer of a DC chemotactic cytokine in a mouse tumor indicates that these molecules indeed have the potential to regulate DC trafficking in vivo, though the possibility that MCP-3 may act via secondary mediators cannot be formally discarded.

Chemokine Receptors in Immature DC

Receptor expression is a crucial determinant of the spectrum of action of chemokines [44–51]. Therefore, the pattern of chemokine receptors present in DC was examined (fig. 1). Northern blot analysis revealed that both mono-DC and CD34-DC express CCR1, CCR5 and CXCR4. These receptors account for the chemotactic response to RANTES, MCP-3, MIP-1α, MIP-1β, MIP-5 and SDF-1. DC also express specific receptors for PAF, fMLP and C5a [24, 26]. In spite of the lack of DC migration to MCP-1 and IL-8, CCR2 and CXCR2 were also found expressed. CCR3, CCR4, CCR7 and CCR8 can be detectable by this assay, however, mRNA for CCR4 and CCR7 were not detected by PCR or RNase protection assay [29, 30, and unpubl. data]. These low levels of receptor expression could account for the chemotactic response of DC to MDC, a CCR4 ligand [25, 52], and to MIP-3β, the ligand of CCR7 [28, 53], observed in vitro. Purified circulating DC were also found to express CCR1, CCR2, CCR3, CCR5 and CXCR4 by PCR analysis [54].

MIP-3α, also known as LARC or Exodus, is the only chemokine which differentiates between mono-DC and CD34-DC. Only CD34-DC, but not mono-DC, migrates in response to this chemokine and expresses CCR6, the MIP-3α receptor (fig. 1) [32, 33]. CCR6, a receptor expressed in resting T lymphocytes [55], is transiently induced in CD34-DC during in vitro culture by

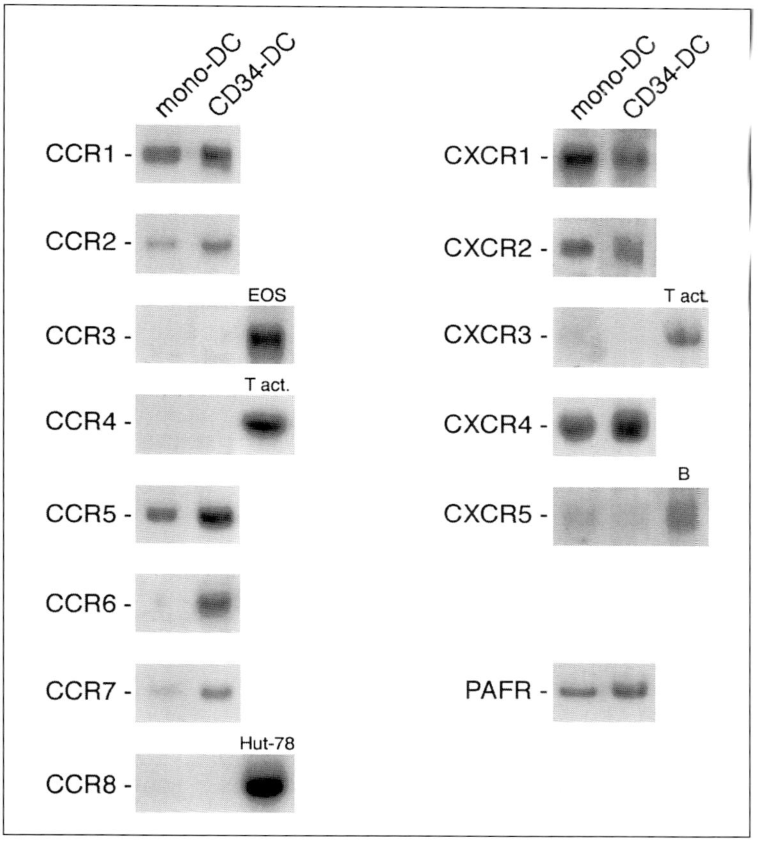

Fig. 1. Chemokine receptor expression in DC subsets. Mono-DC were differentiated from blood monocytes cultured with GM-CSF (50 ng/ml) and IL-13 (20 ng/ml) for 7 days [24]. CD34-DC were differentiated from CD34+ cord blood cultured with GM-CSF (50 ng/ml) stem cell factor (50 ng/ml) and TNF (10 ng/ml) for 12 days [26]. Mono-DC and CD34-DC share the same receptor repertoire with the exception of CCR6, which is selectively expressed in CD34-DC. For receptors not expressed by DC, positive controls are shown: EOS = eosinophils; T act. = PHA-activated T lymphocytes; Hut-78 = T lymphocyte cell line; B = tonsil B lymphocytes.

day 6 and becomes barely detectable by day 14. On the contrary, monocytes and mono-DC do not express CCR6 [29, 32, 33].

Chemokine receptor expression in DC has been recently investigated in relation to HIV infection, as these cells may represent an important port of entry of the virus and a vehicle for HIV-1 transmission [55, 57]. In vitro cultured DC and purified circulating DC express both CCR5 and CXCR4, the two main coreceptors for M-tropic (R5) and T-tropic (X4) strains of the virus, respectively [24, 54, 58]. Immature DC selectively replicate R5 HIV [59], and immature LC express only CCR5 and select R5 HIV strains in vivo [60, 61]. LC and immature DC are present at mucosal sites of virus transmission and selective entry and replication of R5 HIV could explain the restriction of virus phenotype during viral infection before seroconversion.

Differential Regulation of Chemokine Receptor Expression during Maturation

Maturation of DC can be induced in vitro by a variety of factors, in particular by LPS and inflammatory cytokines TNF and IL-1. Engagement of CD40 and of the newly described molecule TRANCE/RANK with their respective ligands expressed on activated T cells, also leads to maturation and activation of DC [3, 62]. In vivo, antigen uptake and the exposure of immature DC to immune and inflammatory agonists cause the rapid mobilization of DC from peripheral nonlymphoid tissues and activate the maturation process in these cells [3, 4].

Previous studies performed with mononuclear phagocytes and lymphocytes have shown that cell activation is often associated with a rearrangement of the repertoire of expressed chemokine receptors. In particular, proinflammatory agonists (e.g. LPS, IL-1 and TNF) induce a downmodulation of certain CC chemokine receptors in monocytes, while anti-inflammatory signals such as IL-10, have an opposite effect [47, 48, 63–65].

Recently it was shown that signals that induce maturation of DC affect also their migratory ability [28–30, 66, 67]. Exposure of DC to LPS, IL-1 and TNF, or culture in the presence of CD40 ligand, induced a rapid (<1 h) inhibition of chemotactic response to MIP-1α, MIP-1β, MIP-3α, RANTES, MCP-3 and fMLP [28, 29]. As previously observed in phagocytes [47, 68], inhibition of chemotaxis was followed, with a slower kinetics, by the reduction of membrane receptors and the downregulation of mRNA receptor expression [28–30, 59, 67]. Concomitantly, in the same experimental conditions, the expression of CCR7 and the migration of its ligand MIP-3β, a chemokine constitutively expressed in lymphoid organs, were strongly upregulated, with a maximal effect at 24 h. Upregulation of CCR7 in DC migrating to secondary lymphoid organs appears biologically relevant, since in situ hybridization analysis has shown that MIP-3β is specifically expressed in T-cell-rich areas of tonsils and spleen, where mature DC home, becoming interdigitating DC [29, 41]. Receptor expression and chemotactic response to other constitutive chemokines, such as SDF-1 (CXCR4) and MDC (CCR4), were increased

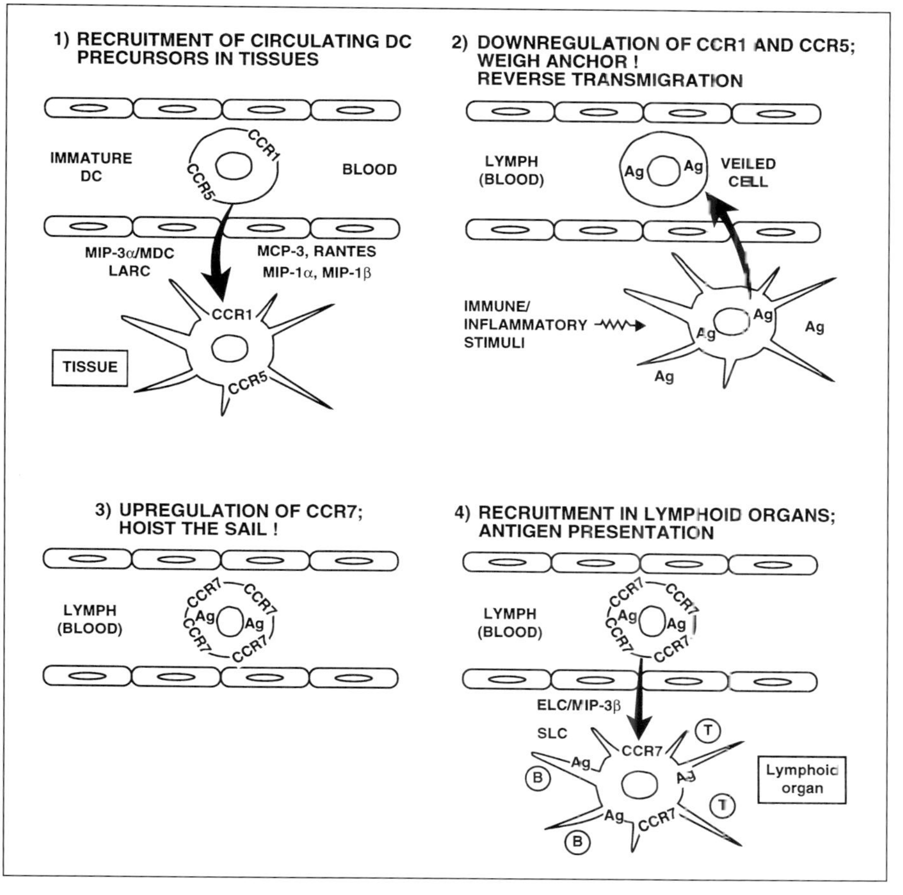

Fig. 2. A model for DC trafficking: 'weigh anchor – hoist the sail'. (1) Inducible chemokines (e.g. MCP-3, RANTES, etc.) acting via CCR1 and CCR5, may function as signals to recruit immature DC precursors. (2) Inflammatory and immune stimuli induce maturation of DC and downregulation of CCR1 and CCR5 (weigh anchor!). Migrating DC reenter circulation by reverse transmigration. (3) Mature DC strongly upregulate CCR7 (hoist the sail!). (4) Recruitment in lymphoid organs is mediated by SLC and MIP-3β (acting via CCR7) constitutively expressed at these sites.

during maturation of DC, in contrast to receptors for inducible chemokines, which were downregulated [30, 34, 67].

Overall, these findings provide a model for DC trafficking, illustrated in figure 2. Inflammatory chemokines acting through CCR1 and CCR5 may function as signals to localize DC precursors to nonlymphoid organs. On the contrary, the loss of responsiveness of DC to the massive production of these chemokines during inflammation and immune reactions may play a permissive role for DC to leave peripheral tissues. Meantime, the slower upregulation for CCR7 prepares the cells to respond to MIP-3β and SLC (another ligand for CCR7) [69], expressed in lymphoid organs. The selective upregulation of CCR7 may not be unique to this receptor inasmuch as similar results were observed with the PAF-R [26] and with a novel orphan receptor [unpubl. results].

Direct and Reverse Transendothelial Migration of DC

During migration from the tissue of residence to afferent lymphatics, DC interact with the extracellular matrix (ECM) and with the endothelial lining of lymphatic and blood vessels [4]. A number of studies have analyzed the expression of adhesion molecules which mediate their binding to endothelial cells (EC) and to ECM.

Mono-DC and CD34-DC express CD31, the β2 integrins LFA-1, Mac-1 and p150,95 the β1 integrin VLA-4 and VLA-5, but were negative for other β1 integrins and for L selectin [70]. In adhesion assays, binding to resting monolayers of umbilical cord vein EC was strongly inhibited by anti-CD11a and CD11b, but not CD11c mAbs. On TNF-activated EC, anti-VLA-4 in concert with anti-CD18 inhibited most of the binding [70]. CD34-DC behaved similarly to mono-DC in terms of expression of adhesive molecules and binding ability [70]

DC effectively transmigrated through EC cultured on porous polycarbonate filters in a transwell system. The proportion of cells spontaneously crossing a monolayer of resting EC in a 1-hour assay was 33% of EC-adherent cells. Activation of EC with TNF or IL-1 increased the net number of transmigrated cells, but the proportion over input cells remained the same [70]. Anti-β2 integrin mAb inhibited adhesion as well as transendothelial migration. In contrast, anti-CD31 did not affect adhesion but partially inhibited transmigration, suggesting an involvement of platelet endothelial cell adhesion molecule (PECAM-1) [70]. The amount of DC transmigrated through EC monolayers was increased 2- to 3-fold in response to chemokines. Active chemokines included MCP-3, MIP-3β, MIP-1β, MIP-5 and SDF-1 (fig. 3) [70]. These data are in line with the response to DC in classical chemotaxis assays [23, 24]. Similar results were confirmed with CD34-derived murine DC cultured with GM-CSF and fLT3L. These cells transmigrated through a microvascular murine endothelial cell line and increased transmigration was observed in response to murine MIP-1α, RANTES and SDF-1 [34].

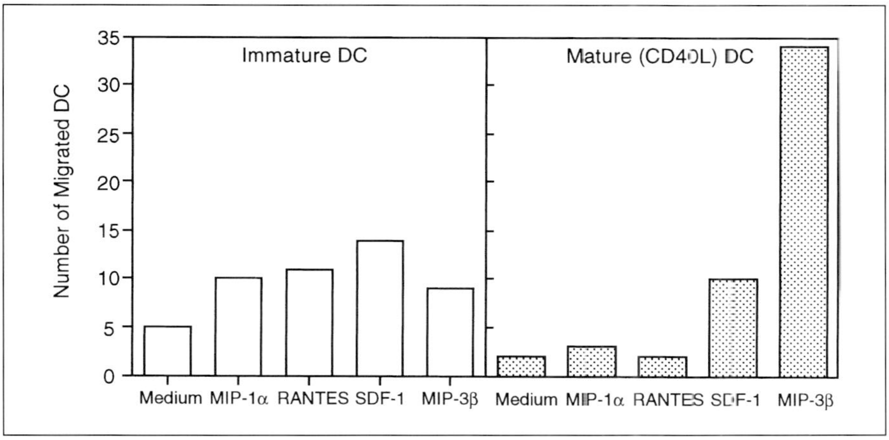

Fig. 3. Transendothelial migration of immature and mature DC. Immature DC were differentiated from blood monocytes by culturing with GM-CSF (50 ng/ml) and IL-13 (20 ng/ml) for 7 days. Maturation of DC was obtained by cocultivation with a CD40-transfected cell line for 48 h. Maturation of DC abrogated the response to MIP-1α and RANTES, migration to SDF-1 was slightly decreased, in contrast the response to MIP-3β was strongly augmented.

Similarly to chemotactic response, treatment of DC with LPS, TNF and CD40L almost abrogated the response of mature DC to MIP-1α and RANTES in transmigration assay. Response to SDF-1 was not significantly affected by maturation. In contrast, a strong response to MIP-3β was induced upon DC maturation (fig. 3). MIP-3β was by far the strongest stimulus in transendothelial migration, inducing a 17-fold increase of mature DC migration, compared to a 2-fold increase in immature DC [28].

Unlike circulating leukocytes, upon transendothelial migration, tissue DC interact with the basal layer of the endothelium. We therefore established an assay to mimic the basal-to-apical migration to DC into lymphatic/blood vessels (reverse transmigration). In this assay an upper filter is coated with ECM, and a lower filter is coated with a monolayer of EC, placed upside down. Mono-DC were able to migrate across the basal membrane and then through the EC monolayer to reach the luminal surface. About 20% of the EC-adherent cells spontaneously crossed the ECM and EC monolayer. This proportion is slightly lower than that observed in the direct transmigration assay (33%) [70].

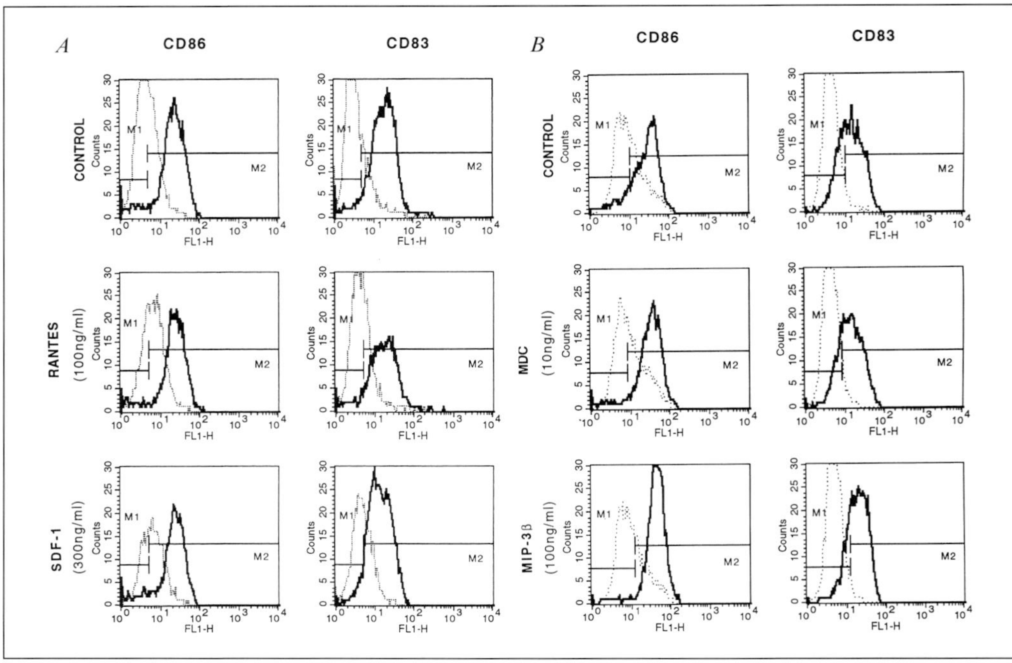

Fig. 4. Effect of chemokines on mono-DC differentiation. Chemokines were added to the culture medium either at the beginning of the culture (*A*) or at day 6 of culture (*B*). Results refer to the membrane phenotype of immature DC cultured for 8 days with GM-CSF (50 ng/ml) and IL-13 (20 ng/ml) (dotted line), and to mature DC receiving at day 6 of culture LPS (10 ng/ml) for 2 days (bold line). The expression of CD86 and CD83 was strongly induced in mature DC and was comparable in cells cultured with and without chemokines. Marker sets (M1 and M2) define cells stained with isotype-matched irrelevant and relevant mAbs, respectively.

Effect of Chemokines in DC Differentiation

Chemokines also have nonchemotactic effects on leukocytes [21, 22]. Therefore, chemokines were tested for their ability to modulate cell functions typically related to DC. Neither short (1 h) nor long (24 h) treatments of mono-DC with a number of chemokines including MCP-3, MIP-1α, MIP-3β, RANTES, MDC and SDF-1 modified the ability of these cells to take up FITC-dextran or activate T lymphocyte proliferation in MLR (data not shown) [24]. The ability of chemokines to interfere with the in vitro cytokine-driven differentiation of monocytes into DC was also investigated. Chemokines were added in the culture medium, together with GM-CSF and IL-13, at the beginning of the 7-day culture. Phenotype analysis of the resulting population revealed no significant effect of RANTES and SDF-1 on DC differentiation as far as the expression of CD86 and CD83 (fig. 4A). Moreover, MDC and MIP-3β did not affect terminal maturation of DC induced by LPS, when added at day 6 of differentiation, together with LPS (fig. 4B). These results indicate that chemokines, at least at the doses optimal for chemotaxis assay, have no relevant effect on DC differentiation from precursors and on their biological functions, other than cell migration.

Chemokines in Polarized Th1 and Th2 Responses

Distinct sets of chemokines are known to control migration of T lymphocytes. Memory or activated T cells mainly express CCR1, CCR2, CCR5 and CXCR3. On the contrary, naive T lymphocytes migrate in response to SDF-1 (CXCR4) and MIP-3β (CCR7) [71, 72], chemokines that are also active on mature DC. T cells can be subdivided in polarized type I and type II cells, depending on the spectrum of cytokines which they are able to produce. T-helper 1 cells (Th1 cells) are characterized by production of TNF and IFN-γ and activate immunity based on macrophage activation and effector functions. At the other extreme of the spectrum, Th2 cells are characterized by IL-4 and IL-5 production and elicit immune responses based on the effector function of mastocytes and eosinophils. The latter cell types are typically involved in allergic inflammation.

Recent results indicate that chemokines are part of the Th1 and Th2 paradigm. It was found that polarized Th1 and Th2 populations differentially express chemokine receptors. In particular, as summarized in figure 5, Th1 cells characteristically express high levels of CCR5 and CXCR3, whereas Th2 cells express CCR4, CCR8 and to a lesser degree, CCR3. Type I and type II CD8+ cells (Tc1 and Tc2, respectively) express a pattern of chemokine receptors very similar to that observed in Th1 and Th2 lymphocytes [51]. In accordance with receptor expression, polarized Th1/Th2, as well as Tc1/Tc2 cells, differentially respond to appropriate agonists for these receptors, including, for Th1/Tc1 cells, MIP-1β and IP-10 and for Th2/Tc2 cells MDC, 1309 and eotaxin [44, 45, 51]. Production of IP-10 and similar CXCR3 agonists such as ITAC, is induced by IFN-γ. Conversely, production of eotaxin and/or MDC is induced by IL-4 and IL-13, typical Th2 cytokines [21, 22, 73]. Thus, chemokines are an essential part of an amplification circuit of polarized type I and type II responses.

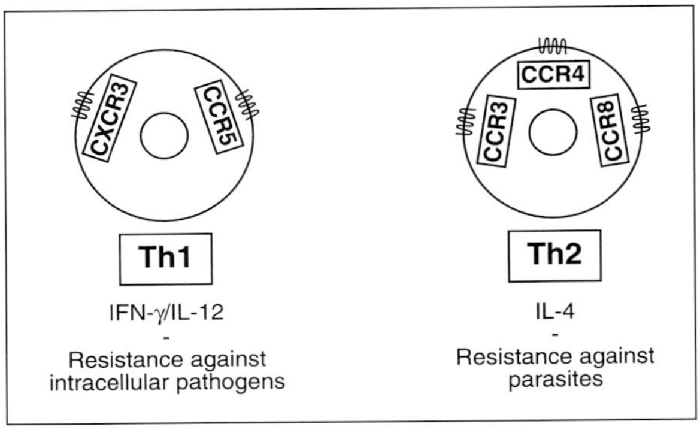

Fig. 5. Differential chemokine receptor expression in polarized Th1 and Th2 lymphocytes. Th1 cells expressed CCR3 and CCR5, while Th2 cells express CCR3, CCR4 and CCR8.

Concluding Remarks

DC trafficking is an essential step in the initiation of specific immune responses. Technical improvements have provided a large number of in vitro differentiation DC for the characterization of the migratory properties of these cells, under controlled and uniform conditions. Moreover, the setting up of convenient assays representative of different steps of DC trafficking, such as reverse transmigration [70, 74], offered tools to begin the dissection of the molecular basis of this complex series of events. Chemokines have emerged as major regulators of DC migration in vitro and, by inference, in vivo. DC are both a target and a source of chemokines. DC respond to a spectrum of molecules which overlaps with, but is distinct from, that active on other leukocyte populations.

In addition, analysis of CCR6 expression has revealed heterogeneity among DC in terms of their repertoire of chemokine receptors and, accordingly, responsiveness. The analysis of how chemokine receptor expression is modulated during maturation of DC has highlighted a pivotal role of CCR7 and provided a comprehensive model for the role of chemokines and their receptors in DC trafficking: 'weigh anchor – host the sail', depicted in figure 2 [28]. The actual relevance of this model will now need to be put to a test in vivo, using for instance gene-modified animals [75].

While the focus has been on chemokines as determinants for DC trafficking, other more classic, lipid or peptide attractants may play a no less important role. The recent finding of upregulation of PAF receptor during maturation [26] raises the important issue of the actual role of this lipid in DC migration in vivo.

DC are considered a powerful target of immunotherapeutic approaches. A better understanding of the molecular basis of DC trafficking may provide molecular and conceptual tools to direct and modulate DC traffic as a strategy to upregulate and orient specific immunity.

Acknowledgments

This study was supported by Associazione Italiana per la Ricerca sul Cancro (AIRC); special project AIDS (40A.0.66) from Istituto Superiore Sanità; National Research Council (CNR) Finalized Project Biotechnology. R.B. is the recipient of a fellowship from Fondazione Italiana per la Ricerca sul Cancro (FIRC).

References

1 Steinman RM: The dendritic cell system and its role in immunogenicity. Annu Rev Immunol 1991; 9:271–296.
2 Hart DNJ: Dendritic cells: Unique leukocyte populations which control the primary immune response. Blood 1997;90:3245–3286.
3 Banchereau J, Steinman RM: Dendritic cells and the control of immunity. Nature 1998;392:245–252.
4 Austyn JM: New insights into the mobilization and phagocytic activity of dendritic cells. J Exp Med 1996;183;1287–1292.
5 Frey JR, Wenk P: Experimental studies on the pathogenesis of contact eczema in the guinea pig. Arch Allergy Appl Immunol 1957;11:81–100.
6 Barker CF, Billingham RE: The role of afferent lymphatics in the rejection of skin homografts. J Exp Med 1968;128:197–221.
7 Macatonia SE, Knight SC, Edwards AJ, Griffiths S, Freyer F: Localization of antigen on lymph node dendritic cells after exposure to the contact sensitizer fluorescein isothiocyanate. Functional and morphological studies. J Exp Med 1987;166:1654–1667.
8 McWilliam AS, Nelson D, Thomas JA, Holt PG: Rapid dendritic cell recruitment is a hallmark of the acute inflammatory response at mucosal surfaces. J Exp Med 1994;179:1331–1336.
9 McWilliam AS, Napoli S, Marsh AM, Pemper FL, Nelson DJ, Pimm CL, Stumbles PA, Wells TNC, Holt PG: Dendritic cells are recruited into the airway epithelium during the inflammatory response to a broad spectrum of stimuli. J Exp Med 1996;184:2429–2432.
10 Macpherson GG, Jenkins CD, Stein MJ, Edwards C: Endotoxin-mediated dendritic cell release from the intestine – Characterization of released dendritic cells and TNF dependence. J Immunol 1995;154:1317–1322.
11 Roake JA, Rao AS, Morris PJ, Larsen CP, Hankins DF, Austyn JM: Dendritic cell loss from nonlymphoid tissues after systemic administration of lipopolysaccharide, tumor necrosis factor, and interleukin-1. J Exp Med 1995;181:2237–2247.
12 De Smedt T, Pajak B, Muraille E, Lespagnard L, Heinen E, Debaetselier P, Urbain J, Leo O, Moser M: Regulation of dendritic cell numbers and maturation by lipopolysaccharide in vivo. J Exp Med 1996;184:1413–1424.
13 Matsuno K, Ezaki T, Kudo S, Uehara Y: A life stage of particle-laden rat dendritic cells in vivo: Their terminal division, active phagocytosis, and translocation from the liver to the draining lymph. J Exp Med 1996;183:1865–1878.
14 Caux C, Dezutter-Dambuyant C, Schmitt D, Banchereau J: GM-CSF and TNF-α cooperate in the generation of dendritic Langerhans' cells. Nature 1992;360:258–261.

15 Romani N, Gruner S, Brang D, Kampgen E, Lenz A, Trockenbacher B, Konwalinka G, Fritsch PO, Steinman RM, Schuler G: Proliferating dendritic cell progenitors in human blood. J Exp Med 1994;180:83–93.

16 Sallusto F, Lanzavecchia A: Efficient presentation of soluble antigen by cultured human dendritic cells is maintained by granulocyte/macrophage colony-stimulating factor plus interleukin-4 and downregulated by tumor necrosis factor-alpha. J Exp Med 1994;179:1109–1118.

17 Rosenzwajg M, Canque B, Gluckman JC: Human dendritic cell differentiation pathway from CD34(+) hematopoietic precursor cells. Blood 1996;87:535–544.

18 Springer TA: Traffic signal of lymphocyte recirculation and leukocyte emigration: The multistep paradigm. Cell 1994;76:301–314.

19 Baggiolini M, Dewald B, Moser B: Human chemokines: An update. Annu Rev Immunol 1997;15: 675–705.

20 Hendrick JA, Zlotnik A: Chemokines and lymphocyte biology. Curr Opin Immunol 1996;8:343–347.

21 Rollins BJ: Chemokines. Blood 1997;90:909–928.

22 Mantovani A, Allavena P, Vecchi A, Sozzani S: Chemokines and chemokine receptors during activation and deactivation of monocytes and dendritic cells and in amplification of Th1 versus Th2 responses. Int J Clin Lab Res 1998;28:77–82.

23 Sozzani S, Sullusto F, Luini W, Zhou D, Piemonti L, Allavena P, Van Damme J, Valitutti S, Lanzavecchia A, Mantovani A: Migration of dendritic cells in response to formyl peptides, C5a and a distinct set of chemokines. J Immunol 1995;155:3292–3295.

24 Sozzani S, Luini W, Borsatti A, Polentarutti N, Zhou D, Piemonti L, D'Amico G, Power CA, Wells TN, Gobbi M, Allavena P, Mantovani A: Receptor expression and responsiveness of human dendritic cells to a defined set of CC and CXC chemokines. J Immunol 1997;159:1993–2000.

25 Godiska R, Chantry D, Raport CJ, Sozzani S, Allavena P, Leviten D, Mantovani A, Gray PW: Human macrophage-derived chemokine (MDC): A novel chemoattractant for monocytes, monocyte-derived dendritic cells, and natural killer cells. J Exp Med 1997;185:1595–1604.

26 Sozzani S, Longoni D, Bonecchi R, Luini W, Bersani L, D'Amico G, Borsatti A, Bussolino F, Allavena P, Montovani A: Human monocyte-derived and CD34+ cell-derived dendritic cells express functional receptors for platelet-activating factor. FEBS Lett 1997;418:98–100.

27 Rubbert A, Combadiere C, Ostrowski M, Arthos J, Dybul M, Machado E, Cohn MA, Hoxie J, Murphy PM, Fauci AS, Weissman D: Dendritic cells express multiple chemokine receptors used as coreceptors for HIV entry. J Immunol 1998;160;3933–3941.

28 Sozzani S, Allavena P, D'Amico G, Luini W, Bianchi G, Kataura M, Imai T, Yoshie O, Bonecchi R, Mantovani A: Cutting edge: Differential regulation of chemokine receptors during dendritic cell maturation: A model for their trafficking properties. J Immunol 1998;161:1083–1086.

29 Dieu MC, Vanbervliet B, Vicari A, Bridon J M, Oldham E, Ait-Yahia S, Briere F, Zlotnik A, Lebecque S, Caux C: Selective recruitment of immature and mature dendritic cells by distinct chemokines expressed in different anatomic sites. J Exp Med 1998;188:373–386.

30 Sallusto F, Schaerli P, Loetscher P, Schaniel C, Lenig D, Mackay CR, Qin S, Lanzavecchia A: Rapid and coordinated switch in chemokine receptor expression during dendritic cell maturation. Eur J Immunol 1998;28:2760–2769.

31 Xu LL, Warren M, Rose WL, Gong WH, Wang JM: Human recombinant monocyte chemotactic protein and other C-C chemokines bind and induce directional migration of dendritic cells in vitro. J Leukoc Biol 1996;60:365–371.

32 Power CA, Church DJ, Meyer A, Alouan S, Proudfoot AEI, Clark-Lewis I, Sozzani S, Mantovani A, Wells TNC: Cloning and characterization of a specific receptor for the novel CC chemokine MIP-3-alpha from lung dendritic cells. J Exp Med 1997;186:825–835.

33 Greaves DR, Wang W, Dairaghi DJ, Dieu MC, de Saint-Vis B, Franz-Bacon K, Rossi D, Caux C, McClanahan T, Gordon S, Zlotnik A, Schall TJ: CCR6, a CC chemokine receptor that interacts with macrophage inflammatory protein-3-alpha and is highly expressed in human dendritic cells. J Exp Med 1997;186:837–844.

34 Vecchi A, Massimiliano L, Ramponi S, Luini W, Bernasconi S, Bonecchi R, Allavena P, Parmentier M, Mantovani A, Sozzani S: Differential responsiveness to constitutive versus inflammatory chemokines of immature and mature mouse dendritic cells. J Leukoc Biol 1999; in press.

35 Nakamura K, Williams IR, Kupper TS: Keratinocyte-derived monocyte chemoattractant protein 1 (MCP-1): Analysis in a transgenic model demonstrates MCP-1 can recruit dendritic and Langerhans' cells to skin. J Invest Dermatol 1995;105:635–643.
36 Mohamadzadeh M, Poltorak AN, Bergstresser PR, Beutler B, Takashima A: Dendritic cells produce macrophage inflammatory protein-1-gamma, a new member of the CC chemokine family. J Immunol 1996;156:3102–3106.
37 Adema GJ, Hartgers F, Verstraten R, deVries E, Marland G, Menon S, Foster J, Xu YM, Nooyen P, McClanahan T, Bacon KB, Figdor CG: A dendritic-cell-derived C-C chemokine that preferentially attracts naive T cells. Nature 1997;387:713–717.
38 Vicari AP, Figueroa DJ, Hedrick JA, Foster JS, Singh KP, Menon S, Copeland NG, Gilbert DJ, Jenkins NA, Bacon KB, Zlotnik A: TECK: A novel CC chemokine specifically expressed by thymic dendritic cells and potentially involved in T-cell development. Immunity 1997;7:291–301.
39 Zhou LJ, Tedder TF: A distinct pattern of cytokine gene expression by human CD83(+) blood dendritic cells. Blood 1995;86:3295–3301.
40 Caux C, Massacrier C, Vanbervliet B, Dubois B, Vankooten C, Durand I, Banchereau J: Activation of human dendritic cells through CD40 cross-linking. J Exp Med 1994;180:1263–1272.
41 Ngo VN, Tang HL, Cyster JG: Epstein-Barr virus-induced molecule 1 ligand chemokine is expressed by dendritic cells in lymphoid tissues and strongly attracts naive T cells and activated B cells. J Exp Med 1998;188:181–191.
42 Fioretti F, Fradelizi D, Stoppacciaro A, Ruco L, Minty A, Sozzani S, Vecchi A, Mantovani A: Reduced tumorigenicity and augmented leukocyte infiltration after MCP-3 gene transfer: Perivascular accumulation of dendritic cells in peritumoral tissue and neutrophil recruitment within the tumor. J Immunol 1998;161:342–346.
43 Goldman SA, Baker E, Weyant RJ, Clarke MR, Myers JN, Lotze MT: Peritumoral CD1a-positive dendritic cells are associated with improved survival in patients with tongue carcinoma. Arch Otolaryngol Head Neck Surg 1998;124:641–646.
44 Bonecchi R, Bainchi G, Bordignon PP, D'Ambrosio D, Lang R, Borsatti A, Sozzani S, Allavena P, Gray PA, Mantovani A, Sinigaglia F: Differential expression of chemokine receptors and chemotactic responsiveness of type 1 T helper cells (Th1) and Th2. J Exp Med 1998;187:129–134.
45 Sallusto F, Mackay CR, Lanzavecchia A: Selective expression of the eotaxin receptor CCR3 by human T helper 2 cells. Science 1997;277:2005–2007.
46 Leotscher P, Uguccioni M, Bordoli L, Baggiolini M, Moser B, Chizzolini C, Dayer JM: CCR5 is characteristic of Th1 lymphocytes. Nature 1998;391:344–345.
47 Sica A, Saccani A, Borsatti A, Power CA, Wells TNC, Luini W, Polentarutti N, Sozzani S, Mantovani A: Bacterial lipopolysaccharide rapidly inhibits expression of C-C chemokine receptors in human monocytes. J Exp Med 1997;185:969–974.
48 Sozzani S, Ghezzi S, Iannolo G, Luini W, Borsatti A, Polentarutti N, Sica A, Locati M, Mackay C, Wells TNC, Biswas P, Vicenzi E, Poli G, Mantovani A: Interleukin-10 increases CCR5 expression and HIV infection in human monocytes. J Exp Med 1998:187:439–444.
49 Polentarutti N, Allavene P, Bianchi G, Giardina G, Basile A, Sozzani S, Mantovani A, Introna M: IL-2 regulated expression of the monocyte chemotactic protein-1 receptor (CCR2) in human NK cells: Characterization of a predominant 3.4 kb transcript containing CCR2B and CCR2A sequences. J Immunol 1997;158:2689–2694.
50 Loetscher P, Seitz M, Baggiolini M, Moser B: Interleukin-2 regulates CC chemokine receptor expression and chemotactic responsiveness in T lymphocytes. J Exp Med 1996;184:569–577.
51 D'Ambrosio D, Iellem A, Bonecchi R, Mazzeo D, Sozzani S, Mantovani A, Sinigaglia F: Cutting edge: Selective upregulation of chemokine receptors CCR4 and CCR8 upon activation of polarized human type 2 T helper cells. J Immunol 1998;161:5111–5115.
52 Imai T, Chantry D, Raport CJ, Wood CL, Nishimura M, Godiska R, Yoshie C. Gray PW: Macrophage-derived chemokine is a functional ligand for the CC chemokine receptor 4. J Biol Chem 1998;273:1764–1768.
53 Yoshida R, Imai T, Hieshima K, Kusuda J, Baba M, Kitaura M, Nishimura M, Kakizaki M, Nomiyama H, Yoshie O: Molecular coloning of a novel human CC chemokine EBI1-ligand chemokine that is a specific functional ligand for EBI1, CCR7. J Biol Chem 1997;272:13803–13809.

54 Ayehnie S, Garcia-Zepeda EA, Hoxie JA, Horuk R, Kupper TS, Luster AD, Ruprecht RM: Human immunodeficiency virus-1 entry into purified blood dendritic cells through CC and CXC chemokine coreceptors. Blood 1997;90:1379–1386.

55 Baba M, Imai T, Nishimura M, Kakizaki M, Takagi S, Hieshima K, Nomiyama H, Yoshie O: Identification of CCR6, the specific receptor for a novel lymphocyte-directed CC chemokine LARC. J Biol Chem 1997;272:14893–14898.

56 Graziosi C, Pantaleo G: The multi-faceted personality of HIV. Nat Med 1998;12:1318–1320.

57 Cameron PU, Freudenthal PS, Barker JM, Gezelter S, Inaba K, Steinman RM: Dendritic cells exposed to human immunodeficiency virus type-1 transmit a vigorous cytopathic infection to CD4+ T cells. Science 1992;257:383–387.

58 Granelli-Piperno A, Moser B, Pope M, Chen DL, Wei Y, Isdell F, O'Doherty U, Paxton W, Koup R, Mojsov S, Bhardwaj N, Clarklewis I, Baggiolini M, Steinman RM: Efficient interaction of HIV-1 with purified dendritic cells via multiple chemokine coreceptors. J Exp Med 1996;184: 2433–2438.

59 Granelli-Piperno A, Delgado E, Finkel V, Paxton W, Steinman RM: Immature dendritic cells selectively replicate macrophagetropic (M-tropic) human immunodeficiency virus type 1, while mature cells efficiently transmit both M- and T-tropic virus to T cells. J Virol 1998;72:2733–2737.

60 Reece JC, Handley AJ, Anstee EJ, Morrison WA, Crowe SM: HIV-1 selection by epidermal dendritic cells during transmission across human skin. J Exp Med 1998;187:1623–1631.

61 Zaitseva M, Blauvelt A, Lee S, Lapham CK, Klaus-Kovtun V, Motowski H, Manischewitz J, Golding H: Expression and function of CCR5 and CXCR4 on human Langerhans' cells and macrophages: Implication for HIV primary infection. Nat Med 1997;3:1369–1375.

62 Cella M, Sallusto F, Lanzavecchia A: Origin, maturation and antigen presenting function of dendritic cells. Curr Opin Immunol 1997;9:10–16.

63 Penton-Rol G, Polentarutti N, Luini W, Borsatti A, Mancinelli R, Sica A, Sozzani S, Mantovani A: Selective inhibition of expression of chemokine receptor CCR2 in human monocytes by IFN-γ. J Immunol 1998:160:3869–3873.

64 Xu L, Rahimpour R, Ran L, Kong C, Biragyn A, Andrews J, Devries M, Wang JM, Kelvin DJ: Regulation of CCR2 chemokine receptor mRNA stability. J Leukoc Biol 1997;62:653–660.

65 Tangirala RK, Murao K, Quehenberger O: Regulation of expression of the human monocyte chemotactic protein-1 receptor (hCCR2) by cytokines. J Biol Chem 1997;272:8050–8056.

66 Yanagihara S, Komura E, Nagafune J, Watarai H, Yamaguchi Y: EBI1/CCR7 is a new member of dendritic cell chemokine receptor that is upregulated upon maturation. J Immunol 1998;161: 3096–3102.

67 Lin CL, Suri RM, Rahdon RA, Austyn JM, Roake JA: Dendritic cell chemotaxis and transendothelial migration are induced by distinct chemokines and are regulated on maturation. Eur J Immunol 1998;28:4114–4122.

68 Lloyd AR, Biragyn A, Johnston JA, Taub DD Xu LL, Michiel D, Sprenger H, Oppenheim JJ, Kelvin DJ: Granulocyte colony-stimulating factor and lipopolysaccharide regulate the expression of interleukin-8 receptors on polymorphonuclear leukocytes. J Biol Chem 1995;270:28188–28192.

69 Gunn MD, Tangemann K, Tam C, Cyster JG, Rosen SD, Williams LT: A chemokine expressed in lymphoid high endothelial venules promotes the adhesion and chemotaxis of naive T lymphocytes. Proc Natl Acad Sci USA 1998;95:258–263.

70 D'Amico G, Bianchi G, Bernasconi S, Bersani L, Piemonti L, Sozzani S, Mantovani A, Allavena P: Adhesion, transendothelial migration, and reverse transmigration of in vitro cultured dendritic cells. Blood 1998;92:207–214.

71 Sallusto F, Lanzavecchia M, Mackay CR: Chemokines and chemokine receptors in T-cell priming and Th1/Th2-mediated responses. Immunol Today 1998;19:568–574.

72 Baggiolini M: Chemokines and leukocyte traffic. Nature 1998;392:565–568.

73 Bonecchi R, Sozzani S, Stine J, Luini W, D'Amico G, Allavena P, Chantry D, Mantovani A: Divergent effects of IL-4 and interferon-gamma on macrophage-derived chemokine (MDC) production: An amplification circuit of polarized T-helper-2 responses. Blood 1998;92:2668–2671.

74 Randolph GJ, Beaulieu S, Pope M, Sugawara I, Hoffman L, Steinman RM, Muller WA: A physiologic function for p-glycoprotein (MDR-1) during the migration of dendritic cells from skin via afferent lymphatic vessels. Proc Natl Acad Sci USA 1998;95:6924–6929.
75 Gunn MD, Kyuwa S, Tam C, Kakiuchi T, Matsuzawa A, Williams LT, Nakano H: Mice lacking expression of secondary lymphoid organ chemokine have defects in lymphocyte homing and dendritic cell localization. J Exp Med 1999;189:451–460.

Dr. Paola Allavena, Istituto di Ricerche Farmacologiche 'Mario Negri',
Via Eritrea 62, I–20157 Milan (Italy)
Tel. +39 02 39014 563, Fax +39 02 3546277, E-Mail allavena@irfmn.mnegri. it

Mantovani A (ed): Chemokines.
Chem Immunol. Basel, Karger, 1999, vol 72, pp 86–101

The Role of CXC Chemokines in the Regulation of Angiogenesis

Michael P. Keane, Robert M. Strieter

Department of Internal Medicine (Division of Pulmonary and Critical Medicine), The University of Michigan Medical School, Ann Arbor, Mich., USA

Angiogenesis is defined as the growth of neovasculature from preexisting vessels. This is an important biological process central to a variety of physiologic and pathologic processes. The regulation of angiogenesis depends upon a dual, yet opposing balance of local factors which promote (angiogenic factors) or inhibit (angiostatic factors) neovascularization. For example, the rate of normal capillary endothelial cell turnover in adults is typically measured in months or years, suggesting the potential of an equivalent balance in the presence of both angiogenic and angiostatic factors under homeostatic conditions. By contrast, during wound repair and development of granulation tissue, this balance shifts in favor of a predominance of angiogenic factors leading to establishment of new functioning capillaries within a matter of days. Wound-associated angiogenesis is locally controlled and transient. As rapidly as neovascularization occurs in the wound, these neovessels virtually disappear, returning the tissue vasculature to a homeostatic environment. This abrupt termination of angiogenesis in the context of the resolution of wound repair supports the notion that the following occurs in the local environment: a marked reduction in the elaboration of angiogenic factors and/or a simultaneous increase in the levels of factors that inhibit neovascularization. In contrast to the precise regulation of angiogenesis of wound repair, dysregulation of angiogenesis can lead to an imbalance in the relationship of angiogenic and angiostatic factors that favors persistent *net* angiogenesis that contributes to the pathogenesis of chronic inflammation and solid tumor growth.

The complement of angiogenic and angiostatic factors may vary among different physiologic and pathologic settings. However, the recognition of this dual mechanism of control is critical in order to gain insight into this complex process and understand the regulation of angiogenesis. The list of factors that can regulate angiogenesis is extensive (table 1). However, the purpose of this chapter will be to introduce the topic of angiogenesis and focus on the CXC chemokine family, as these cytokines are a unique family of molecules that can behave in a disparate manner in the regulation of angiogenesis.

Angiogenesis

The process of angiogenesis is initiated in the postcapillary venule. The initial angiogenic response is associated with a change in cellular adhesive interactions between adjacent endothelial cells, pericytes, and smooth muscle cells. Activated endothelial cells reorganize their cytoskeletal elements, express cell surface adhesion molecules (e.g. integrins and selectins), and generate extracellular matrix. Endothelial cells produce a variety of proteolytic enzymes aiding in degradation of the basement membrane and migration into the surrounding extracellular matrix. This event is followed by the formation of capillary buds, which can proceed in the absence of endothelial proliferation. Subsequent phases of angiogenesis leading to the formation of microvessels requires continual exposure to angiogenic mediators that are either released from depots in the extracellular matrix or produced in the local environment. These angiogenic factors function in either an autocrine and/or paracrine manner to induce endothelial cell migration, proliferation, elongation, orientation, and differentiation leading to reestablishment of the basement membrane, lumen formation, and anastomosis with other neovessels or preexisting vessels. Depending on the balance in expression of angiogenic and angiostatic factors in the local environment, the neovasculature may persist as capillaries, differentiate into mature venules or arterioles, or undergo regression. The factors responsible for this latter event are now being identified and may either function to initiate apoptosis or induce cell cycle arrest of endothelial cells. Thus, the process of angiogenesis is a complex interaction of extracellular matrix with activated endothelial cells undergoing migration, proliferation, and tube formation in response to an imbalance in the presence of angiogenic, as compared to angiostatic factors in their local environment.

A dual, yet opposing system of angiogenic and angiostatic factors regulate net angiogenesis. Angiogenic factors are molecules that induce endothelial cell migration, proliferation, and differentiation into tubular structures. These molecules are produced by an array of cells and function as ligands in an autocrine and paracrine manner to facilitate endothelial cell activation. While angiogenic factors can directly stimulate angiogenesis by interacting with

Table 1. Inhibitors (angiostatic factors) and promoters (angiogenic factors) of angiogenesis

Inhibitors of angiogenesis	Promoters of angiogenesis
Proteins and peptides	Cytokines
Angiostatin	Acidic fibroblast growth factor (aFGF)
Endostatin	Basic fibroblast growth factor (bFGF)
Eosinophilic major basic protein	Epidermal growth factor (EGF)
High-molecular-weight hyaluronan	Interleukin-1 (IL-1)
Interferon-α	Interleukin-2 (IL-2)
Interferon-β	Scatter factor/hepatocyte growth factor (SF/HGF)
Interferon-γ	Transforming growth factor α (TGF-α)
ELR^- CXC chemokines	Transforming growth factor β (TGF-β)
Interleukin-1	Tumor necrosis factor α (TNF-α)
Interleukin-4	Vascular endothelial growth factor (VEGF)
Interleukin-12	ELR^+ CXC chemokines
Laminin and fibronectin peptides	
Placental RNAase (angiogenin) inhibitor	Carbohydrates and lipids
Somatostatin	12(R)-hydroxyeicosatrienoic acid (Compound D)
Substance P	Hyaluronan fragments
Thrombospondin-1	Lactic acid
Tissue inhibitor of metalloproteinases (TIMPs)	Monobutyrin
	Prostaglandins E_1 and E_2
Lipids	
Angiostatic steroids	Other proteins and peptides
Retinoids	Angiogenin
Vitamin A	Angiotensin II
	Ceruloplasm
Others	Fibrin
Nitric oxide	Human angiogenic factor
Vitreous fluids	Plasminogen activator
Prostaglandin synthetase inhibitor	Polyamines
	Urokinase
	Others
	Adenosine
	Angiotropin
	Copper
	Heparin
	Nicatinamide
	ESAF

specific receptors on endothelial cells, other molecules in the local environment may be important for indirectly promoting angiogenesis by attracting and activating accessory cells, such as macrophages and fibroblasts, that produce additional angiogenic factors. In addition, various molecules can function as cofactors for the promotion of angiogenesis. For example, proteases can lead to the release of active angiogenic factors. Moreover, heparin, a glycosaminogylcan sequestered in the extracellular matrix, can play a key role in stabilizing and/or enhancing the function of angiogenic molecules.

A role for angiostatic factors in the control of angiogenesis was first observed when hyaline cartilage was found to be resistant to vascular invasion. Studies demonstrated that a heat-labile guanidium chloride extract prepared from cartilage contained an inhibitor of neovascularization. Other angiostatic factors have been reported from cell and tissue extracts and for a variety of natural and artificial agents including: inhibitors of basement membrane biosynthesis, placental ribonuclease inhibitor, lymphotoxin, interferons, prostaglandin synthetase inhibitors, heparin-binding fragments of fibronectin, protamine, angiostatic steroids, several antineoplastic and anti-inflammatory agents, platelet factor-4 (PF4), interferon-γ-inducible protein 10 (IP-10), monokine induced by interferon-γ (MIG), thrombospondin-1, angiostatin, endostatin and antagonists of the integrin $\alpha_v\beta_3$. Although speculation may exist as to whether angiogenic or angiostatic factors are tissue- or process-specific (e.g. embryogenesis vs. wound repair), the shear redundancy of positive and negative factors that regulate neovascularization affirms the fundamental nature of this process.

The CXC Chemokine Family of Cytokines

A variety of factors have been described that promote angiogenesis (table 1). Perhaps the best studied of the angiogenic factors are VEGF and bFGF. In contrast, both angiostatin and endostatin have been found to display marked inhibition of angiogenesis. While these factors are important in the regulation of angiogenesis in both physiological and pathophysiological processes, these molecules do not fully account for all the neovascular response in pathological conditions, such as tumorigenesis. The CXC chemokine family consists of polypeptides that are < 10 kD, and are characteristically heparin-binding proteins. On the structural level, this family displays four highly conserved cysteine amino acid residues, with the first two cysteines separated by one nonconserved amino acid residue, hence the name CXC. Although the CXC motif distinguishes this family from other chemokine families, a second structural domain within this family dictates their angiogenic potential. The

Table 2. ELR^+ and ELR^- CXC chemokines are angiogenic and angiostatic factors, respectively

Angiogenic CXC chemokines containing the ELR motif (ELR^+)
Interleukin-8 (IL-8)
Epithelial neutrophil-activating protein-78 (ENA-78)
Growth-related oncogene α (GRO-α)
Growth-related oncogene β (GRO-β)
Growth-related oncogene γ (GRO-γ)
Granulocyte chemotactic protein-2 (GCP-2)
Platelet basic protein (PBP)
Connective tissue-activating protein-III (CTAP-III)
β-Thromboglobulin (β-TG)
Neutrophil-activating protein-2 (NAP-2)
Angiostatic CXC chemokines that lack the ELR motif (ELR^-)
Platelet factor-4 (PF4)
Interferon-γ-inducible protein-10 (IP-10)
Monokine induced by interferon-γ (MIG)

NH_2-terminus of the majority of the CXC chemokines contains three amino acid residues (Glu-Leu-Arg: the 'ELR' motif) which precedes the first cysteine amino acid residue of the primary structure of these chemokines. The family members that contain the 'ELR' motif (ELR^+) are potent promoters of angiogenesis in physiological concentrations of 1–10 n*M*. In contrast, members that lack the ELR motif (ELR^-) are potent inhibitors of angiogenesis in physiological concentrations of 500 p*M* to 1 n*M*. This suggests on a structural/functional level that members of the CXC chemokine family are unique cytokines in their ability to behave in a disparate manner in the regulation of angiogenesis. The angiogenic members include interleukin (IL-8), epithelial neutrophil-activating protein-78 (ENA-78), growth-related oncogenes (GRO-α, -β and -γ), granulocyte chemotactic protein-2 (GCP-2), and NH_2-terminal truncated forms of platelet basic protein (PBP), which are generated by proteolytic cleavage with monocyte-derived proteases and include connective tissue activating protein-III (CTAP-III), β-thromboglobulin (β-TG), and neutrophil activating protein-2 (NAP-2). GRO-α, -β, and -γ are closely related CXC chemokines, with GRO-α originally described for its melanoma growth stimulatory activity (table 2). IL-8, ENA-78 and GCP-2 were all initially identified on the basis of neutrophil activation and chemotaxis.

The angiostatic (ELR^-) members of the CXC chemokine family include PF4, which was originally described for its ability to bind heparin and inactivate heparin's anticoagulation function. Other angiostatic ELR^- CXC chemokines include MIG and IP-10 (table 2). Stromal cell-derived factor (SDF-1) has

Table 3. Stimulus specificity for the expression and production of CXC chemokines

CXC chemokines	Stimulus			
	LPS	TNF	IL-1	IFN-γ
IL-8	++++	++++	++++	----
ENA-78	+++	+++	+++	----
GRO-α	+++	+++	+++	----
IP-10	+	+	+	+++
MIG	–	–	–	+++

recently gained notoriety when it was shown that SDF-1 induces lymphocyte migration and prevents infection of T cells by lymphotropic strains of HIV-1. Although SDF-1 is another ELR$^-$ CXC chemokine, it remains unclear whether it inhibits angiogenesis. SDF-1 was found to induce in vitro migration of human umbilical vein endothelial cells, whereas, in another study, SDF-1 was found to attenuate the in vivo angiogenic activity of either ELR$^+$ CXC chemokines, bFGF, or VEGF using the rat cornea micropocket assay of neovascularization [1]. IP-10 can be induced by all three interferons (IFN-α, -β and -γ). MIG is unique in that it is only induced by IFN-γ. In addition, IL-12 and IL-18, via the induction of IFN-γ, have been found to induce the expression of IP-10 and MIG [2]. While interferons induce the production of the angiostatic CXC chemokines, IP-10 and MIG, they attenuate the expression of the angiogenic CXC chemokines IL-8, GRO-α and ENA-78 (table 3). This differential regulation of angiostatic versus angiogenic CXC chemokines by interferons is likely to account for their previously documented inhibitory effect on angiogenesis.

CXC Chemokines Are Potent Regulators of Angiogenesis

PF4 (ELR$^-$) was the first CXC chemokine to be reported to have a role in the regulation of angiogenesis. Recombinant PF4 has been found to inhibit bFGF-induced angiogenesis and attenuate growth of melanoma and colon carcinomas in murine models of tumorigenesis. In contrast, IL-8 (ELR$^+$) was the first CXC chemokine to be found to induce angiogenesis. IL-8 was shown to mediate both in vitro endothelial cell chemotactic and proliferative activity, as well as in vivo angiogenesis in the absence of preceding inflammation using bioassays of angiogenesis [3]. These findings have been substantiated by other investigations that have shown that IL-8, similar to bFGF or VEGF induces endothelial cell tubular formation in vitro and angiogenesis in vivo in the rat mesenteric-window angiogenesis assay. These experiments prove that IL-8 has a direct effect on the endothelial cell, and that this angiogenic activity was distinct from its ability to recruit neutrophils and induce inflammation. These findings suggested that members of the CXC chemokine family function in a disparate manner, and can behave as either potent angiogenic or angiostatic factors in regulating net neovascularization.

Based on these findings, our laboratory hypothesized that the highly conserved 'ELR' motif of several members of the CXC chemokine family is a structural/functional domain that dictates their angiogenic activity. To test this postulate we found that ELR^+ CXC chemokines were potent angiogenic factors, inducing both in vitro endothelial chemotaxis and in vivo corneal neovascularization [4]. In contrast, the ELR^- CXC chemokines, PF4, IP-10, and MIG, not only failed to induce significant in vitro endothelial cell chemotaxis or in vivo corneal neovascularization, but were found to be potent angiostatic factors in the presence of either ELR^+ CXC chemokines or the unrelated angiogenic factors, bFGF and VEGF [4]. Additionally, mutant IL-8 proteins lacking the 'ELR' motif demonstrated potent angiostatic effects in the presence of either ELR^+ CXC chemokines or bFGF [4]. In contrast, a mutant of MIG containing the 'ELR' motif was found to induce in vivo angiogenic activity [4]. These findings suggest a functional role of the 'ELR' motif in determining the angiogenic or angiostatic potential of CXC chemokines, supporting the hypothesis that the net biological balance between angiogenic and angiostatic CXC chemokines may play an important role in regulating overall angiogenesis.

Putative Endothelial Cell CXC Chemokine Receptors That Bind Angiogenic and Angiostatic CXC Chemokines

Evidence would suggest that the endothelial receptor for ELR^+ CXC chemokines is the CXC chemokine receptor, CXCR2. In support of this contention are the following data: (1) both IL-8 and NAP-2 (ELR^+ CXC chemokines) have been shown to bind to endothelial cells; (2) CXCR2 is the putative receptor for all ELR^+ CXC chemokines on neutrophils, and all ELR^+ CXC chemokines are angiogenic [4]; (3) while the Duffy antigen receptor for chemokines (DARC) has been identified on postcapillary venule endothelial cells, this receptor binds not only ELR^+ CXC chemokines, but also a variety of CC chemokines without apparent signal-coupling [5]; (4) expression of CXCR2 in human burn wound (granulation tissue) is found in association with capillary endothelial cells in areas of neovascularization [6]; (5) expression of CXCR2 in human melanoma is associated with both melanoma cells and microvessels within the tumor [7]; (6) the expression of CXCR2 is present on microvascular endothelial cells associated with breast cancer and head and neck squamous cell carcinoma [8, 9]; (7) human Kaposi's sarcoma herpesvirus (KSHV) encodes a G-protein-coupled receptor structurally homologous to CXCR2 that is constitutively active and linked to cellular proliferation [10]; this suggests that a CXCR2-like receptor may facilitate tumorigenesis of this angiosarcoma; (8) recent findings from our laboratory have demonstrated that neutralizing antibodies to murine CXCR2 attenuate the angiogenic activity of murine KC, murine MIP-2, and human IL-8 in the rat CMP bioassay, without inhibiting the angiogenic activity of either bFGF or VEGF [unpubl. observ.]. These observations support the notion that CXCR2 may be an important target to attenuate the angiogenic activity of ELR$^+$ CXC chemokines.

In contrast to ELR$^+$ CXC chemokines, IP-10 appears to bind to a specific cell surface site on endothelial cells [11]. This receptor appears to be a heparin sulfate proteoglycan-associated receptor, as either heparin together with IP-10 or heparinase pretreatment of endothelial cells attenuates IP-10 binding [11]. This binding site is specific for IP-10, as neither ELR$^+$ CXC chemokines nor various CC chemokines compete for binding on this site. In addition, binding of IP-10 to endothelial cells resulted in an inhibition of proliferation that was independent of calcium flux and apoptosis, and dependent on reversible cell cycle arrest. While it is not clear whether this receptor represents the recently identified receptor for IP-10/MIG (CXCR3), these findings suggest that IP-10 and potentially MIG are unique members of the CXC chemokine family that share a heparin sulfate proteoglycan component of their receptor that accounts, in part, for their binding to endothelial cells and subsequent angiostatic activity.

CXC Chemokines Promote Angiogenesis Associated with Tumorigenesis

IL-8 been found to be significantly elevated in non-small cell lung cancer (NSCLC) [12]. In addition, IL-8 was determined to be a major angiogenic factor contributing to overall tumor-derived angiogenic activity in NSCLC [13]. These studies were extended to an in vivo model system of human tumorigenesis, which employed a human NSCLC/SCID mouse chimera by injecting human NSCLC cell lines into SCID mice [13]. This model system demonstrated a progressive increase in tumor size that was directly correlated with tumor-derived IL-8 [13] in both tumor homogenates and plasma. To ascertain whether IL-8 contributes to tumorigenesis of human NSCLC in

SCID mice, animals were subjected to a strategy of IL-8 depletion. Tumor-bearing animals treated with neutralizing antibodies to IL-8 demonstrated a >40% reduction in tumor growth, that was paralleled by a trend toward a reduction in spontaneous metastases to the lung [13]. The attenuation of tumor growth and metastases was directly correlated with reduced tumor-derived angiogenic activity and vessel density from the tumors of animals passively immunized with neutralizing anti-IL-8 antibodies. These finding have been corroborated by another study that found a majority of NSCLC cell lines constitutively expressed IL-8, and when grown in nude mice, neutralizing anti-IL-8 antibodies inhibited a significant portion of their angiogenic activity [14]. These studies demonstrated that a significant angiogenic signal for NSCLC neovascularization in vivo is directly mediated by tumor-associated IL-8.

Similar to NSCLC, the progression and growth of ovarian carcinoma is dependent on successful angiogenesis. To determine whether expression of specific angiogenic factors was associated with tumorigenesis and survival of nude mice with intraperitoneal human ovarian carcinomas, Yoneda et al. [15] examined the expression of IL-8, bFGF and VEGF. Five different tumor cell lines were used in this study [13]. All cell lines in vitro expressed similar levels of bFGF, however, these cell lines expressed either high or low levels of IL-8 or VEGF. When implanted into the peritoneum, the high expressing IL-8 and VEGF tumors were associated with either all mice dying <51 days or with a mean survival of 48 days, respectively [13]. In contrast, the low expressing IL-8 and VEGF tumors were associated with all mice surviving beyond 80 days [13]. The more aggressive tumors that resulted in increased mortality were highly associated with evidence of neovascularization [13]. Interestingly, the expression of IL-8 was inversely correlated with survival, whereas VEGF expression was only associated with production of ascites [13]. No correlation was found for the expression of bFGF with either tumor neovascularization or survival [13]. These studies have also been substantiated in primary cutaneous melanoma, where the expression of IL-8 correlates wiith both tumorigenicity and metastatic properties of these tumors [16].

To satisfy Koch's law, the specificity of the pathogenic agent must be present in all cases of the disease, inoculations of the agent must produce the same disease in animals, and isolation of the agent must be propagate in culture. The CXC chemokines clearly satisfy Koch's law as important mediators of tumorigenesis related to their angiogenic properties. Although GRO-β has been recently reported to inhibit angiogenesis [17], the concentration used in this study was 1,000-fold higher (1–10 μ*M*) than what was found for its angiogenic activity (1–10 n*M*). This would suggest that superphysiological concentrations of GRO-β could 'desensitize' the angiogenic response. Moreover, studies in melanoma support that all GROs play a significant role in mediating tumorigenesis related to both their mitogenic and angiogenic activities. The melanoma's ability to utilize a molecule for both autocrine growth and paracrine angiogenesis correlates with the potential aggressive phenotype of this carcinoma. For example, GRO-α, -β and -γ are all found to be highly expressed in human melanoma specimens [7]. To determine the biological significance of the presence of these ELR⁺ CXC chemokines in melanoma, human GRO-α, -β and -γ genes were transfected into immortalized murine melanocytes [7]. The continuous expression of any of these GROs transformed their phenotypic behavior to allow them to both form large colonies in soft agar in vitro and to generate tumors in vivo in both nude and SCID mice [7]. The tumors that formed were highly vascular and similar to the vascularity of B16 melanoma controls [7]. When tumor-bearing animals were passively immunized with specific anti-GRO antibodies there was a marked attenuation of tumor growth that was associated with a reduction in tumor angiogenic activity and vessel density [7]. These findings support the notion that the ELR⁺ CXC chemokines, such as GRO-α, -β and -γ, have the unique ability in melanoma to act in both an autocrine (mitogen) and paracrine (angiogenic factor) manner to promote tumorigenesis. The above studies suggest that ELR⁺ CXC chemokines play a major role in mediating angiogenesis in support of tumor growth.

ELR⁻ CXC Chemokines Attenuate Angiogenesis Associated with Tumorigenesis

The antithesis of ELR⁺ is the function of ELR⁻ CXC chemokines in regulating angiogenesis. Burkitt's lymphoma cell lines have been found to give rise to significant tumors in nude mice. Angiogenesis in this Epstein-Barr virus (EBV)-associated lymphoproliferative disorder appears to be essential to tumorigenesis of these lymphomas analogous to carcinomas. To determine whether IP-10 or MIG were contributing to the angiogenic activity of EBV-associated lymphomas, Sgadari et al. [18] implanted several of these tumor cell lines in nude mice. The expression of IP-10 was higher in the tumors that demonstrated spontaneous regression, as compared to those tumors with significant growth in nude mice. The regression of the tumors was directly related to evidence of reduced angiogenesis, increased tumor vascular damage and tissue necrosis. To determine whether this effect was related to IP-10, EBV-associated lymphoma cell lines that grew in nude mice were subjected to either intratumor inoculation with IP-10 or the cells were engineered to constitutively express high levels of IP-10 and injected into nude mice [18]. Both conditions resulted in marked reduction in angiogenesis associated with vascular damage and tissue necrosis. In a subsequent study, this same group demonstrated similar findings for MIG in this model system [19, 20]. The expression of MIG was found to be markedly higher in tumor cell lines that underwent spontaneous regression in nude mice [19, 20]. In contrast, tumor cell lines that demonstrated lower levels of constitutive expression of MIG grew large tumors in nude mice. Intratumor inoculation of recombinant MIG resulted in attenuation of angiogenesis, augmented vascular damage and tissue necrosis of these tumors to the same magnitude as what was seen with IP-10 [19, 20]. Although both IP-10 and MIG have been demonstrated to induce mononuclear recruitment via the interaction with their putative CXC chemokine receptor (CXCR3), the ability of both of these ELR^- CXC chemokines to inhibit angiogenesis and induce tumor regression in the above studies in nude mice support that these chemokines mediate their effect in a T-cell-independent manner.

Our laboratory has examined the role of IP-10 in regulating angiogenesis associated with NSCLC [21]. The levels of IP-10 from human surgical tumor specimens were significantly higher than in normal lung tissue. The increase in IP-10 from human NSCLC tissue was entirely attributable to the higher levels of IP-10 present in squamous cell carcinoma, as compared to adenocarcinoma. Moreover, depletion of IP-10 from human surgical squamous cell carcinoma specimens resulted in augmented angiogenic activity as measured by endothelial chemotaxis and the corneal micropocket model (CMP) bioassay of neovascularization [21]. The marked difference in the levels and bioactivity of IP-10 associated with squamous cell carcinoma, as compared to adenocarcinoma, is pathophysiologically relevant and represents a possible mechanism for the biologic differences of these two cell types of NSCLC. Patient survival is lower, metastatic potential is higher, and evidence of angiogenesisis greater for adenocarcinoma, as compared to squamous cell carcinoma of the lung [22, 23]. These studies were extended to a SCID mouse system to examine the effect of IP-10 in human NSCLC cell line tumor growth in a T- and B-cell-independent manner. SCID mice were inoculated with either A549 (adenocarcinoma) or Calu 1 (squamous cell carcinoma) cells [21]. The production of IP-10 from A549 and Calu 1 tumors was inversely correlated with tumor growth [21]. However, IP-10 levels were significantly higher in the Calu 1 (squamous), as compared to A549 (adenocarcinoma) tumors. The appearance of spontaneous lung metastases in SCID mice bearing A549 tumors occurred after IP-10 levels from either the primary tumor or plasma reached a nadir. In subsequent experiments, SCID mice bearing Calu 1 tumors were treated with either neutralizing anti-IP-10 or control antibodies, whereas animals bearing A549 tumors were treated with intratumor IP-10. Depletion of IP-10 in Calu 1 tumors resulted in a 2-fold increase in their size at 10 weeks. In contrast, 'reconstitution' of intratumor IP-10 in A549 tumors reduced both their size by >40% and metastatic potential, that was attributable to attenuation of tumor-associated angiogenic activity and vessel density.

Angiogenesis Contributes to the Pathology of Chronic Angiogenic/Fibroproliferative Diseases

Several lines of evidence suggest that an imbalance in the production of promoters and inhibitors of angiogenesis contributes to the pathogenesis of several angiogenesis-dependent disorders. For example, in rheumatoid arthritis the unrestrained proliferation of fibroblasts and capillary blood vessels leads to the formation of prolonged and persistent granulation tissue of the pannus whose degradative enzymes contribute to profound destruction of joint spaces. Koch and coworkers [24] have shown that a subpopulation of macrophages isolated from rheumatoid synovium produce factors that are potentially angiogenic in vivo and chemotactic for capillary endothelial cells in vitro. Psoriasis, a common genetic skin disease, is a well-known angiogenesis-dependent disorder that is characterized by marked dermal neovascularization. Keratinocytes isolated from psoriatic plaques demonstrate a greater production of angiogenic activity, as compared to normal keratinocytes. Interestingly, this aberrant phenotype is due, in part, to a combined defect in the overproduction of the angiogenic cytokine IL-8, and a deficiency in the production of the angiogenesis inhibitor, thrombospondin-1, resulting in a proangiogenic environment.

The Role of CXC Chemokines in Pulmonary Fibrosis

Interstitial pulmonary fibrosis (IPF) is a disease of unknown etiology that is characterized by the accumulation of neutrophils and mononuclear cells, followed by the progressive deposition of collagen within the interstitium and subsequent destruction of lung airspaces.

While studies have suggested an importance for IL-8 in mediating neutrophil recruitment, CXC chemokines have been found to exert disparate effects in regulating angiogenesis [25]. This latter issue is relevant to IPF, as the pathology of IPF demonstrates features of dysregulated and abnormal repair with exaggerated angiogenesis, fibroproliferation, and deposition of extracellular matrix, leading to progressive fibrosis and loss of lung function. The existence of neovascularization in IPF was originally identified by Turner-Warwick, who examined the lungs of patients with widespread IPF, and demonstrated neovascularization leading to anastomoses between the systemic and pulmonary microvasculature [26]. Further evidence of neovascularization during the pathogenesis of pulmonary fibrosis has been demonstrated in bleomycin-induced pulmonary fibrosis [27]. Peao et al. [27] perfused the vascular tree of rat lungs with methacrylate resin at a time of maximal bleomycin-induced pulmonary fibrosis. Using scanning electron microscopy, these investigators demonstrated major vascular modifications that included neovascularization of an elaborate network of microvasculature located in the peribronchial regions of the lungs, and distortion of the architecture of the alveolar capillaries. The location of neovascularization was closely associated with regions of pulmonary fibrosis, similar to the findings for human lungs [26], and this neovascularization appeared to lead to the formation of systemic-pulmonary anastomoses [27]. Although these studies supported the presence of angiogenesis, there have been limited investigations to delineate factors that may be involved in the regulation of this angiogenic activity during pulmonary fibrosis.

We have recently demonstrated that in IPF lung tissue there is an imbalance in the presence of CXC chemokines that behave as either promoters of angiogenesis (IL-8) or inhibitors of angiogenesis (IP-10) [28]. This imbalance favors augmented net angiogenic activity [28]. Lung tissue from IPF patients have elevated levels of IL-8, as compared to control lung tissue, and demonstrate in vivo angiogenic activity that can be significantly attenuated in the presence of neutralizing IL-8 antibodies [28]. Immunolocalization of IL-8 demonstrated that the pulmonary fibroblast was the predominant interstitial cellular source of this chemokine, and areas of IL-8 expression were essentially devoid of neutrophil infiltration [28]. This would seem to be discordant with the previous observations of augmented BALF IL-8 in IPF, in association with BALF neutrophilia [29]. However this disparity may be explained by the different compartments analyzed in these studies, i.e. BALF vs. lung interstitium, moreover BALF neutrophilia may simply be a marker of disease without their involvement in the pathogenesis of IPF. In further support of IL-8's role as an angiogenic factor is its association with the regulation of angiogenic activity in psoriasis, rheumatoid arthritis, and non-small cell lung cancer [12, 13, 24, 30]. This supports an alternative biological role for IL-8 or other ELR^+ CXC chemokines in the interstitium of IPF lung tissue.

The pulmonary fibroblast is the predominant cellular source of IL-8 in the interstitium of IPF, supporting the notion that the pulmonary fibroblast has a pivotal role in mediating the angiogenic activity during the pathogenesis of IPF [28]. This was confirmed by the in vivo angiogenic activity of pulmonary fibroblast-conditioned media, which was significantly inhibited by anti-IL-8 antibodies [28]. The difference in expression of IL-8 and IP-10 between IPF and control pulmonary fibroblasts lends further support to the notion of a phenotypic difference between IPF and normal pulmonary fibroblasts. Relative bioactive levels of IL-8 and IP-10 from IPF pulmonary fibroblast conditioned media demonstrated a significant imbalance favoring IL-8-induced-angiogenic activity, whereas normal pulmonary fibroblasts had greater levels of bioactive IP-10 and the imbalance of IL-8 and IP-10 from control pulmonary fibroblasts favored a net inhibition of angiogenesis [28].

In contrast to the increased angiogenic activity attributable to IL-8, we found a deficiency of the production of the angiostatic factor, IP-10, in IPF, as compared to controls [28]. The angiogenic activity from pulmonary fibroblast-conditioned media and lung tissue from either IPF or controls was augmented in the presence of neutralizing IP-10 antibodies [28]. This finding is similar to our previous studies of IP-10 in the regulation of angiogenesis in association with tumorigenesis of human non-small cell lung carcinoma, and its potential to inhibit tumor growth and metastases via its angiostatic activity [21]. Interestingly, IFN-γ, a major inducer of IP-10 from a number of cells, is a known inhibitor of wound repair, in part, due to its angiostatic properties [31], and has been shown to attenuate fibrosis in bleomycin-induced pulmonary fibrosis [32]. We have found that the angiostatic properties of IFN-γ may, in part, be attributable to IP-10. This supports the notion that the distal mediator of the affect of IFN-γ is IP-10 (and potentially MIG), and an imbalance in the expression of this angiostatic CXC chemokine is found in IPF. These results suggest that attenuation of the angiogenic (IL-8) or augmentation of the angiostatic (IP-10) CXC chemokines may represent a viable therapeutic option for the treatment of IPF.

Conclusion

Angiogenesis is regulated by an opposing balance of angiogenic and angiostatic factors. For example, the magnitude of the expression of angiogenic and angiostatic factors in a primary tumor correlates with both tumor growth and potential of spontaneous metastases. The above studies have demonstrated that as a family, the CXC chemokines behave as either angiogenic or angiostatic factors, depending on the presence of the 'ELR' motif that immediately precedes the first cysteine amino acid residue of the primary structure of these cytokines. In addition, CXC chemokines are important endogenous factors that regulate tumor-derived angiogenic activity, neovascularization, and spontaneous metastases of NSCLC. Furthermore, these chemokines are important regulators of angiogenic activity in pulmonary fibrosis. These findings represent proof of principle that therapy directed at either inhibition of angiogenic or augmentation of angiostatic CXC chemokines may be a novel approach in the treatment of solid tumors, and chronic fibroproliferative disorders.

Acknowledgments

This work was supported, in part, by NIH grants CA66180, P50 HL56402, and P50 HL60289 (R.M.S.) and KO8 HL03906 (M.P.K.).

References

1 Arenberg DA, Polverini PJ, Kunkel SL, Shanafelt A, Strieter RM: In vitro and in vivo systems to assess the role of C-X-C chemokines in the regulation of angiogenesis. Methods Enzymol 1997; 288:190–220.

2 Coughlin CM, Salhany KE, Wysocka M, Aruga E, Kurzawa H, Chang AE, Hunter CA, Fox JC, Trinchieri G, Lee WMF: Interleukin-12 and interleukin-18 synergistically induce murine tumor regression which involves inhibition of angiogenesis. J Clin Invest 1998;101:1441–1452.

3 Strieter RM, Kunkel SL, Elner VM, Martonyi CL, Koch AE, Polverini PJ, Elner SG: Interleukin-8. A corneal factor that induces neovascularization. Am J Pathol 1992;141:1279–1284.

4 Strieter RM, Polverini PJ, Kunkel SL, Arenberg DA, Burdick MD, Kasper J, Dzuiba J, Van Damme J, Walz A, Marriott D, Chan S, Roczniak S, Shanafelt A: The functional role of the ELR motif in CXC chemokine-mediated angiogenesis. J Biol Chem 1995;270:27348–27357.

5 Neote K, Darbonne W, Ogez J, Horuk R, Schall T: Identification of a promiscuous inflammatory peptide receptor on the surface of red blood cells. J Biol Chem 1993;268:985–991.

6 Nanney LB, Mueller SG, Bueno R, Peiper SC, Richmond A: Distributions of melanoma growth stimulatory activity or growth-related gene and the interleukin-8 receptor type B in human wound repair. Am J Pathol 1995;147:1248–1260.

7 Luan J, Shattuck-Brandt R, Haghnegahdar H, Owen JD, Strieter R, Burdick M, Nirodi C, Beauchamp D, Johnson KN, Richmond A: Mechanism and biological significance of constitutive expression of MGSA/GRO chemokines in malignant melanoma tumor progression. J Leukoc Biol 1997; 62:588–597.

8 Miller LJ, Kurtzman SH, Wang Y, Anderson KH, Lindquist RR, Kreutzer DL: Expression of interleukin-8 receptors on tumor cells and vascular endothelial cells in human breast cancer tissue. Anticancer Res 1998;18:77–81.

9 Richards BL, Eisma RJ, Spiro JD, Lindquist RL, Kreutzer DL: Coexpression of interleukin-8 receptors in head and neck squamous cell carcinoma. Am J Surg 1997;174:507–512.

10 Arvanitakis L, Geras-Raaka E, Varma A, Gershengorn MC, Cesarman E: Human herpesvirus KSHV encodes a constitutively active G-protein-coupled receptor linked to cell proliferation. Nature 1997;385:347–350.

11 Luster AD, Greenberg SM, Leder P: The IP-10 chemokine binds to a specific cell surface heparin sulfate site shared with platelet factor 4 and inhibits endothelial cell proliferation. J Exp Med 1995; 182:219–231.

12 Smith DR, Polverini PJ, Kunkel SL, Orringer MB, Whyte RI, Burdick MD, Wilke CA, Strieter RM: Inhibition of interleukin-8 attenuates angiogenesis in bronchogenic carcinoma. J Exp Med 1994;179:1409–1415.

13 Arenberg DA, Kunkel SL, Burdick MD, Polverini PJ, Strieter RM: Treatment with anti-IL-8 inhibits non-small cell lung cancer tumor growth (abstract). J Invest Med 1995;43(suppl 3):479A.

14 Yatsunami J, Tsuruta N, Ogata K, Wakamatsu K, Takayama K, Kkawasaki M, Nakanishi Y, Hara N, Hayashi S: Interleukin-8 participates in angiogenesis in non-small cell, but not small cell carcinoma of the lung. Cancer Lett 1997;120:101–108.

15 Yoneda J, Kuniyasu H, Crispens MA, Price JE, Bucana CD, Fidler IJ: Expression of angiogenesis-related genes and progression of human ovarian carcinomas in nude mice. J Natl Cancer Inst 1998; 90:447–454.

16 Singh RK, Gutman M, Radinsky R, Bucana CD, Fidler IJ: Expression of interleukin-8 correlates with the metastatic potential of human melanoma cells in nude mice. Cancer Res 1994;54:3242–3247.

17 Cao Y, Chen C, Weatherbee JA, Tsang M, Folkman J: Gro-beta, a C-X-C-chemokine, is an angiogenesis inhibitor that suppresses the growth of Lewis lung cacinoma in mice. J Exp Med 1995;182:2069–2077.
18 Sgadari C, Angiolillo AL, Cherney BW, Pike SE, Farber JM, Koniaris LG, Vanguri P, Burd PR, Sheikh N, Gupta G, Teruya-Feldstein J, Tosato G: Interferon-inducible protein-10 identified as a mediator of tumor necrosis in vivo. Proc Natl Acad Sci USA 1996;93:13791–13796.
19 Teruya-Feldstein J, Jaffe ES, Burd PR, Kanegane H, Kingma DW, Wilson WH, Longo DL, Tosato G: The role of Mig, the monokine induced by interferon-gamma, and IP-10, the interferon-gamma-inducible protein-10, in tissue necrosis and vascular damage associated with Epstein-Barr virus-positive lymphoproliferative disease. Blood 1997;90:4099–4105.
20 Sgadari C, Farber JM, Angiolillo AL, Liao F, Teruya-Feldstein J, Burd PR, Yao L, Gupta G, Kanegane C, Tosato G: Mig, the monokine induced by interferon-gamma, promotes tumor necrosis in vivo. Blood 1997;89:2635–2643.
21 Arenberg DA, Kunkel SL, Polverini PJ, Morris SB, Burdick MD, Glass MC, Taub DT, Iannettoni MD, Whyte RI, Strieter RM: Interferon-γ-inducible protein 10 (IP-10) is an angiostatic factor that inhibits human non-small cell lung cancer (NSCLC) tumorigenesis and spontaneous metastases. J Exp Med 1996;184:981–992.
22 Carney DN: Cancers of the lungs; in Fishman AP (ed): Pulmonary Diseases and Disorders, ed 2. New York, McGraw-Hill, 1988, pp 1885–2068.
23 Yuan A, Yang PC, Yu CJ, Lee YC, Yao YT, Chen CL, Lee LN, Kuo SH, Luh KT: Tumor angiogenesis correlates with histologic type and metastasis in non-small cell lung cancer. Am J Respir Crit Care Med 1995;152:2157–2162.
24 Nickoloff BJ, Mitra RS, Varani J, Dixit VM, Polverini PJ: Aberrant production of interleukin-8 and thrombospondin-1 by psoriatic keratinocytes mediates angiogenesis. Am J Pathol 1994;144:820–828.
25 Strieter RM, Polverini PJ, Arenberg DA, Kunkel SL: The role of CXC chemokines as regulators of angiogenesis. Shock 1995;4:155–160.
26 Turner-Warwick M: Precapillary systemic-pulmonary anastomoses. Thorax 1963:18:225–237.
27 Peao MND, Aguas AP, DeSa CM, Grande NR: Neoformation of blood vessels in association with rat lung fibrosis induced by bleomycin. Anat Rec 1994;238:57–67.
28 Keane MP, Arenberg DA, Lynch JP, Whyte RI, Iannettoni MD, Burdick MD, Wilke CA, Morris SB, Glass MC, DiGiovine B, Kunkel SL, Strieter RM: The CXC chemokines, IL-8 and IP-10, regulate angiogenic activity in idiopathic pulmonary fibrosis. J Immunol 1997;159:1437–1443.
29 Lynch JP, Standiford TJ, Kunkel SL, Rolfe MW, Strieter RM: Neutrophilic alveolitis in idiopathic pulmonary fibrosis: The role of interleukin-8. Am Rev Respir Dis 1992;145:1433–1438.
30 Koch AE, Leibovich SJ, Polverini PJ: Stimulation of neovascularization by human rheumatoid synovial tissue macrophages. Arthritis Rheum 1986;29:471–479.
31 Stout AJ, Gresser I, Thompson WD: Inhibition of wound healing in mice by local interferon alpha/beta injection. Int J Exp Pathol 1993;74:79–85.
32 Hyde DM, Henderson TS, Giri SN, Tyler NK, Stovall MY: Effect of murine gamma interferon on the cellular responses to bleomycin in mice. Exp Lung Res 1988;14:687–695.

Robert M. Strieter, MD, Department of Internal Medicine,
Division of Pulmonary and Critical Care,
1150 W Medical Center Drive, 6200 MSRB III, Ann Arbor, MI 48109-0642 (USA)
Tel. +1 734 936 2612, Fax +1 734 764 4556, E-Mail rstriete@umich.edu

Mantovani A (ed): Chemokines.
Chem Immunol. Basel, Karger, 1999, vol 72, pp 102–120

Chemokines: Function, Regulation and Alteration of Inflammatory Responses

Nicholas W. Lukacs, Cory Hogaboam, Emma Campbell, Steven L. Kunkel

Department of Pathology, University of Michigan Medical School, Ann Arbor, Mich., USA

Historically, chemokines have been viewed as leukocyte chemoattractants that regulate cellular movement from circulation into inflamed tissue. However, as investigators continue to examine the function of chemokines in both disease and hemostatic environments, one finds a complex regulation of function, and interaction with multiple cell types. Chemokines have been primarily divided into two main families based upon their sequence homology and the position of the first two cysteine residues, C-x-C (α) and C-C (β) [1–3]. This group of chemoattractants continues to grow at a staggering pace through broad-based searches for sequence homology in EST databases. However, as this 'mining for chemokines' continues, the function of all of these members must be characterized in order to determine their individual role in the inflamed and noninflamed environment. Two other distinct families are the C family and the C-x-x-x-C family. Both of these latter families have only a single member thus far, lymphotactin and neurotactin (fractalkine), respectively. In addition to the continuously growing family of chemokines, their receptors are only now being identified through the cloning and characterization of numerous 'orphan' receptors.

The C-x-C or α chemokine family can be further subdivided depending upon whether the chemokines have an amino acid E-L-R motif within its sequence in the N-terminal region (table 1). This consensus sequence appears to determine whether the chemokines have the ability to induce chemotaxis of neutrophils and also determines whether the C-x-C chemokine is angiogenic (ELR) or angiostatic (non-ELR). Both of these processes likely depend upon specific receptor usage of the chemokines. For many years the function of the C-x-C chemokines was hypothesized to center only around neutrophil

Table 1. Chemokine families

C-x-C (α)	C-C (β)	C	Cx3C
IL-8	MCP-1, 2, 3, 4, 5	Lymphotactin	Fractalkine
GROα, β, γ	MIP-1α, β, γ		(Neurotactin)
ENA-78	RANTES		
GCP-2	Eotaxin		
NAP-2	HCC-1, 2, 3, 4		
CTAP III	Eotaxin-2		
SDF-1	SLC		
IP-10	ELC		
MIG	TARC		
	LARC		
	I-309		

migration, however, more recently the C-x-C chemokines and especially the non-ELR containing members have been shown to be potent lymphocyte chemoattractants. These findings may suggest an additional regulation point in determining the type of leukocyte that migrates into the site of inflammation.

The CC or β chemokine family is the fastest growing group of chemokines with new members being reported through EST database searches. This family was traditionally viewed as mononuclear cell chemoattractants and associated with chronic inflammation. However, as the family grew and new members were discovered, it soon became apparent that the members of this family were also important in directing the migration of not only monocytes and lymphocytes, but also basophils, eosinophils, NK cells and mast cells. In addition, the members of this family may also play a functional role in leukocyte hematopoiesis in the local environment of the bone marrow and as regulators of immune function through alteration of cytokine profiles. These latter functions will be covered more thoroughly in this review.

The production and function of the two smaller families of chemokines, C and C-x-x-x-C, is unclear. However, the limited organ distribution may give a clue as to their relative function. Lymphotactin, the only C family ligand, is produced in several tissues, but has substantially higher expression in the thymus where it appears to recruit immature T lymphocytes from the bone marrow [4]. However, little is yet known about the function of this cytokine during immune/inflammatory events. Fractalkine (a.k.a.- neurotactin), the only member of the CX3C family, has a significantly different morphologic distribution than the other families [5–9] This latter chemokine is displayed on the surface of cells (particularly those within the CNS) anchored by an adhesion molecule-like stalk with a transmembrane domain and a cytoplasmic tail. It appears that the chemotactic region of this molecule can be cleaved off and remains active in its soluble form. Fractalkine may be the first of several of the members of this family that may serve a function during both cell-to-cell interactions and as a soluble factor.

Chemokine Receptors

Although the number of chemokine receptors has grown over the past several years, the function and cellular expression patterns are still relatively unknown. Some would predict that the number of chemokine receptors may be nearly as daunting as the number of chemokines themselves [10–12]. The C-x-C family of chemokines has five receptors described to date, C-x-CR1 to C-x-CR5. In general, the C-x-CR1 and R2 appear to be primarily displayed on neutrophils, whereas C-x-CR3 and R4 are displayed on mononuclear cells. This pattern follows the specificity and chemoattractant function of the specific ligands for these receptors as the ELR-containing C-x-C chemokines bind to C-x-CR1 and 2, whereas the non-ELR containing chemokines bind to C-x-CR3 and SDF binds to C-x-CR4. A fifth C-x-C receptor has been recently identified with specificity for B lymphocytes (BLR1) and appears to have specificity for only those cells.

The CC chemokine receptors have also expanded over the past several years [13]. There are now at least nine different receptors and their ligand specificity has not completely been identified. The newer receptors of this family (CCR6 thru CCR9) have been less well characterized compared to the first five receptors. The first receptor, CCR1, was shown to bind MIP-1α, MCP-3 and RANTES and appears to be expressed on most leukocytes. CCR2 was originally shown to bind MCP-1 and subsequently appears to bind all of the MCP family members (1 thru 5). CCR3 is highly expressed on eosinophils, is associated with allergic responses and binds RANTES, eotaxin, MCP-3, MCP-4, eotaxin-2 (and MIP-1α in murine systems). All of these latter chemokines that bind to CCR3 have been implicated in eosinophil accumulation during allergic responses, such as asthma. There have been mixed reports on the CC chemokines which bind to CCR4. It appears that TARC is the main ligand, while RANTES and MIP-1α have a lesser affinity for the receptor. Perhaps the best characterized receptor is CCR5 due to its use as a coreceptor for HIV infectivity. This receptor binds MIP-1α MIP-1β, and RANTES and when ligated with these chemokines, can inhibit HIV infectivity in vitro. Although the ligands for many of these receptors are now known, their regulation of expression has not been well characterized. The contents of this review will summarize accumulated data from several laboratories that demonstrate that these chemokines and their receptors are not only involved in chemotaxis of leukocytes but can also alter and regulate their function.

Chemokines and Effector Cell Activation

Neutrophils

Over the past several years it has become apparent that the members of the chemokine family are not only chemotactic for leukocytes but also have a role in activation and regulation of effector functions [14–19]. This was first realized by those reseachers studying neutrophil activation during disease pathogenesis. In these early studies, it appeared that IL-8 was a potent neutrophil chemoattractant and the level of its production dictated the level of neutrophil activation. Subsequently, several investigators demonstrated that IL-8 can directly induce neutrophil activation and degranulation. In addition to IL-8, other ELR-containing C-x-C chemokines also appear to have the ability to induce neutrophil activation and degranulation, including ENA-78 and GROα, β, γ [20–26]. Although these responses may best be elicited in coordination of other signals, these findings may have important implications during disease progression. The ability of C-x-C chemokines to induce these responses suggests that during certain chronic diseases which have continuous neutrophil infiltration and activation, such as cystic fibrosis, neutralization of these chemokines may have a beneficial effect.

Mast Cells and Basophils

The ability of chemokines to initiate and maintain cellular recruitment and activation during the initial stages of inflammation and immune reaction may be critical to the evolution of an effective response. Several studies have now shown that injection of chemokines into the skin induces an immediate-type inflammatory response, suggesting a role for chemokines in activation of local cell populations. In particular, MCP-1 appears to be a potent inducer of these immediate-type responses in skin of rats [27–32] and can induce the activation and degranulation of mature mast cell populations. Furthermore, one of the earliest cells to traffic to the site of inflammatory responses is the basophil. Seminal studies by several laboratories have demonstrated that multiple CC chemokines, including MCP-1, MIP-1α, and RANTES, cannot only recruit basophils to a site of inflammation, but also can directly cause the cells to degranulate and release inflammatory mediators, such as histamine and leukotrienes. In addition to the original chemokines that were shown to activate basophils, it appears that any chemokine which binds to CCR3, which is highly expressed on basophils [33], can cause activation and degranulation, such as eotaxin and MCP-4 [34]. Chemokine activation of mast cells and basophils may play an important role in the initiation of responses but may also be involved in detrimental responses in human diseases due to the mediators released by these cell populations.

In recent unpublished studies from our laboratory, we have identified that instillation of MCP-1 (but not any other CC chemokine) into the airways of normal mice induces an immediate histamine release and airway hyperreactivity response by 1 h postinstillation [unpubl. data]. This response is accompanied by a significant increase in leukotriene B_4 in the bronchoalveolar lavage (BAL) fluid from these mice. Most importantly, the airway hyperreactivity is not transient, but is maintained at 24 h postinstillation. These studies correlate well with our initial observations that inhibition of MCP-1 significantly attenuated airway hyperreactivity in a murine model of allergic airway inflammation [35]. In studies of patients with human asthma, a significant increase in MCP-1 is associated with allergen challenge and airway hyperreactivity and appeared to localize within the airway epithelial cells [36–39]. Thus, the production of MCP-1 during asthmatic responses may be detrimental through its ability to activate mast cells and basophils, further inducing the release of mediators, such as leukotrienes and histamine that can alter airway function.

Eosinophils

Over the past several years a considerable effort has been initiated to identify chemokines that are involved in eosinophil recruitment and activation. These cells have been identified as effector cells in a number of parasitic infections [40, 41] appear to be the cell responsible for damage in asthma [42–44] and may play a significant role in development of fibrotic tissue during chronic inflammatory disease [45–47]. One of the original chemokines that was identified to promote eosinophil recruitment in vitro is RANTES [48–50]. The addition of RANTES to cultures of eosinophils can cause direct activation and degranulation of the cells, which may correlate to its function during disease. The production of RANTES can be found in multiple cell types including: lymphocytes, macrophages, epithelial cells, and fibroblasts, with substantial amounts prepackaged in platelets [2, 51]. In studies related to human asthma, increased production and function of RANTES has not been thoroughly studied. When recombinant RANTES was instilled down the airways of guinea pigs [52] or rate [53], primarily a monocytic infiltrate was observed with no eosinophils, possibly suggesting a specified function for RANTES. However, in an allergic hyperreactive airway model in mice, antibodies directed against RANTES specifically decreased eosinophilia with no effect on mononuclear cell infiltration or airway hyperreactivity responses [35]. Altogether, these studies suggest that during specific disease situations RANTES may have a significant role in eosinophil and/or mononuclear cell accumulation during disease development.

Over the past several years a number of CC chemokines have been identified which induce eosinophil recruitment. However, the identification of eotaxin as the first chemokine with preferential ability to recruit eosinophils has focused researchers of allergic responses on this molecule. Eotaxin was first discovered in the BAL fluid of guinea pigs after an allergen challengs [54–56]. It has since been cloned in human, mouse and rat, and appears to have similar functions, although a paucity of data still exists [54, 57]. Eotaxin binds to a single receptor, CCR3, which is highly expressed on eosinophils and therefore likely explains the specificity and intensity of the recruitment response [57–59]. In addition to recruiting eosinophils, eotaxin has the ability to cause eosinophils to degranulate [55, 60–62], which may be a crucial step in the developing pathogenesis of asthmatic inflammation. These latter data may be the most critical aspect of eotaxin's functions during allergic inflammation, given the fact that eotaxin can be localized primarily to airway epithelial cells during an allergic response in the lung [63, 64]. This localized production may preferentially target eosinophils to this area and further cause them to degranulate and damage this area of the lung. Studies in eotaxin 'knockout' mice have not demonstrated a dependence upon eotaxin, as only a modest reduction in eosinophil accumulation at a single early time point (but not at later time points) afler allergen challenge was observed [65]. In additional studies in our laboratory, we have found that eotaxin plays a significant role in eosinophil accumulation and activation as well as airway hyperreactivity during persistent or chronic allergen challenge but not in acute exacerbations (single allergen challenge) [unpubl. data]. Thess latter data would be consistent with an earlier publication which suggests that eotaxin may be important for eosinophil accumulation into the airway after multiple allergen exposures [66].

Other C-C chemokines may also be important in the development of eosinophilic airway inflammation. MCP-3 binds to CCR1, 2 and 3, and may have effects on multiple cell populations [13, 67, 68]. Depletion of MCP-3 in allergic airway models has demonstrated a significant role for this molecule on eosinophil recruitment to the airways [69]. In addition, MIP-1α has a preferential role in eosinophil recruitment during the initial phases of Th2-type allergic airway inflammation, but not during chronic airway inflammation in mice [35, 70, 71]. The expression of CC chemokines in human asthma has clearly shown a relationship between allergen challenge and disease and their presence may play multiple activational and leukocyte recruitment roles.

NK and Cytotoxic Cells

During specific inflammatory/immune responses, NK cells rapidly accumulate in tissues. The chemokines that are responsible for their localization to the tissue are likely those that are produced early during a response. The primary role for NK cells during a response appears to be nonspecific killing of foreign pathogens by the release of destructive enzymes and proteins. Initial studies demonstrated that members of both the C-x-C (IP-10) and C-C (RANTES, MCP-1, 2, 3 and MIP-1β) chemokine families had the ability to cause chemotaxis of NK cells, suggesting the expression of multiple functional chemokine receptors [72–74]. In addition, these studies demonstrated that the chemokines could enhance the release of serine esterases and cytotoxic responses of NK cells but not for LAK or ADCC-mediated killing. Subsequently, further investigations demonstrated that lymphotactin, a member of the C family, was also a chemoattractant for NK cells, but does not augment adhesion of the cells to activated endothelium as does other NK cell activators, such as IL-12 [74, 75]. Chemokines may also be involved in the maturation and generation of NK cells from CD56+ cell populations [76]. In addition to affecting the activation of nonspecific NK cell killing, a number of chemokines have also been shown to increase antigen specific granule release and killing by cytotoxic T cells [77]. These later results likely have important consequences in viral diseases such as HIV, where the pathogen spends most of its life cycle intracellularly and specific cytotoxic destruction of the infected cell is necessary.

Lymphocyte Regulation by Chemokines

Over the past several years an appreciation of chemokines as not only chemotactic agents but as immune regulators has been established. The regulation and activation of CD4+ T lymphocytes and their cytokine production may be the most critical issue for alteration of immune responses. Several laboratories have begun investigating whether chemokines can direct the immune system toward a specific response. Early studies have demonstrated that CC, but not ELR-containing C-x-C, chemokines could augment T-lymphocyte reactivity and IL-2 production both in vitro and in vivo [78]. In seminal studies by Bacon et al. [78, 80], RANTES was shown to not only induce intracellular signals capable of activating T cells (Ca^{2+} flux) but also was shown to upregulate IL-2 receptors on the surface of these cells, an event that is critical for lymphocyte proliferation. Although the levels of RANTES were rather high, the latter studies demonstrated that chemokines likely have a direct role in T-lymphocyte activation. In subsequent studies in other laboratories, the role of CC family chemokines in regulation of lymphokines has elucidated interesting differences in the role of these cytokines in the immune response. Using a TCR transgenic mouse strain that responded to ovalbumin, it was identified that co-incubation of MCP-1 in vitro could skew the response toward a Th2-like, IL-4-producing response, whereas MIP-1α upregulated IFN-γ and a Th1-like immune response [81]. Similar results were also observed using antigen-specific lymphocyte populations from immunized mice in vitro, where MCP-1 upregulated and MIP-1α downregulated IL-4 production [82]. In a more recent study, MCP-1 production from fibroblasts was able to downregulate antigen-specific T-lymphocyte responses (proliferation and IFN-γ production) during fibroblast:CD4+ lymphocyte coculture [83]. In studies designed to determine the role of eotaxin during Th1- and Th2-type granuloma development, both neutralization of eotaxin in vivo and addition of eotaxin in vitro demonstrated that eotaxin could regulate Th1-type IFN-γ production. It is not clear in any of the above studies whether the chemokines are driving the lymphocytes to differentiation or merely regulating cytokine production. In any event, these studies demonstrate that CC family chemokines have the ability to aid in the direction and intensity of the immune response.

A novel area of investigation is the expression of chemokine receptors on T-lymphocyte subsets that have been differentiated toward Th1- or Th2-type cytokine production. In seminal studies, it was demonstrated that a subset of cells that were differentiated toward IL-4 production (Th2) express high levels of CCR3 on their surface [84]. In subsequent studies, other CC chemokine receptors were found to be differentially expressed on T-lymphocyte subsets which were of Th1 or Th2 phenotypes. In particular, CCR4 was found to be more highly expressed than CCR3 on Th2-type cells, possibly suggesting that this receptor may help to identify T lymphocytes that express Th2-type cytokines [85, 86]. The expression of CCR8, the receptor for I–309, has also been identified as a possible marker for Th2-type cells [87–89]. The T lymphocytes from Th1-type responses appear to preferentially express CCR1 and CCR5, coordinating with the data that MIP-1α and RANTES may help to promote these responses [85, 86]. The relevance of these in vitro observations has not been fully evaluated and the correlation and impact of these data in vivo during disease progression need to be investigated in future experiments.

Chemokine Activation of Nonimmune Cells

The primary role of chemokines appears to be for recruitment and activation of leukocytes to a site of inflammation or immune response. Structural cell populations, such as epithelial cells, fibroblasts, and smooth muscle cells, likely play a significant role in producing these factors for localization of leukocytes to the inflamed tissue. However, recent evidence has demonstrated that chemokines may play a direct role on the function of structural cell populations. In particular, information on fibroblast activation by MCP-1 appears to be the strongest. Significant levels of MCP-1 can be found in fibrotic lesions and those undergoing overt scarring, such as in burn wounds [90–96]. However, a significant body of information is now accumulating that indicates that MCP-1 may have direct effects on fibroblast activation and matrix protein production. In the mouse, JE (mMCP-1) was first described as an immediate, early competence factor after PDGF activation of fibroblasts [97]. Further studies indicate that MCP-1 can directly induce TGF-β and collagen in isolate fibroblast populations through a specific receptor [98]. Perhaps the best evidence of a role for MCP-1 in fibrosis comes from an in vivo model of crescentic nephritis [90, 91]. In this model neutralization of MCP-1 resulted in a dramatic decrease in glomerular crescent formation and deposition of type I collagen. These latter observations lend to the idea that MCP-1 production during fibrotic diseases may help to promote maintenance of the responses and exacerbate disease progression. In recent studies in our laboratory, it appears that fibroblasts grown from fibrotic lesions produce significantly higher levels of MCP-1 and have a significant expression of CCR2 on their surface [unpubl. data]. The neutralization of MCP-1 significantly attenuates the relatively high constitutive levels of TGF-β in these 'Th2-type' fibroblasts compared to fibroblasts from normal, nonfibrotic tissue, thus supporting the aforementioned studies.

In addition to fibroblast activation, chemokines also activate other cell populations and induce proliferation. In particular, IL–8 has mitogenic and chemotactic properties for both smooth muscle cells and endothelial cells [99]. This mechanism of activation is likely important not only in disease progression, as in atherosclerosis, but also in the normal growth of vessels. In fact, the role of C-x-C chemokines in general for angiogenesis may be of utmost importance in progression of fibrotic, cancerous and other proliferative diseases [100]. The CC chemokines also appear to induce smooth muscle cell activation as MCP-1 induces rat vascular smooth cell activation and proliferation [101]. Other studies have identified CC chemokine receptors, CCR1 and CCR2, on human smooth muscle cells, which correlates well with chemokine activation of these cells [102]. Thus, a number of cell populations associated with normal tissue growth, as well as those involved in disease progression, are affected by chemokines.

Other specialized cell populations may also be directly affected by chemokines. In recent studies by Colletti and Strieter [unpubl. data], the C-x-C, ELR-containing chemokines appear to induce the proliferation of hepatocytes in vitro. These observations were also translated into an in vivo model of necrotic liver damage and regeneration using acetaminophen-induced injury. During the acetaminophen-induced injury several C-C and C-x-C chemokines were produced, but the neutralization of MIP-2, a C-x-C, ELR-containing chemokine, demonstrated an effect to the response [unpubl. data]. Those mice that were passively immunized with antibodies specific to MIP-2 had a significant increase in mortality compared to control antibody, anti-MIP-1α or anti-MCP-1-treated animals. These animals further demonstrated increased necrosis of the liver and retarded regeneration. Exogenous administration of MIP-2 by either intravenous injection of recombinant MIP-2 or by local administration of an adenovirus overexpressing MIP-2 significantly decreased mortality and accelerated the regeneration of the liver tissue. The role of additional C-x-C chemokines in liver regeneration are now being examined. These studies demonstrated striking results that indicated that the C-x-C chemokines may be involved in growth-related functions within the liver and may be a therapeutic modality for patients with acute and chronic liver damage.

Chemokine Production and Function during Disease Progression

In order to identify the role of individual chemokines during disease progression, a thorough evaluation of production and function must be performed using animal models and translating the findings into a clinical setting. A number of animal models of disease have been utilized in order to evaluate the role of chemokines during disease pathogenesis.

Sepsis

Perhaps one of the most detrimental and difficult diseases to treat is sepsis leading to multiorgan failure. This syndrome can be induced by multiple mechanisms including trauma, burn and bacterial infection. The common factor in all of these situations is the overexpression of cytokines/chemokines. There is no doubt that the early response cytokines, TNF and IL-1, may be the most detrimental mediators produced during this response [103, 104]. Evidence over the past several years has demonstrated a role for chemokines in both the activation and regulation of the disease process [105, 106]. One of the first chemokines identified in patients undergoing septic responses was IL-8. This chemokine appears to be central to the neutrophil accumulation and activation in various organs and leads to end-stage disease development. The correlation of IL-8 and sepsis was not only observed in the patient population, but also in nonhuman primate models of septic responses. In addition to IL-8, numerous other C-x-C and C-C chemokines have been described during septic responses.

In animal models of septic shock, several chemokines have been identified as potential targets for therapy, including IL-8, GROα MIP-1α, and RANTES [107–110]. Furthermore, certain chemokines may have a beneficial effect during septic responses. In particular, recent data has indicated that MCP-1, which is produced in a later time course compared to other chemokines, may be protective against the detrimental effects of inflammatory cytokines [111]. The inhibition of MCP-1 in endotoxin or cecal ligation and puncture models of sepsis significantly increased the mortality, whereas exogenous administration of recombinant MCP-1 significantly decreased mortality [112]. Upon examination of inflammatory cytokines, TNF, IFN-γ and IL-12 were found to be regulated by MCP-1 during the endotoxic/septic response. Thus, MCP-1 appears to regulate inflammatory cytokines produced during endotoxic shock. It is not clear whether these observations are mediated by MCP-1 directly through a single cell or indirectly via multiple cell populations. These later data correlate well with recent findings for MCP-1 in the induction of oral tolerance, downregulating a Th1-type response in an EAE model [113]. Thus, a potential role for chemokines in regulation of inflammatory responses is suggested by these results.

Granuloma Formation

One of the first chronic models of inflammation used to examine the role of chemokines was a model of inflammatory granuloma formation initiated by embolization of parasite *(Schistosoma mansoni)* eggs to the lungs of mice. Through a series of studies which included specific neutralization of individual chemokines, a pattern of chemokine usage was identified, depending upon the stage and immune type of granuloma that was formed. During primary, Th1-type granuloma formation, the neutralization of MIP-1α significantly decrease the granuloma formation, whereas neutralization of MCP-1 had little or no effect [114]. In contrast, when the secondary or Th2-type granuloma forrnation was examined (initiated in presensitized mice) the neutralization of MCP-1, but not MIP-1α, attenuated the granuloma formation [115]. These studies correlate well with the earlier mentioned in vitro results demonstrating the relationship of MIP-1α with IFN-γ production and MCP-1 with IL-4 production [81, 82]. In other studies, IL-4 has been identified as an inducer of the pathological fibrotic responses associated with Th2-type lesions [116]. The overexpression of IL-4 using an adenoviral vector during the formation of nonfibrotic Th1-type pulmonary granulomas significantly increased lesion size, induced eosinophil accumulation, and exacerbated the expression of procollagen mRNA within the lung. In addition, when the chemokines were examined during this process ~10-fold increase in MCP-1 production was observed. The correlation of MCP-1 and increase in granuloma formation and induction of collagen expression correlates well with the previously mentioned studies on the role of MCP-1 in fibrosis and TGF-β production.

Autoimmune Encephalomyelitis

Chemokines have been described in other disease models and to play differential roles in disease progression and leukocyte activation. In experimental autoimmune encephalomyelitis (EAE), a model for multiple sclerosis, mRNA for a number of C-x-C and C-C chemokines were originally described and expressed prior to disease induction [117] and following leukocyte accumulation [118]. In an attempt to identify the important chemokines that are involved in the induction of a relapsing EAE response, diseased animals were treated with neutralizing antibodies to MIP-1α or MCP-1 prior to induction of the disease [119]. Only anti-MIP-1α attenuated the induction and relapse of the disease through the reduced recruitment of mononuclear cells to the CNS. Even though anti-MCP-1 had no effect on the induction of EAE, it became clear that it was expressed in the CNS during established disease development [120]. Subsequent studies examined the relapsing EAE response by treating animals with neutralizing antibodies to MIP-1α and MCP-1 during remission, prior to the initial relapse of the disease. In contrast to the induction phase, only anti-MCP-1 blocked the relapsing stage during established disease [121]. The source of the different chemokinss during disease likely determines the relevance of each of the chemokines and the phase in which they participate. The expression of MIP-1α and RANTES was detected in infiltrating mononuclear cells, correlating to early disease progression [122]. In contrast, MCP-1 and IP-10 appear to be produced primarily by astrocytes and glial cells within the CNS, possibly explaining their involvement in chronic stages of the disease [118, 123]. Examining the chemokine receptors that are expressed during disease progression of EAE, it was found that CCR2, CCR5, CxCR4 and CX3CR1 were all upregulated during induction of EAE in an acute rat model [124]. However, in human multiple sclerosis, generic studies have demonstrated no protection from disease in patients with a CCR5 deletion [125]. Thus, in this model of autoimmune disease, it appears that multiple chemokines and specific receptors may participate in responses at different stages of disease progression. Other animal models are also being utilized to dissect the role of chemokines in disease progression and will no doubt elucidate novel mechanisms of action.

Conclusion

The field of chemokine biology has expanded greatly over the past several years. Not only are the chemokine families growing, but their individual func-

Table 2. Characterized functions of chemokines

Chemokine	Family	Cell specificity	Known function
IL-8, ENA, GRO	C-x-C (ELR)	Neutrophils	Chemotaxis, activation
		Endothelial cells	Proliferation (angiogenic)
		Smooth muscle	Proliferation
		Hepatocytes [unpubl. data]	Proliferation
IP-10, MIG	C-x-C (non-ELR)	T lymphocytes	Chemotaxis, IFN production
		Monocytes	Chemotaxis
		Endothelial cells	Angiostatic
MCP-1	C-C	Monocyte	Chemotaxis, activation
		T lymphocyte	Chemotaxis, IL-4 production
		Fibroblast	TGF-β and collagen production
		Smooth muscle	Proliferation
		Basophil/mast cell	Activation
MIP-1α	C-C	Monocyte	Chemotaxis, activation
		T lymphocyte	Chemotaxis, IFN production
		Basophil	Activation
Eotaxin	C-C	Eosinophil	Activation, chemotaxis
RANTES	C-C	Monocyte	Chemotaxis
		T lymphocyte	Chemotaxis, activation
		Eosinophil	Chemotaxis, activation
		Basophil	Activation

tions are beginning to be defined with specific cell populations. The traditional view of chemokines as mediators of leukocyte accumulation at a site of inflammation is still valid, however, the differential role and activation of immune and nonimmune cell populations has given many of the chemokines a more extended role during disease progression (table 2). Future studies in chemokine biology as well as expression and activation of receptors will help to define the overall function of the chemokines during homeostatic and disease circumstances.

References

1 Moser B, Loetscher M, Piali L, Loetscher P: Lymphocyte responses to chemokines. Int Rev Immunol 1998;16:323–344.

2 Baggiolini M, Dewald B, Moser B: Human chemokines: An update. Annu Rev Immunol 1997;15: 675–705.

3 Taub DD: Chemokine-leukocyte interactions. The voodoo that they do so well. Cytokine Growth Factor Rev 1996;7:355–376.

4 Kennedy J, Kelner GS, Kleyensteuber S, Schall TJ, Weiss MC, Yssel H, Schneider PV, Cocks BG, Bacon KB, Zlotnik A: Molecular cloning and functional characterization of human lymphotactin. J Immunol 1995;155:203–209.

5 Nishiyori A, Minami M, Ohtani Y, Takami S, Yamamoto J, Kawaguchi N, Kume T, Akaike A, Satoh M: Localization of fractalkine and CX3CR1 mRNAs in rat brain: Does fractalkine play a role in signaling from neuron to microglia? FEBS Lett 1998;429:167–172.

6 Rossi DL, Hardiman G, Copeland NG, Gilbert DJ, Jenkins N, Zlotnik A, Bazan JF: Cloning and characterization of a new type of mouse chemokine. Genomics 1998;47:163–170.

7 Imai T, Hieshima K, Haskell C, Baba M, Nagira M, Nishimura M, Kakizaki M, Takagi S, Nomiyama H, Schall TJ, Yoshie O: Identification and molecular characterization of fractalkine receptor CX3CR1, which mediates both leukocyte migration and adhesion. Cell 1997;91:521–530.

8 Schall T: Fractalkine – A strange attractor in the chemokine landscape. Immunol Today 1997;18:147.

9 Pan Y, Lloyd C, Zhou H, Dolich S, Deeds J, Gonzalo JA, Vath J, Gosselin M, Ma J, Dussault B, Woolf E, Alperin G, Culpepper J, Gutierrez-Ramos JC, Gearing D: Neurotactin, a membrane-anchored chemokine upregulated in brain inflammation. Nature 1997;387:611–617. Erratum in Nature 1997;389:100.

10 Baggiolini M, Moser B: Blocking chemokine receptors. J Exp Med 1997;186:1189–1191.

11 Baggiolini M: Chemokines and leukocyte traffic. Nature 1998;392:565–568.

12 Littman DR: Chemokine receptors: Keys to AIDS pathogenesis? Cell 1998;93:677–680.

13 Premack BA, Schall TJ: Chemokine receptors: Gateways to inflammation and infection. Nat Med 1996;2:1174–1178.

14 Teran LM, Johnston SL, Schroder JM, Church MK, Holgate ST: Role of nasal interleukin-8 in neutrophil recruitment and activation in children with virus-induced asthma. Am J Respir Crit Care Med 1997;155:1362–1366.

15 Lowman HB, Slagle PH, DeForge LE, Wirth CM, Gillece-Castro BL, Bourell JH, Fairbrother WJ: Exchanging interleukin-8 and melanoma growth-stimulating activity receptor binding specificities. J Biol Chem 1996;271:14344–14352.

16 Baggiolini M, Loetscher P, Moser B: Interleukin-8 and the chemokine family. Int J Immunopharmacol 1995;17:103–108.

17 Yagisawa M, Yuo A, Kitagawa S, Yazaki Y, Togawa A, Takaku F: Stimulation and priming of human neutrophils by IL-1-alpha and IL-1-beta: Complete inhibition by IL-1 receptor antagonist and no interaction with other cytokines. Exp Hematol 1995;23:603–608.

18 Cale AR, Katzmann JA, Tazelaar HD, Miller VM, McGregor CG: Activation of polymorphonuclear leukocyte oxygen radical production during acute lung rejection in dogs: Inhibition by an antiadhesion molecule monoclonal antibody. J Heart Lung Transplant 1993;12:948–955.

19 Kapp A, Zeck-Kapp G: Activation of the oxidative metabolism in human polymorphonuclear neutrophilic granulocytes: The role of immunomodulating cytokines. J Invest Dermatol 1990;95:94S–99S.

20 Lukacs NW, Hogaboam CM, Kunkel SL, Chensue SW, Burdick MD, Evanoff HL, Strieter RM: Mast cells produce ENA-78, which can function as a potent neutrophil chemoattractant during allergic airway inflammation. J Leukoc Biol 1998;63:746–751.

21 Wuyts A, Haelens A, Proost P, Lenaerts JP, Conings R, Opdenakker G, Van Damme J: Identification of mouse granulocyte chemotactic protein-2 from fibroblasts and epithelial cells. Functional comparison with natural KC and macrophage inflammatory protein-2. J Immunol 1996;157:1736–1743.

22 Magazin M, Vita N, Cavrois E, Lefort S, Guilemot JC, Ferrara P: The biological activities of gro beta and IL-8 on human neutrophils are overlapping but not identical. Eur Cytokine Netw 1992;3:461–467.

23 Suzuki H, Suematsu M, Miura S, Liu YY, Watanabe K, Miyasaka M, Tsurufuji S, Tsuchiya M: Rat CINC/gro: A novel mediator for locomotive and secretagogue activation of neutrophils in vivo. J Leukoc Biol 1994;55:652–657.

24 Metzner B, Elsner J, Dobos G, Kownatzki E, Parlow F, Schraufstatter I, Norgauer J: $[Ca^{2+}]_i$-transients and actin polymerization in human neutrophils under stimulation with GRO alpha and complement fragment C5a. Agents Actions 1994;42:101–106.

25 Walz A, Burgener R, Car B, Baggiolini M, Kunkel SL, Strieter RM: Structure and neutrophil-activating properties of a novel inflammatory peptide (ENA-78) with homology to interleukin-8. J Exp Med 1991;174:1355–1362.

26 Walz A, Strieter RM, Schnyder S: Neutrophil-activating peptide ENA-78. Adv Exp Med Biol 1993;351:129–137.
27 Conti P, Pang X, Boucher W, Letourneau R, Reale M, Barbacane RC, Thibault J, Theoharides TC: Impact of Rantes and MCP-1 chemokines on in vivo basophilic cell recruitment in rat skin injection model and their role in modifying the protein and mRNA levels for histidine decarboxylase. Blood 1997;89:4120–4127.
28 Matsumori A, Furukawa Y, Hashimoto T, Yoshida A, Ono K, Shioi T, Okada M, Iwasaki A, Nishio R, Matsushima K, Sasayama S: Plasma levels of the monocyte chemotactic and activating factor/monocyte chemoattractant protein-1 are elevated in patients with acute myocardial infarction. J Mol Cell Cardiol 1997;29:419–423.
29 Nitschke M, Sohn K, Dieckmann D, Gibbs BF, Wolff HH, Amon U: Effects of basophil-priming and stimulating cytokines on histamine release from isolated human skin mast cells. Arch Dermatol Res 1996;288:463–468.
30 Kaplan AP, Kuna P, Reddigari SR: Chemokines as allergic mediators – Relationship to histamine-releasing factors. Allergy 1994;49:495–501.
31 Conti P, Boucher W, Letourneau R, Feliciani C, Reale M, Barbacane RC, Vlagopoulos P, Bruneau G, Thibault J, Theoharides TC: Monocyte chemotactic protein-1 provokes mast cell aggregation and [^{3}H]5HT release. Immunology 1995;86:434–440.
32 Alam R, Forsythe P, Stafford S, Heinrich J, Bravo R, Proost P, Van Damme J: Monocyte chemotactic protein-2, monocyte chemotactic protein-3, and fibroblast-induced cytokine. Three new chemokines induce chemotaxis and activation of basophils. J Immunol 1994;153:3155–3159.
33 Uguccioni M, Mackay CR, Ochensberger B, Loetscher P, Rhis S, LaRosa GJ, Rao P, Ponath PD, Baggiolini M, Dahinder CA: High expression of the chemokine receptor CCR3 in human blood basophils. Role in activation by eotaxin, MCP-4, and other chemokines. J Clin Invest 1997;100:1137–1143.
34 Stellato C, Collins P, Ponath PD, Soler D, Newman W, La Rosa G, Li H, White J, Schwiebert LM, Bickel C, Liu M, Bochner BS, Williams T, Schleimer RP: Production of the novel C-C chemokine MCP-4 by airway cells and comparison of its biological activity to other C-C chemokines. J Clin Invest 1997;99:926–936.
35 Lukacs NW, Strieter RM, Warmington K, Lincoln P, Chensue SW, Kunkel SL: Differential recruitment of leukocyte populations and alteration of airway hyperreactivity by C-C family chemokines in allergic airway inflammation. J Immunol 1997;158:4398–4404.
36 Sousa AR, Lane SJ, Nakhosteen JA, Yoshimura T, Lee TH, Poston RN: Increased expression of the monocyte chemoattractant protein-1 in bronchial tissue from asthmatic subjects. Am J Respir Cell Mol Biol 1994;10:142–147.
37 Holgate ST, Bodey KS, Janezic A, Frew AJ, Kaplan AP, Teran LM: Release of RANTES, MIP-1-alpha, and MCP-1 into asthmatic airways following endobronchial allergen challenge. Am J Respir Crit Care Med 1997;156:1377–1383.
38 Jahnz-Rozyk KM, Kuna P, Pirozynska E: Monocyte chemotactic and activating factor/monocyte chemoattractant protein (MCAF/MCP-1) in bronchoalveolar lavage fluid from patients with atopic asthma and chronic bronchitis. J Invest Allergol Clin Immunol 1997;7:254–259.
39 Kurashima K, Mukaida N, Fujimura M, Schroder JM, Matsuda T, Matsushima K: Increase of chemokine levels in sputum precedes exacerbation of acute asthma attacks. J Leukoc Biol 1996;59:313–316.
40 Boros DL: The role of cytokines in the formation of the schistosome egg granuloma. Immunobiology 1994;191:441–450.
41 Weller PF: Human eosinophils. J Allergy Clin Immunol 1997;100:283–287.
42 Corrigan CJ, Kay AB: T-cell/eosinophil interactions in the induction of asthma. Eur Respir J Suppl 1996;22:72–78.
43 Hogan SP, Foster PS: Cellular and molecular mechanisms involved in the regulation of eosinophil trafficking in vivo. Med Res Rev 1996;16:407–432.
44 Kay AB, Barata L, Meng Q, Durham SR, Ying S: Eosinophils and eosinophil-associated cytokines in allergic inflammation. Int Arch Allergy Immunol 1997;113:196–199.
45 Minshall EM, Leung DY, Martin RJ, Song YL, Cameron L, Ernst P, Hamid Q: Eosinophil-associated TGF-beta-1 mRNA expression and airways fibrosis in bronchial asthma. Am J Respir Cell Mol Biol 1997;17:326–333.

46 Peterson MW, Monick M, Hunninghake GW: Prognostic role of eosinophils in pulmonary fibrosis. Chest 1987;92:51–56.
47 Zhang K, Gharaee-Kermani M, McGarry B, Remick D, Phan SH: TNF-alpha-mediated lung cytokine networking and eosinophil recruitment in pulmonary fibrosis. J Immunol 1997;158:954–959.
48 Kakazu T, Chihara J, Saito A, Nakajima S: Effect of RANTES on eosinophil adhesion to plates coated with recombinant soluble intercellular adhesion molecule-1 and expression of beta-2-integrin adhesion molecules on eosinophils. Int Arch Allergy Immunol 1995;108:(suppl 1):9–11.
49 Alam R, Stafford S, Forsythe P, Harrison R, Faubion D, Lett-Brown MA, Grant JA: RANTES is a chemotactic and activating factor for human eosinophils. J Immunol 1993;150:3442–3451.
50 Yamada H, Matsukura M, Yudate T, Chihara J, Stingl G, Tezuka T: Enhanced production of RANTES, an eosinophil chemoattractant factor, by cytokine-stimulated epidermal keratinocytes. Int Arch Allergy Immunol 1997;114(suppl 1):28–32.
51 Hirai K, Miyamasu M, Takaishi T, Morita Y: Regulation of the function of eosinophils and basophils. Crit Rev Immunol 1997;17:325–352.
52 Campbell EM, Proudfoot AE, Yoshimura T, Allet B, Wells TN, White AM, Westwick J, Watson ML: Recombinant guinea pig and human RANTES activate macrophages but not eosinophils in the guinea pig. J Immunol 1997;159:1482–1489.
53 Braciak TA, Bacon K, Xing Z, Torry DJ, Graham FL, Schall TJ, Richards CD, Croitoru K, Gauldie J: Overexpression of RANTES using a recombinant adenovirus vector induces the tissue-directed recruitment of monocytes to the lung. J Immunol 1996;157:5076–5084.
54 Jose PJ, Adcock IM, Griffiths-Johnson DA, Berkman N, Wells TN, Williams TJ, Power CA: Eotaxin: Cloning of an eosinophil chemoattractant cytokine and increased mRNA expression in allergen-challenged guinea-pig lungs. Biochem Biophys Res Commun 1994;205:788–794.
55 Jose PJ, Griffiths-Johnson DA, Collins PD, Walsh DT, Moqbel R, Totty NF, Truong O, Hsuan JJ, Williams TJ: Eotaxin: A potent eosinophil chemoattractant cytokine detected in a guinea pig model of allergic airways inflammation. J Exp Med 1994;179:881–887.
56 Griffiths-Johnson DA, Collins PD, Rossi AG, Jose PJ, Williams TJ: The chemokine, eotaxin, activates guinea-pig eosinophils in vitro and causes their accumulation into the lung in vivo. Biochem Biophys Res Commun 1993;197:1167–1172.
57 Ponath PD, Qin S, Ringler DJ, Clark-Lewis I, Wang J, Kassam N, Smith H, Shi X, Gonzalo JA, Newman W, Gutierrez-Ramos JC, Mackay CR: Cloning of the human eosinophil chemoattractant, eotaxin. Expression, receptor binding, and functional properties suggest a mechanism for the selective recruitment of eosinophils. J Clin Invest 1996;97:604–612.
58 Heath H, Qin S, Rao P, Wu L, LaRosa G, Kassam N, Ponath PD, Mackay CR: Chemokine receptor usage by human eosinophils. The importance of CCR3 demonstrated using an antagonistic monoclonal antibody. J Clin Invest 1997;99:178–184.
59 Daugherty BL, Siciliano SJ, DeMartino JA, Malkowitz L, Sirotina A, Springer MS: Cloning, expression, and characterization of the human eosinophil eotaxin receptor. J Exp Med 1996;183: 2349–2354.
60 Rothenberg ME, Ownbey R, Mehlhop PD, Loiselle PM, van de Rijn M, Bonventre JV, Oettgen HC, Leder P, Luster AD: Eotaxin triggers eosinophil-selective chemotaxis and calcium flux via a distinct receptor and induces pulmonary eosinophilia in the presence of interleukin-5 in mice. Mol Med 1996;2:334–348.
61 Elsner J, Hochstetter R, Kimmig D, Kapp A: Human eotaxin represents a potent activator of the respiratory burst of human eosinophils. Eur J Immunol 1996;26:1919–1925.
62 Rothenberg ME, Luster AD, Leder P: Murine eotaxin: An eosinophil chemoattractant inducible in endothelial cells and in interleukin 4-induced tumor suppression. Proc Natl Acad Sci USA 1995; 92:8960–8964.
63 Lilly CM, Nakamura H, Kesselman H, Nagler-Anderson C, Asano K, Garcia-Zepeda EA, Rothenberg ME, Drazen JM, Luster AD: Expression of eotaxin by human lung epithelial cells: Induction by cytokines and inhibition by glucocorticoids. J Clin Invest 1997;99:1767–1773.
64 Li D, Wang D, Griffiths-Johnson DA, Wells TN, Williams TJ, Jose PJ, Jeffery PK: Eotaxin protein and gene expression in guinea-pig lungs: Constitutive expression and upregulation after allergen challenge. Eur Respir J 1997;10:1946–1954.

65 Rothenberg ME, MacLean JA, Pearlman E, Luster AD, Leder P: Targeted disruption of the chemokine eotaxin partially reduces antigen-induced tissue eosinophilia. J Exp Med 1997;185:785–790.

66 Gonzalo JA, Lloyd CM, Kremer L, Finger E, Martinez AC, Siegelman MH, Cybulsky M, Gutierrez-Ramos JC: Eosinophil recruitment to the lung in a murine model of allergic inflammation. The role of T cells, chemokines, and adhesion receptors. J Clin Invest 1996;98:2332–2345.

67 Sarau HM, Rush JA, Foley JJ, Brawner ME, Schmidt DB, White JR, Barnette MS: Characterization of functional chemokine receptors (CCR1 and CCR2) on EoL-3 cells: A model system to examine the role of chemokines in cell function. J Pharmacol Exp Ther 1997;283:411–418.

68 Polentarutti N, Introna M, Sozzani S, Mancinelli R, Mantovani G, Mantovani A: Expression of monocyte chemotactic protein-3 in human monocytes and endothelial cells. Eur Cytokine Netw 1997;8:271–274.

69 Stafford S, Li H, Forsythe PA, Ryan M, Bravo R, Alam R: Monocyte chemotactic protein-3 (MCP-3)/fibroblast-induced cytokine (FIC) in eosinophilic inflammation of the airways and the inhibitory effects of an anti-MCP-3/FIC antibody. J Immunol 1997;158:4953–4960.

70 Lukacs NW, Standiford TJ, Chensue SW, Kunkel RG, Strieter RM, Kunkel SL: C-C chemokine-induced eosinophil chemotaxis during allergic airway inflammation. J Leukoc Biol 1996;60:573–578.

71 Lukacs NW, Strieter RM, Shaklee CL, Chensue SW, Kunkel SL: Macrophage inflammatory protein-1-alpha influences eosinophil recruitment in antigen-specific airway inflammation. Eur J Immunol 1995;25:245–251.

72 Taub DD, Sayers TJ, Carter CR, Ortaldo JR: Alpha and beta chemokines induce NK cell migration and enhance NK-mediated cytolysis. J Immunol 1995;155:3877–3888.

73 Allavena P, Bianchi G, Zhou D, van Damme J, Jilek P, Sozzani S, Mantovani A: Induction of natural killer cell migration by monocyte chemotactic protein-1, -2 and -3. Eur J Immunol 1994;24:3233–3236.

74 Maghazachi AA, Skalhegg BS, Rolstad B, Al-Aoukaty A: Interferon-inducible protein-10 and lymphotactin induce the chemotaxis and mobilization of intracellular calcium in natural killer cells through pertussis toxin-sensitive and -insensitive heterotrimeric G-proteins. FASEB J 1997;11:765–774.

75 Giancarlo B, Silvano S, Albert Z, Mantovani A, Allavena P: Migratory response of human natural killer cells to lymphotactin. Eur J Immunol 1996;26:3238–3241.

76 Maghazachi AA, Al-Aoukaty A, Schall TJ: CC chemokines induce the generation of killer cells from CD56+ cells. Eur J Immunol 1996;26:315–319.

77 Taub DD, Ortaldo JR, Turcovski-Corrales SM, Key ML, Longo DL, Murphy WJ: Beta chemokines costimulate lymphocyte cytolysis, proliferation, and lymphokine production. J Leukoc Biol 1996;59:81–89.

78 Taub DD, Turcovski-Corrales SM, Key ML, Longo DL, Murphy WJ: Chemokines and T lymphocyte activation. I. Beta chemokines costimulate human T lymphocyte activation in vitro. J Immunol 1996;156:2095–2103.

79 Dairaghi DJ, Soo KS, Oldham ER, Premack BA, Kitamura T, Bacon KB, Schall TJ: RANTES-induced T cell activation correlates with CD3 expression. J Immunol 1998;160:426–433.

80 Bacon KB, Premack BA, Gardner P, Schall TJ: Activation of dual T cell signaling pathways by the chemokine RANTES. Science 1995;269:1727–1730.

81 Karpus WJ, Lukacs NW, Kennedy KJ, Smith WS, Hurst SD, Barrett TA: Differential CC chemokine-induced enhancement of T helper cell cytokine production. J Immunol 1997;158:4129–4136.

82 Lukacs NW, Chensue SW, Karpus WJ, Lincoln P, Keefer C, Strieter RM, Kunkel SL: C-C chemokines differentially alter interleukin-4 production from lymphocytes. Am J Pathol 1997;150:1861–1868.

83 Hogaboam CM, Lukacs NW, Chensue SW, Strieter RM, Kunkel SL: Monocyte chemoattractant protein-1 synthesis by murine lung fibroblasts modulates CD4+ T cell activation. J Immunol 1998;160:4606–4614.

84 Sallusto F, Mackay CR, Lanzavecchia A: Selective expression of the eotaxin receptor CCR3 by human T helper 2 cells. Science 1997;277:2005–2007.

85 Bonecchi R, Bianchi G, Bordignon PP, D'Ambrosio D, Lang R, Borsatti A, Sozzani S, Allavena P, Gray PA, Mantovani A, Sinigaglia F: Differential expression of chemokine receptors and chemotactic responsiveness of type 1 T helper cells (Th1s) and Th2s. J Exp Med 1998;187:129–134.

86 Sallusto F, Lenig D, Mackay CR, Lanzavecchia A: Flexible programs of chemokine receptor expression on human polarized T helper 1 and 2 lymphocytes. J Exp Med 1998;187:875–883.
87 Zingoni A, Soto H, Hedrick JA, Stoppacciaro A, Storlazzi CT, Sinigaglia F, D'Ambrosio D, O'Garra A, Robinson D, Rocchi M, Santoni A, Zlotnik A, Napolitano M: The chemokine receptor CCR8 is preferentially expressed in Th2 but not Th1 cells. J Immunol 1998;161:547–551.
88 Roos RS, Loetscher M, Legler DF, Clark-Lewis I, Baggiolini M, Moser B: Identification of CCR8, the receptor for the human CC chemokine I-309. J Biol Chem 1997;272:17251–17254.
89 Goya I, Gutierrez J, Varona R, Kremer L, Zaballos A, Marquez G: Identification of CCR8 as the specific receptor for the human beta-chemokine I-309: Cloning and molecular characterization of murine CCR8 as the receptor for TCA-3. J Immunol 1998;160:1975–1981.
90 Lloyd CM, Minto AW, Dorf ME, Proudfoot A, Wells TN, Salant DJ, Gutierrez-Ramos JC: RANTES and monocyte chemoattractant protein-1 (MCP-1) play an important role in the inflammatory phase of crescentic nephritis, but only MCP-1 is involved in crescent formation and interstitial fibrosis. J Exp Med 1997;185:1371–1380.
91 Lloyd CM, Dorf ME, Proudfoot A, Salant DJ, Gutierrez-Ramos JC: Role of MCP-1 and RANTES in inflammation and progression to fibrosis during murine crescentic nephritis. J Leukoc Biol 1997;62: 676–680.
92 Car BD, Meloni F, Luisetti M, Semenzato G, Gialdroni-Grassi G, Walz A: Elevated IL-8 and MCP-1 in the bronchoalveolar lavage fluid of patients with idiopathic pulmonary fibrosis and pulmonary sarcoidosis. Am J Respir Crit Care Med 1994;149:655–659.
93 Smith RE: Chemotactic cytokines mediate leukocyte recruitment in fibrotic lung disease. Biol Signals 1996;5:223–231.
94 Smith RE, Strieter RM, Zhang K, Phan SH, Standiford TJ, Lukacs NW, Kunkel SL: A role for C-C chemokines in fibrotic lung disease. J Leukoc Biol 1995;57:782–787.
95 Lukacs NW, Chensue SW, Smith RE, Strieter RM, Warmington K, Wilke C, Kunkel SL: Production of monocyte chemoattractant protein-1 and macrophage inflammatory protein-1-alpha by inflammatory granuloma fibroblasts. Am J Pathol 1994;144:711–718.
96 Gibran NS, Ferguson M, Heimbach DM, Isik FF: Monocyte chemoattractant protein-1 mRNA expression in the human burn wound. J Surg Res 1997;70:1–6.
97 Rollins BJ, Morrison ED, Stiles CD: Cloning and expression of JE, a gene inducible by platelet-derived growth factor and whose product has cytokine-like properties. Proc Natl Acad Sci USA 1988;85:3738–3742.
98 Gharaee-Kermani M, Denholm EM, Phan SH: Costimulation of fibroblast collagen and transforming growth factor-beta-1 gene expression by monocyte chemoattractant protein-1 via specific receptors. J Biol Chem 1996;271:17779–17784.
99 Yue TL, Wang X, Sung CP, Olson B, McKenna PJ, Gu JL, Feuerstein GZ: Interleukin-8. A mitogen and chemoattractant for vascular smooth muscle cells. Circ Res 1994;75:1–7.
100 Strieter RM, Polverini PJ, Arenberg DA, Kunkel SL: The role of CXC chemokines as regulators of angiogenesis. Shock 1995;4:155–160.
101 Porreca E, Di Febbo C, Reale M, Castellani ML, Baccante G, Barbacane R, Conti P, Cuccurullo F, Poggi A: Monocyte chemotactic protein 1 (MCP-1) is a mitogen for cultured rat vascular smooth muscle cells. J Vasc Res 1997;34:58–65.
102 Hayes IM, Jordan NJ, Towers S, Smith G, Paterson JR, Earnshaw JJ, Roach AG, Westwick J, Williams RJ: Human vascular smooth muscle cells express receptors for CC chemokines. Arterioscler Thromb Vasc Biol 1998;18:397–403.
103 Bone RC, Fischer CJ, Clemmer TP, Slotman GJ, Metz CA, Balk RA: Sepsis syndrome: A valid clinical entity. Crit Care Med 1989;17:389–393.
104 Hack CE, Aarden LA, Thijs LG: Role of cytokines in sepsis. Adv Immunol 1997;66:101–195.
105 Hack CE, Hart M, Strack-van Schijndel RJM, Eerenberg AJM, Nuijens JH, Thijs LG, Aarden LA: Interleukin-8 in sepsis: Relation to shock and inflammatory mediators. Infect Immun 1992;60:2835–2842.
106 Bossink AW, Paemen L, Jansen PM, Hack CE, Thijs LG, Van Damme J: Plasma levels of the chemokines monocyte chemotactic proteins-1 and -2 are elevated in human sepsis. Blood 1995;86:3841–3847.
107 Kunkel SL, Standiford TJ, Kasahara K, Strieter RM: Interleukin-8: The major neutrophil chemotactic factor in the lung. Exp Lung Res 1991;17:17–21.

108 Lynch IJP, Standiford TJ, Kunkel SL, Rolfe MW, Strieter RM: Neutrophilic alveolitis in idiopathic pulmonary fibrosis: The role of interleukin-8. Am Rev Respir Dis 1992;145:1433–1438.
109 Strieter RM, Standiford TJ, Colletti LM, Kunkel SL: Neutrophil recruitment in acute lung injury: The interplay of early response cytokines, adhesion molecules; and CXC chemokines; in Koch AE, Strieter R (eds): Chemokines in Disease. Austin, Landes, 1996, pp 135–150.
110 Xing Z, Jordana M, Braciak T, Ohtoshi T, Gauldie J: Lipopolysaccharide induces expression of granulocyte/macrophage colony-stimulating factor, interleukin-8, and interleukin-6 in human nasal, but not lung, fibroblasts: Evidence for heterogeneity within the respiratory tract. Am J Respir Cell Mol Biol 1993;9:255–263.
111 Walley KR, Lukacs NW, Standiford TJ, Strieter RM, Kunkel SL: Elevated levels of macrophage inflammatory protein 2 in severe murine peritonitis increase neutrophil recruitment and mortality. Infect Immun 1997;65:3847–3851.
112 Zisman DA, Kunkel SL, Strieter RM, Tsai WC, Bucknell K, Wilkowski J, Standiford TJ: MCP-1 protects mice in lethal endotoxemia. J Clin Invest 1997;99:2832–2836.
113 Karpus WJ, Kennedy KJ, Kunkel SL, Lukacs NW: Monocyte chemotactic protein 1 regulates oral tolerance induction by inhibition of T-helper cell 1-related cytokines. J Exp Med 1998;187:733–741.
114 Lukacs NW, Kunkel SL, Strieter RM, Warmington K, Chensue SW: The role of MIP-1-alpha in *S. mansoni* egg induced granulomatous inflammation. J Exp Med 1993;177:1551–1559.
115 Chensue SW, Warmington KS, Lukacs NW, Lincoln PM, Burdick MD, Strieter RM, Kunkel SL: Monocyte chemotactic protein expression during schistosome egg granuloma formation. Sequence of production, localization, contribution, and regulation. Am J Pathol 1995;146:130–138.
116 Lukacs NW, Addison CL, Gauldie J, Graham F, Simpson K, Strieter RM, Warmington K, Chensue SW, Kunkel SL: Transgene-induced production of IL-4 alters the development and collagen expression of T helper cell 1-type pulmonary granulomas. J Immunol 1997;158:4478–4484.
117 Godiska R, Chantry D, Dietsch GN, Gray PW: Chemokine expression in murine experimental allergic encephalomyelitis. J Neuroimmunol 1995;58:167–176.
118 Glabinski AR, Tani M, Strieter RM, Tuohy VK, Ransohoff RM: Synchronous synthesis of alpha- and beta-chemokines by cells of diverse lineage in the central nervous system of mice with relapses of chronic experimental autoimmune encephalomyelitis. Am J Pathol 1997;150:617–630.
119 Karpus WJ, Lukacs NW, McRae BL, Strieter RM, Kunkel SL, Miller SD: An important role for the chemokine macrophage inflammatory protein-1-alpha in the pathogenesis of the T-cell-mediated autoimmune disease, experimental autoimmune encephalomyelitis. J Immunol 1995;155:5003–5010.
120 Berman JW, Guida MP, Warren J, Amat J, Brosnan CF: Localization of monocyte chemoattractant peptide-1 expression in the central nervous system in experimental autoimmune encephalomyelitis and trauma in the rat. J Immunol 1996;156:3017–3023.
121 Karpus WJ, Kennedy KJ: MIP-1-alpha and MCP-1 differentially regulate acute and relapsing autoimmune encephalomyelitis as well as Th1/Th2 lymphocyte differentiation. J Leukoc Biol 1997;62:681–687.
122 Miyagishi R, Kikuchi S, Takayama C, Inoue Y, Tashiro K: Identification of cell types producing RANTES, MIP-1-alpha and MIP-1-beta in rat experimental autoimmune encephalomyelitis by in situ hybridization. J Neuroimmunol 1997;77:17–26.
123 Hayashi M, Luo Y, Laning J, Strieter RM, Dorf ME: Production and function of monocyte chemoattractant protein-1 and other beta-chemokines in murine glial cells. J Neuroimmunol 1995;60:143–150.
124 Jiang Y, Salafranca MN, Adhikari S, Xia Y, Feng L, Sonntag MK, deFiebre CM, Pennell NA, Streit WJ, Harrison JK: Chemokine receptor expression in cultured glia and rat experimental allergic encephalomyelitis. J Neuroimmunol 1998;86:1–12.
125 Bennetts BH, Teutsch SM, Buhler MM, Heard RN, Stewart GJ: The CCR5 deletion mutation fails to protect against multiple sclerosis. Hum Immunol 1997;58:52–59.

Nicholas W. Lukacs, PhD, Department of Pathology, University of Michigan Medical School, 1301 Catherine, Ann Arbor, MI 48109-0602 (USA)

Mantovani A (ed): Chemokines.
Chem Immunol. Basel, Karger, 1999, vol 72, pp 121–140

Chemokines and the Human Immunodeficiency Virus

Guido Poli

AIDS Immunophathogenesis Unit, DiBiT, San Raffaele Scientific Institute, Milano, Italy

Pathogenesis of HIV Infection

The human immunodeficiency virus (HIV) is a human pathogenic retrovirus causing a syndrome characterized by a profound immunodeficiency leading to death in the great majority of infected individuals. HIV displays a peculiar affinity for immune cells bearing the CD4 molecule on their cell surface, namely a subset of T lymphocytes with 'helper' function and mononuclear phagocytes (MP). Upon in vitro infection, CD4+ T cells rapidly die either by single cell death or after formation of syncytia. In vivo, while CD4+ T cells undergo a progressive depletion, along with a severe impairment of their functions, MP are mostly responsible for spreading and maintaining the infection in privileged sites and organs, such as the brain, that may become true sanctuaries of HIV. After approximately 10 years of silent infection (with the exclusion of the primary HIV infection during which organs are seeded with virus concomitantly with constitutional symptoms and lymphadenopathy) opportunistic infections (OI) and/or tumors such as B-cell lymphomas and Kaposi's sarcoma emerge and cause the death of infected individuals. This terminal stage goes under the name of acquired immunodeficiency syndrome (AIDS) [1].

At the cellular level, docking of the HIV envelope (Env) glycoprotein gp120 to CD4 was known to allow a conformational change in the second fusogenic Env molecule gp41. Insertion of gp41 into the target cell plasma membrane allows the injection of the inner component of HIV particles, a ribonucleoprotein complex containing the preintegration complex, among

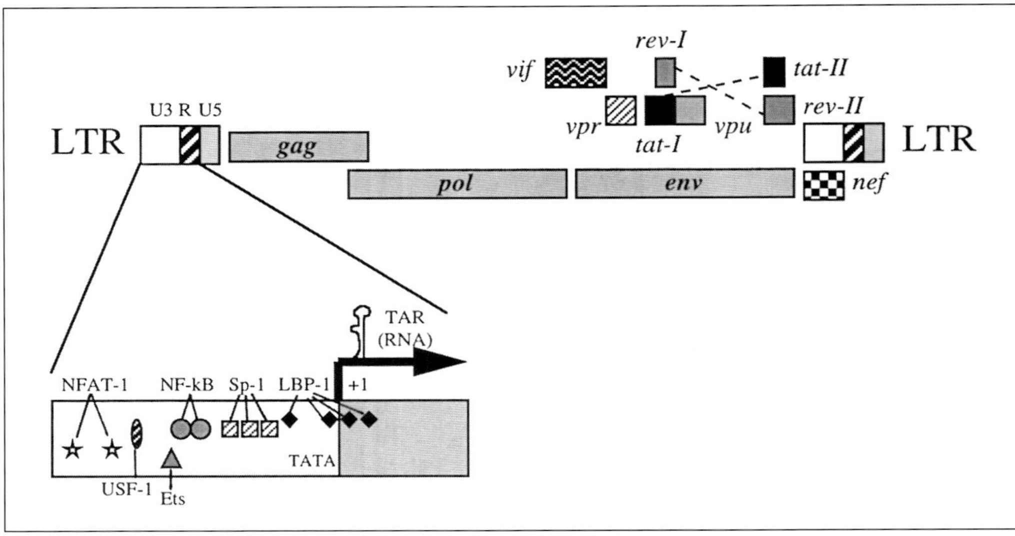

Fig. 1. HIV proviral DNA. In addition to the structural genes (*gag, pol, env*) a set of accessory genes regulate HIV expression and pathogenicity [2, 14]. The viral LTRs, repeated identically at 5′ and 3′ of the genome, encompass several binding sites for cellular transcription factors, particularly in the U3 region (some of which are represented here), whereas the R portion contains the Tat-binding domain known as TAR region.

other, two copies of the viral RNA and the reverse transcriptase, the enzyme responsible for making a cDNA version of the viral RNA that will be integrated into the host genome in coincidence, at least in T cells, with cell division [2]. During reverse transcription, two identical copies of the viral promoter, named long terminal repeats (LTRs), are synthesized at 5′ and 3′ and encompass the structural genes (*gag, pol, env*) which consitute the retrovirus backbone, plus a set of accessory genes (*tat, rev, vif, vpr, vpu* and *nef*) present in the 3′ portion of the provirus adding complexity to the regulation of HIV expression (fig. 1). Once integrated, expression of HIV genes, and their consequent assembly into new progeny viral particles (virions) becomes dependent from the cellular RNA poll I and from signals affecting either its transcription or regulating the efficiency of viral protein synthesis at posttranscriptional level. Complex glycosylation of its Env occurs in the Golgi apparatus and plays a major role in the ability of HIV to interact with cell surface molecules and receptors.

Although the fundamental characteristics of HIV and of several viral genes have been rapidly delineated after its discovery as the causative agent of AIDS in the early 1980s, the mechanism(s) involved in the ability of the virus to cause a progressive immunodeficiency remains the object of strong debate and divergent opinions. Despite unsuspected high levels of HIV replication have recently been demonstrated [3], several aspects of HIV-associated immune dysfunction cannot be accounted for by a direct infection of CD4+ cells. Indirect mechanisms of HIV-induced immune dysfunction encompass autoimmune-like cross-reactivity between some HIV genes and MHC genes, shedding of Env and/or other HIV proteins (i.e. Tat), killing or profound functional impairment of bone marrow-derived progenitor cells, and impairment of thymic or postthymic T-cell renewal [1].

At the cellular level, unlike CD4+ T cells, MP are substantially resistant to HIV-induced killing, although features of cytopathicity (including formation of syncytia) may occur in vitro [4, 5]. Infected MP synthesize and accumulate HIV particles in their Golgi apparatus, suggestive of their role as 'Trojan horses' of HIV infection [4, 5]; of note, this feature has been observed also in vivo [6]. In general, monocyte-derived macrophages (MDM), the most common model of in vitro infection of MP, are triggered to produce inflammatory cytokines and related molecules shortly after infection. Several of these effects have been reproduced by MDM incubation with HIV gp120 or anti-CD4 monoclonal antibodies (mAb) [7, 8]. In vivo, circulating monocytes are rarely infected [9], whereas tissue macrophages residing in different organs such as the brain, the lungs, liver, spleen, etc. have been repeatedly documented to carry and express HIV [6]. Dysfunctions of monocytes, however, have been highlighted soon after the description of CD4+ T cells as cellular targets for HIV. Of interest, defective chemotactic responses to classic agents such as f-Met-Leu-Phe, C5a, or crude cytokine-enriched culture supernatants have been early described as typical mononuclear and polymorphonuclear leukocytes of infected individuals before the discovery of chemokines [10–13].

HIV-Suppressive Cytokines and CD8-Dependent Nonlytic Suppression of HIV Replication

As a retrovirus, HIV can lead to acute infection rapidly followed by cell death or to a state of chronic infection as integrated provirus [2]. In this scenario, residual cells surviving the acute phase of infection become often chronically infected cells and carry one or two copies of integrated proviral genomes; in addition they have downmodulated the CD4 molecule on their cell surface as a result of multiple interactions with HIV Env [1, 14]. In addition, these cells are frequently, although not invariably, characterized by a state of relative latency susceptible to the regulatory effects exerted by viral proteins such as Tat or Rev, or by host factors such as cytokines, UV light, and chemical agents such as phorbol esters [1, 14]. The ability of tumor necrosis factor-α/-β (TNF-α/-β) to upregulate HIV transcription has been elegantly linked to the activation of the cellular transcription factor NF-κB that binds to two consensus sequences present in the HIV LTR just upstream a TATA box and the transcription start site [15] (fig. 1). Models of HIV replication driven by autocrine/paracrine secretion of TNF-α or other proinflammatory cytokines including interleukin (IL)-1β, IL-6, and IFN-γ have been reported and have served as paradigm of the ability of HIV to take advantage of the complex host regulatory network of cytokine and related signals (including CD3, CD28, CD30, CD40 and their ligands) to spread from latently infected cells [1, 14]. Although the existence of latent cells in vivo has been questioned in the past, recent studies have definitively proven their relevance in terms of persistent infection and reignition of viral replication after suspension of antiviral therapy [16–18].

In contrast to an abundant literature describing HIV-inducing cytokines and related factors, only a few molecules have been demonstrated to have clear-cut inhibitory or suppressive effects on HIV expression and/or replication. Neutralization of IFN-α/-β has been shown to augment HIV replication during in vivo infection or after ex vivo culture of patients peripheral blood mononuclear cells (PBMC) [19–21]. The mechanism of action of IFN-α/-β has been shown to be complex and potentially capable of affecting multiple steps of the HIV life cycle, from reverse transcription to budding and release of new virions from the plasma membrane of infected cells [22, 23]. Anti-inflammatory cytokines and related molecules including transforming growth factor-β (TGF-β), IL-4, IL-10, IL-13, and the IL-1 receptor antagonist (IL-1ra) have been shown to act as potent inhibitors of HIV replication in different models of chronic infection of T cells and/or MP [14]. In the case of TGF-β, inhibition of HIV transcription has been formally demonstrated [24]. However, all these molecules (with the potential exception of IL-13 and IL-1ra) have also shown HIV-inductive capacity as a function of either the different model systems or of whether cells were stimulated before or after infection with HIV [6, 14], revealing a degree of plasticity of HIV to the human immune system even higher than initially suspected. These results also highlight the difficulty to elaborate a cytokine-based intervention in HIV disease aimed either at suppressing viral replication or at triggering HIV expression from latently infected cells in order to facilitate their elimination by specific effectors of the immune system.

In this scenario, depletion of CD8+ T cells from PBMC of infected individuals allowed better viral replication and, in some instances, was the only method resulting in HIV isolation from these cells [25]. This observation, subsequently confirmed by several investigators, was followed by the formal demonstration that CD8+ T cells were acting independently from their well-known capacity to kill infected cells in a MHC-restricted manner as cytotoxic T lymphocytes (CTL) [26]. In the face of its reproducibility, the search for the cellular soluble factor(s) responsible for such a nonlytic suppression of viral replication has remained elusive for several years; the activity, also become known as CD8 antiviral factor (CAF), has been negatively defined through the years as a growing list of factors (mostly based on experiments involving anticytokine neutralizing Ab) not responsible for the described effect [26]. Unlike most recombinant cytokines shown to act in different in vivo systems of infection, CAF has retained a high level of interest as a candidate of a 'truly suppressive' factor(s) acting in vivo. In this regard, evidence has been reported that CAF inhibits transcription, essentially resulting in or favoring the persistence of a state of latent HIV infection [26].

HIV-Suppressive Chemokines: RANTES, MIP-1α, MIP-1β

At the end of 1995, a claim was made that the true nature of CAF had been uncovered. Based on a model of a T-cell line (PM-1) susceptible to both T-cell tropic and macrophage-tropic HIV strains, culture supernatants derived from CD8+ T-cell clones immortalized by the human T-lymphotropic virus type-1 (HTLV-1) revealed potent HIV-inhibitory activity. Repeated cycles of purification and testing in the PM-1 system led to the identification of three CC chemokines previously discovered but not linked to HIV: regulated upon activation normal T cell expressed and secreted (RANTES), macrophage inflammatory protein-1α (MIP-1α) and MIP-1β [27]. These chemokines, either alone or added together, revealed HIV-inhibitory activity whereas only their simultaneous neutralization resulted in the reversal of effect, i.e. HIV replication in cultures of PBMC of infected individuals [27]. The mechanism of action of these chemokines was not originally discussed. However, the spectrum of action of the three chemokines was suggestive of their relative prevailing activity against macrophage (M)-tropic HIV strains in that the prototypic T-cell-tropic strain LAI/IIIB was not inhibited (although the replication of another T-cell-tropic strain, MN, was impaired) [27]. At the time, the basis for chemokine selectivity of action was unclear, although it was known that major determinants of T- vs. M-tropisms were residing in the region of gp120 Env encompassing the V3 hypervariable loop [28].

Shortly after, the identification of a 7-transmembrane domain receptor, the ligand of which was unknown, resembling chemokine receptors was reported to confer HIV-dependent fusogenic properties to cells simultaneously cotransfected with the human CD4. The molecule, previously identified and named LESTR or HUMSTR, was renamed 'fusin' because of this property [29]. Of interest, fusin made cells susceptible to gp120 Env-dependent fusion or infection only by T-cell-tropic, but not by M-tropic HIVs [29], implying that similar molecules would act as coreceptors together with CD4 for this second group of viruses. A chemokine receptor, CCR5, was then shown to act as coreceptor for M-tropic HIVs [30, 31]. This molecule was independently discovered to be the receptor for RANTES, MIP-1α and MIP-1β, the three chemokines previously reported to induce preferential inhibitory effects on M-tropic HIV strains [27]. Finally, the fusin ligand was identified in the molecule named stromal cell-derived factor-1 (SDF-1) [33–35] that, as predictable, showed restricted inhibitory effects on T-cell-tropic viruses [33, 35]. At this point a general model could be formulated (fig. 2). HIV-1 could be defined by its phenotypic growth into M-tropic vs. T-lymphotropic viruses. These two group of HIVs also fit their respective capacity or inability to replicate and cause syncytia in the CD4+ MT-2 transformed T-cell line [36]. Both SI and NSI viruses bound CD4 as primary cell surface receptor, however they differed in their usage of the type of chemokine receptor utilized for infecting their target cells. M-tropic/NSI viruses used CCR5, whereas T-cell tropic/SI viruses utilized CXCR4. Conversely, the respective chemokine receptor ligands (RANTES, MIP-1α and MIP-1β for CCR5, and SDF-1 for CXCR4, respectively) acted as inhibitors of the binding of HIV to the chemokine coreceptor molecules, likely without interfering with its interaction with CD4 (fig. 2). Indeed, it was demonstrated that interaction between gp120 and CD4 is the first obligatory step in viral entry, inducing conformational changes indispensable for its subsequent binding to the chemokine receptor [37, 38]. After the formation of a complex between gp120 Env, CD4, and the chemokine receptor, the fusogenic component of HIV Env, gp41, undergoes a conformational change similar to that of a jackknife that allows its insertion into the target cell membrane and the fusion of the virion and the cell [37] (fig. 2).

In support of this model, synthetic truncated molecules capable of binding but not of transducing signals in terms of Ca^{2+} fluxes or chemotaxis could inhibit CCR5-dependent HIV infection [39], and chemokine analogs, such as and particularly AOP-RANTES, showed comparable and even greater potency as chemokine receptor antagonists [40]. Studies involving the constructions of chimeric chemokine receptors have shed further light on the requirements for cell signaling and inhibition of HIV infection. In essence, these studies have indicated that the sites involved in ligand binding and HIV entry are not identical [41, 42], supporting the possibility of developing selective antagonists for HIV infection that virtually would not perturb the interaction of chemokines with their receptors during inflammatory responses.

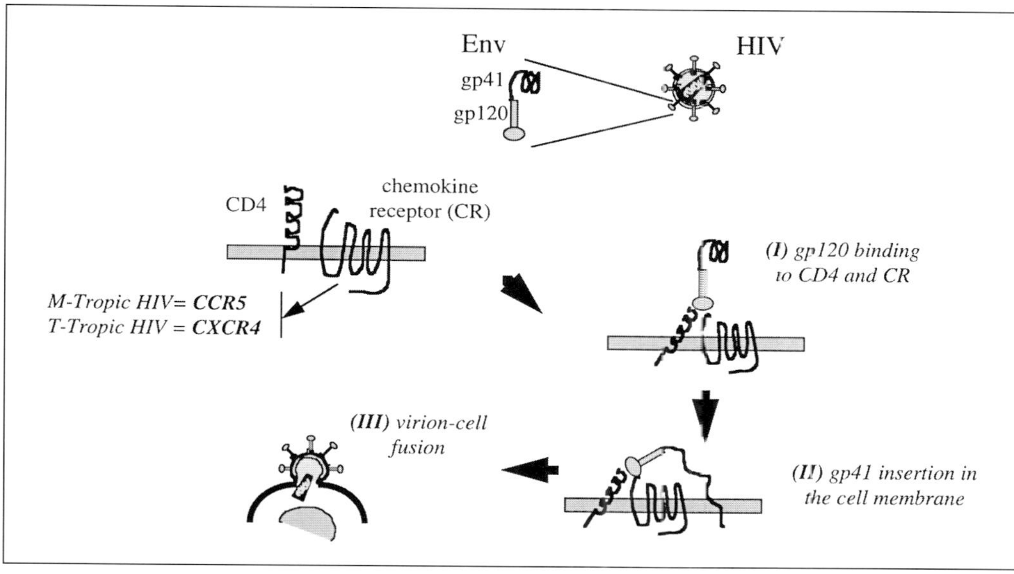

Fig. 2. Sequential events leading to HIV-CD4+ cell fusion. After interaction of HIV gp120 Env with CD4, a conformational change leads to a second interaction with a chemokine receptor and formation of a complex. This step is intermediate to the springing of the fusogenic gp41 Env into the plasma cell membrane, thus allowing the injection of the core into the cytoplasm of the target cell.

Other HIV-Relevant Chemokines

An outburst of excellent scientific reports have extended the paradigm of obligatory chemokine receptor usage by HIV beyond CCR5 and CXCR4, CCR2B, CCR3 and CCR8 have been subsequently shown to act as coreceptors for viral entry in surrogate systems generally represented by nonhuman cell lines (constitutively resistant to HIV infection) becoming susceptible to the virus after cotransfection of human CD4 and one of the candidate chemokine receptors [43–48]. The in vivo utilization of these coreceptors is usually linked to HIV disease progression, in that, independently from the modality of infection (through sexual contact, blood transfusion or vertical transmission), the great majority of the viruses isolated early after infection are CCR5-monotropic viruses (recently defined as R5 HIV [49]) [50, 51]. Evolution of HIV in the infected individual leading to a progressive state of immunodeficiency is associated frequently, although not invariably, with the expansion of the number of chemokine receptors that can be utilized by the virus CD4+ cells. In

Table 1. Chemokine receptors serving as HIV-1 coreceptors for entry

Receptor	Ligands	Comments	Reference(s)
CCR2b	MCP-1, -2, -3, -4	Rare	45, 53, 54, 62
CCR3	Eotaxin, RANTES, MCP-2, -3, -4	Rare (Microglia)	43, 45, 56
CCR5	RANTES, MIP-1α, MIP-1β	Main HIV receptor (early disease)	27, 30, 31, 39, 40, 80
CCR8	I-309, TARC, MIP-1β	Rare?	46, 55
CXCR4	SDF-1	Common (late disease)	29, 33, 35, 87
US28	RANTES, MCP-1	CMV gene	61, 62
Bob		Rare	112
Bonzo		Rare	112

approximately 50% of infected individuals, before or during transition to AIDS, acquisition of the ability to use CXCR4 occurs and coincides with the previously defined switch from NSI to SI viruses [50, 51]. It should be underscored, however, both that such a switch is not an obligatory process for disease progression (approximately 50% of individuals die of AIDS with M-tropic/NSI viruses) [36], and that the loss of CCR5 usage is rarely observed in HIV isolates obtained from AIDS patients [Poli, unpubl. observations]. The selection mechanisms resulting from behind the fact that most viruses isolated from infected individuals during early HIV disease are R5 monotropic are essentially unknown, although it has been proposed that poor expression of CXCR4 on the cell surface of mucosal dendritic cells may contribute to the selection process [52].

As predictable by the general model, ligands of the chemokine receptors serving as HIV entry cofactors usually inhibit the infection of Env-matched viruses. Eotaxin, uniquely binding to CCR3, as well as monocyte chemotactic protein-2 (MCP-2) and MCP-3 (binding to CCR2 and to CCR2 and CCR3, respectively), and I-309 or TARC (binding to CCR8) can inhibit HIV replication [43, 45, 48, 53–55] (table 1). In addition, CCR3 and its ligands are likely to play an important role in HIV infection of the central nervous system (CNS), in that expression of this chemokine receptor is relevant for infection of the microglial (the resident brain macrophages which are primary targets and reserviors of infection in the CNS) [56].

Less clear is the role played by MCP-1, a prototypic CC chemokine, which binds exclusively to CCR2. Although HIV inhibition by MCP-1 and/or anti-CCR2b mAb has been reported [54], it is unlikely that this effect occurs via the 'classic' inhibition of viral entry, as supported by the fact that the viruses studied did not use CCR2 as coreceptor for entry [54]. In addition,

MCP-1 may play an important role in HIV disease particularly in the pathogenesis of HIV infection of the CNS leading to the clinical condition known as AIDS-associated dementia which is sustained at the tissue level by a HIV-induced encephalitis (HIVE). A selective accumulation of MCP-1, but not of other chemokines, has been demonstrated in the cerebrospinal fluid (CSF) of AIDS patients affected by AIDS-associated dementia [57] or HIVE [58]. A positive correlation was found betweeen MCP-1 and HIV RNA levels in the CNS, but not in the plasma, of these individuals, suggesting a functional link between virus replication in the CNS and MCP-1 accumulation [58]. At the cellular level, infection by HIV of astrocytes, another cell type infected in vivo by HIV, has been demonstrated to induce MCP-1 [57], whereas infection of MDM has been shown to induce MCP-1 [58, 113], but also MIP-1α and MIP-1β secretion [59, 60], thus providing a potential model for recruitment of monocytes from the bloodstream into the CNS. In addition to HIVE, only cytomegalovirus encephalitis (CMVE), but not other major OI or tumors (primary lymphomas) of the CNS, has been associated with increased MCP-1 levels in the CSF [61]. Of interest, CMV encodes a gene (US28) codifying for a functional chemokine receptor capable of both binding MCP-1 and RANTES and of acting as HIV coreceptor [62], suggesting the possibility that autocrine/paracrine mechanisms driven by virus-induced MCP-1 may play a role in the pathogenesis of CMV disease in the CNS, and that coinfection by CMV and HIV may also occur at the cellular level.

In contrast to the general model, RANTES, MCP-1 and MCP-3 have been reported to inhibit also X4 HIV replication in T lymphocytes [53, 62], although their antiviral mechanism was not defined. Similar results were obtained with macrophage-derived chemokine (MDC). This chemokine was originally defined as chemotactic for several cell types, and particularly for natural killer cells and dendritic cells [63]. The receptor for MDC was subsequently known to be CCR4 [64], a molecule not demonstrated to be used as entry receptor, at least for HIV type 1. A variant of MDC lacking the initial two amino acids at the N-terminus [(–2)MDC], named native MDC, was purified with a procedure similar to that which successfully led to the identification of RANTES, MIP-1α and MIP-1β as HIV inhibitory molecules [65]. This molecule showed broad-spectrum inhibitory activity against the replication of several HIV strains, including X4 and R5 viruses, in CD8-depleted PBMC [65]. Although its mechanism of antiviral action was not elucidated, this spectrum of bioactivity made unlikely inhibition of viral entry by selective occupancy of chemokine receptors. Although a recent report has confirmed a modest (30–40%) inhibitory capacity of both MDC and [(–2)MDC] towards R5 and X4 HIV replication [66], other investigators have not confirmed these original findings [67, 68]. Finally, we have recently analyzed the efficacy of MDC against HIV and observed a selective inhibition of R5 viruses in MDM, but not in activated T lymphocytes. In addition, we could formally prove that MDC inhibited HIV replication at a postentry level, in that the accumulation of HIV DNA as a result of virion-associated reverse transcription was unaffected by the chemokine [unpubl. observations]. Thus it is conceivable that MDC or some of its derivatives may represent a noncanonical HIV inhibitory chemokine acting with a mechanism resembling that of anti-inflammatory cytokines or interferons [14, 23], perhaps via binding to a receptor different from CCR4 [66].

Do Chemokines Enhance HIV Replication?

The paradigm of chemokines blocking HIV entry at the cell surface via binding to chemokine receptors does not involve a role for a chemokine-mediated signaling. This simple model, sustained by the lack of interference of pertussis toxin with viral inhibition by chemokines [38] and by the demonstration that peptidic antagonists can exert a similar function when devoid of the capacity to transduce cell activation signals [39], however, has been challenged by other observations. First, interaction between HIV Env and the chemokine receptor was demonstrated capable of transducing a cell activation signal [69]; similar results have been independently described in terms of activation of the Pyk-2-dependent pathway [70]. In addition, although aminooxypentane (AOP)-RANTES, an agent potently blocking HIV infection [40], lacks chemotactic capacity, it retains Ca^{2+}-inducing activity [71]. This effect has been linked to the peculiarity of AOP-RANTES, compared to RANTES or Met-RANTES, to permanently downregulate CCR5 from the cell surface, a mechanism earlier suggested of crucial importance in chemokine-mediated inhibition of viral entry [72].

One fundamental concern regarding the potential use of chemokines or chemokine analogs in the therapy or prevention of HIV infection is the possibility that these agents may favor the emergence of more aggressive T-cell-tropic/SI viruses. In this regard, chemokine-mediated selective pressure leading to the emergence of X4 viruses has been reported in ex vivo experiments using PBMC obtained from infected individuals [73]. Unlike their HIV-inhibitory effects, enhancement of HIV replication by CCR5 binding chemokines was pertussis toxin sensitive, implying a role for cellular activation [73]. Similar conclusions were previoulsy drawn with HIV infection of MDM [74]. Enhancement of R5 HIV replication has been then described in both monocytes and MDM that had been pretreated up to 24 h with RANTES, MIP-1α, or MIP-1β before infection, whereas inhibition of HIV replication was observed in the same cells if incubation with chemokines was performed after infection [75]. Increased HIV replication in T lymphocytes stimulated with RANTES or other chemokines has been also reported and correlated to increase CXCR4 expression [76]. Finally, we have observed that MCP-1 can act as enhancer of HIV replication in cultures of PBMC obtained from infected individuals and depleted of CD8+ T cells [unpubl. observations].

Chemokine Receptor Genes and HIV Infection

The importance of chemokine receptors (and indirectly of their ligands) for HIV infection has been impressively highlighted by the observation that individuals carrying an homozygous deletion of 32 bp in their CCR5 gene (Δccr5/Δccr5) are virtually protected from HIV infection [77–79]. Their cells were still infectable in vitro by X4 HIV, but were totally resistant to R5 HIV [77–79]. This gene variant, causing the retention of a truncated protein in the cytoplasm without expression at the cell surface [80], is apparently compatible with a normal life and immune response capacity, whereas only a few individuals have been reported thus far infected despite their homozygosity for Δ-32 ccr5 [81]. The gene is present in Caucasians, but not in Asian or African populations [77]; because highly exposed uninfected (EU) individuals are present also in these regions of the world, protective factors of yet undefined origin and different for Δccr5 must exist. Expression of CCR5 on the cell surface of immune cells is crucial for virus 'engraftment' soon after transmission. As mentioned, regardless either to which quasispecies predominates in the transmitter or to the modality of transmission (sexual, via blood exchange, or vertically), the initial strain of HIV is almost invariably CCR5-dependent [50, 51].

Heterozygosity for Δccr5 does not confer protection from HIV infection either in vitro or in vivo; however, this condition is associated with a lack of a slower disease progression (long-term nonprogressors, LTNP) [77–79]. Because only approximately 33% of LTNP are Δccr5, other related mutations have been searched in this subset of infected individuals accounting for 1–5% of the entire infected population. A conservative mutation of a single AA in the transmembrane region of CCR2 (CCR2-64I), a gene located in close proximity to the CCR5 gene on the host chromosome encoding the receptor for MCP-1 through MC-4, has been found in some [82–84], but not all [85] cohorts of LTNP. In one study, the combined prevalence of CCR5 Δ-32 and CCR2-64I accounted for more than 70% of LTNP [84], suggesting that this relatively benign outcome of infection is largely accounted for by the genetic makeup of the host. Finally, a mutation in the 3′ untranslated region of SDF-1, the ligand for CXCR4, has also been linked to a delayed disease progression

[86]. Unlike CCR5 Δ-32 [80], the biological correlates of CCR2 and SDF-1 mutations are unclear. One attractive hypothesis is that these mutations are 'flags' of concomitant mutations in linkage dysequilibrium present in the CCR5 promoter [83], therefore resulting in diminished expression of this HIV coreceptor on the surface of immune cells.

Conclusions and Perspectives

Chemokine and their receptors have only recently entered the arena of AIDS pathogenesis, but they have already substantially improved our knowledge of the pathogenesis of this disease and has opened new possibilities of intervention. The dogma that CD4 is the primary receptor for HIV is currently being challenged by the observation that some HIV strains can infect CD4-negative cells via chemokine receptors [87, 88]. According to this hypothesis, CD4 together with cell surface sugars would serve as recruiting molecules, whereas the chemokine receptor would act as the actual entry receptor [88, 89]. The epidemiological genetics has revealed that absence of CCR5 is an almost universal correlate of protection from HIV infection; however, the fact that this mutation is not present in vast areas of the world where HIV is highly prevalent indicates that other genes or factors play a similar role. In this regard, a mutation in the CCR5 gene linked invariably to Δ-32 hetrozygosity has been found in EU individuals and it has been correlated to in vitro resistance to R5 HIV infection [90]. A number of allelic variants of CCR5 have been recently discovered [91], and their role in HIV infection is under investigation.

The demonstration that chemokines such as RANTES, MIP-1α, MIP-1β, eotaxin and others can block entry of HIV into CD4+ cells has, to some extent, completed the paridigm that the entire HIV life cycle is under the influence of the cytokine network [1, 14] and emphasizes the degree of adaption of HIV to the human immune system. The possibility of translating this important concept in the development of novel therapeutic or preventive strategies is a current challenge for both scientists and the pharmaceutical industry. The feasibility of developing agents capable of interfering with 7-transmembrane domain receptors, such as the chemokine receptors, has been successful before. Compounds such as AOP-RANTES [40, 71], the CXCR4 antagonists AMD3100 [92, 93], ALXCL [94] and T22 [95], as well as naturally truncated chemokines generated after cleavage at the cell surface by the dipeptidyl-peptidase IV (CD26) [96, 97], illustrate the concept that it is possible to develop receptor anatagonists with greater binding affinity and/or altered biology. Some of these molecules may affect intracellular pathways of chemokine receptors [71, 72, 97, 98] ultimately resulting in greater anti-HIV potency.

Finally, chemokine-related trapping of chemokine receptors as a mechanism of preventing access to HIV has been formally demonstrated [99, 100]. The observation that chemokines and HIV bind to different domains of the receptor [41, 42] should facilitate the search of selectivity for these agents.

The possibility to induce high levels of chemokine production in order to cause a state of resistance to HIV infection has been suggested. A minority of EU individuals have indeed shown increased in vitro production of CCR5-binding chemokines that were also responsible for the in vitro resistance of their PBMC [101], an observation that has been extended in part to some EU hemophiliacs who have received large amounts of contaminated factor VIII before 1985 [102]. Subsequently, antigen-driven chemokine production from T-cell clones of EU, but not of infected individuals [103], or stimulation of macrophages by lipopolysaccaride [104] or by CD40 ligand [105] resulted in production of CC chemokines to an extent capable of blocking entry of R5 HIV in vitro. In vivo, macaques that were rectally inoculated and subsequently became resistant to challenge by the HIV-related pathogenic simian immunodeficiency virus (SIV) were shown to produce high local levels of RANTES, MIP-1α and MIP-1β [106].

Although these results are exciting in terms of their potential implications for modern vaccinology and strategies of HIV infection curtailment, they should also be viewed with caution. One of the reasons derives from the reported in vitro ability of chemokines to potentiate HIV replication and, eventually, favor the selection of more aggressive X4 variants, as discussed above [73–76]. It is likely that these HIV-potentiating effects are the result of the physiologic activation of immune cells consequent to chemokine stimulation, an activity that may compete with the ability of some chemokines to interfere with HIV binding at the cell surface. In addition, chemokines may act synergistically with other pro- and anti-inflammatory cytokines in the activation of HIV expression, although this hypothesis has not been thoroughly investigated. In this regard, IL-10, an anti-inflammatory molecule previously shown to exert dichotomous effects on HIV replication [14], could facilitate HIV infection of monocytes via upregulation of the levels of CCR5 expression on their cell surface [107]. IL-4, a benchmark of the Th2 CD4+ lymphocytes, has been recently shown to increase CXCR4 expression and X4-dependent HIV replication [108, 109, 114], but also inhibition of R5 viral production [109]. This dual effect was correlated to an opposite regulatory effect on CXCR4 vs. CCR5 expression, as well as to enhancement of HIV transcription [109]. Similar results were observed after infection of subclones of the U937 cell line that inefficiently supported HIV replication in the presence of the myeloid-differentiating agent 1,25-bihydroxyvitamin D_3 that enhanced viral replication, at least in part, by upregulating the levels of CXCR4 expression [110].

In conclusion, chemokines have given us a fresh new perspective in the investigation of the mechanisms underlying the factors and mechanisms in HIV spreading in vivo, and have also indicated potential new strategies for curtailment or prevention of the AIDS pandemia. The concurrent impressive progress in the potential management of the infection by the combination of potent antiviral agents targeting different key factors in the HIV life cycle (such as reverse transcriptase and protease), either alone or in combination with immune-based therapies such as IL-2 [111], sheds an optimistic light on the possibility of definitively conquering this disease soon after the beginning of the new millennium.

Acknowledgments

I wish to thank Priscilla Biswas, Chiara Bovolenta, and Elisa Vicenzi for their dedication to AIDS research and for critical reading of the manuscript. This work was supported by grants of the National AIDS Project of Istituto Superiore di Sanità, Rome, Italy.

References

1 Fauci AS: Host factors and the pathogenesis of HIV-induced disease. Nature 1996;384;529–534.
2 Emerman M, Malim MH: HIV-1 regulatory/accessory genes: Keys to unraveling viral and host cell biology. Science 1998;280:1880–1884.
3 Ho DD, Neumann AU, Perelson AS, Chen W, Leonard JM, Markowitz M: Rapid turn-over of plasma virions an CD4 lymphocytes in HIV-1 infection. Nature 1995;373:123–126.
4 Gartner S, Markovits P, Markovitz DM, Kaplan MH, Gallo RC, Popovic M: The role of mononuclear phagocytes in HTLV-III/LAV infection. Science 1986;233:215–219.
5 Gendelman HE, Orenstein JM, Martin MA, Ferrua C, Mitra R, Phipps T, Wahl LA, Lane HC, Fauci AS, Burke DS, Skilllman D, Meltzer MS: Efficient isolation and propagation of human immunodeficiency virus on recombinant colony-stimulating factor 1-treated monocytes. J Exp Med 1988;167:1428–1441.
6 Poli G, Fauci AS: The role of monocyte/macrophages and cytokines in the pathogenesis of HIV infection. Pathobiology 1992;60:246–251.
7 Clouse KA, Robbins PB, Fernie B, Ostrove JM, Fauci AS: Viral antigen stimulation of the production of human monokines capable of regulating HIV-1 expression. J Immunol 1989;143:470–475.
8 Merrill JE, Koyanagi Y, Chen ISY: Interleukin-1 and tumor necrosis factor χ can be induced from mononuclear phagocytes by human immunodeficiency virus type 1 binding to the CD4 receptor. J Virol 1989;63:4404–4408.
9 Massari FE, Poli G, Schnittman SM, Psallidopoulos MC, Davey V, Fauci AS: In vivo T lymphocyte origin of macrophage-tropic strains of HIV: Role of monocytes during in vitro isolation and in vivo infection. J Immunol 1990;144:4628–4632
10 Smith PD, Ohura K, Masur H, Lane HC, Fauci AS, Wahl SM: Monocyte function in the acquired immune deficiency syndrome. Defective chemotaxis. J Clin Invest 1984;74:2121–2128.
11 Ras GJ, Eftychis HA, Anderson R, van der Walt I: Mononuclear and polymorphonuclear leucocyte dyfunction in male homosexuals with the acquired immunodeficiency syndrome (AIDS). South Afr Med J 1984;66:806–809.

12 Poli G, Bottazzi B, Acero R, Bersani L, Rossi V, Introna M, Lazzarin A, Galli M, Mantovani A: Monocyte function in intravenous drug abusers with lymphadenopathy and in patients with acquired immunodeficiency syndrome: Selective impairment of chemotaxis. Clin Exp Immunol 1985;62: 136–142.

13 Lazzarin A, Uberti Foppa C, Galli M, Mantovani A, Poli G, Franzetti F, Novati R: Impairment of polymorphonuclear leukocyte function in patients with acquired immunodeficiency syndrome and with lymphadenopathy syndrome. Clin Exp Immunol 1986;65:105–11[illegible].

14 Vicenzi E, Biswas P, Mengozzi M, Poli G: Role of pro-inflammatory cytokines and β-chemokines in controlling HIV replication. J Leukoc Biol 1997;62:34–40.

15 Siebenlist U, Franzoso G, Brown K: Structure, regulation and function of NF-κB. Annu Rev Cell Biol 1994;10:405–455.

16 Finzi D, Hermankova M, Pierson T, Carruth LM, Buck C, Chaisson RE, Quinn TC, Chadwick K, Margolick J, Brookmeyer R, Gallant J, Markowitz M, Ho DD, Richman DD, Siliciano RF: Identification of a reservoir for HIV-1 in patients on highly active antiretroviral therapy. Science 1997;278:1295–1300.

17 Wong JK, Hezareh M, Gunthard HF, Havlir DV, Ignacio CC, Spina CA, Richman DD Recovery of replication-competent HIV despite prolonged suppression of plasma viremia. Science 1997;278: 1291–1295.

18 Chun TW, Stuyver L, Mizell SB, Ehler LA, Mican JA, Baseler M, Lloyd AL, Norwak MA, Fauci AS: Presence of an inducible HIV-1 latent reservior during highly active antiretroviral therapy. Proc Natl Acad Sci USA 1997;94;13193–13197.

19 Gallo RC, Sarin PS, Gelmann EP, Robert-Guroff M, Richardson E, Kalyanaraman VS, Mann D, Sidhu GD, Stahl RE, Zolla-Pazner S, Leibowitch J, Popovic M: Isolation of human T-cell leukemia virus in acquired immune deficiency syndrome (AIDS). Science 1983;220:865–867.

20 Barre-Sinoussi F, Chermann, JC, Rey F, Nugeyre MT, Chamaret S, Gruest J, Dauguet C, Axler-Blin C, Vezinet-Brun F, Rouzioux C, Rozenbaum W, Montagnier L: Isolation of a T-lymphotropic retrovirus from a patient at risk for acquired deficiency syndrome (AIDS). Science 1983;220:868–871.

21 Markham PD, Salahuddin SZ, Veren K, Orndorff SH, Gallo RC: Hydrocortisone and some other hormones enhance the expression of HTLV-III. Int J Cancer 1986;37:67–72.

22 Poli G, Kinter A, Folks TM, Fauci AS: Interferon alpha but not AZT suppresses HIV expression in chronically infected cell lines. Science 1989;244:575–577.

23 Poli G, Biswas P, Fauci AS: Interferons in the pathogenesis and treatment of human immunodeficiency virus infection. Antiviral Res 1994;24:221–233.

24 Poli G, Kinter AL, Justement JC, Bressler P, Kehrl JH, Fauci AS: Transforming growth factor-β suppresses human immunodeficiency virus expression and replication in infected cells of the monocyte/macrophage lineage. J Exp Med 1991;173:589–597.

25 Walker CM, Moody DJ, Stites DP, Levy JA: CD8+ lymphocytes can control HIV infection in vitro by suppressing virus replication. Science 1986;234:1563–1566.

26 Levy JA, Mackewicz CE, Barker E: Controlling HIV pathogenesis: The role of the noncytotoxic anti-HIV response of CD8+ T cells. Immunol Today 1996;17:217–224.

27 Cocchi F, DeVico AL, Garzino Demo A, Arya SK, Gallo R, Lusso P: Identification of RANTES, MIP-1α and MIP-1β as the major HIV-suppressive factor produced by CD8+ T cells. Science 1995;270:1811–1815.

28 Hwang SS, Boyle TJ, Lyerly HK, Cullen BR: Identification of the envelope V3 loop as the primary determinant of cell tropism in HIV-1. Science 1991;253:7[illegible]–73.

29 Feng Y, Broder CC, Kennedy PE, Berger EA: HIV-1 entry cofactor; Cloning of a seven-transmembrane G protein-coupled receptor. Science 1996;272:872–877.

30 Dragic T, Litwin V, Allaway GP, Martin SR, Huang Y, Nagashima KA, Cayanan C, Maddon PJ, Koup RA, Moore JP, Paxton WA: HIV-1 entry into CD4+ cells is mediated by the chemokine receptor CC-CKR-5. Nature 1996;381:667–673.

31 Alkhatib G, Combadiere C, Broder CC, Feng Y, Kennedy PE, Murphy PM, Berger EA: CC CKR5: A RANTES, MIP-1α, MIP-1β receptor as a fusion cofactor for macrophage-tropic HIV-1. Science 1996;272:1955–1958.

32 Samson M, Labbe O, Mollereau C, Vassart G, Parmentier M: Molecular cloning and functional expression of a new human CC-chemokine receptor gene. Biochemistry 1996;35:3362–3367.

33 Bleul C, Farzan M, Choe H, Parolin C, Clark-Lewis I, Sodroski J, Springer TA: The lymphocyte chemoattractant SDF-1 is a ligand for LESTR/fusin and blocks HIV-1 entry. Nature 1996;382: 829–833.

34 Nagasawa T, Hirota S, Tachibana K, Takakura N, Nishikawa S, Kitamura Y, Yoshida N, Kikutani H, Kishimoto T: Defects of B-cell lymphopoiesis and bone-marrow myelopoiesis in mice lacking the CXC chemokine PBSF/SDF-1. Nature 1996;382:635–638.

35 Oberlin E, Amara A, Bachelerie F, Bessia C, Virelizier JL, Arenzana-Seisdedos F, Schwartz O, Heard JM, Clark-Lewis I, Legler DF, Loetscher M, Baggiolini M, Moser B: The CXC chemokine SDF-1 is the ligand for LESTR/fusin and prevents infection by T-cell-line adapted HIV-1. Nature 1996;382:833–835.

36 Koot M, Vos AV, Keet RPM, De Goede REY, Dercksen W, Terpstra FG, Coutinho RA, Miedema F, Tersmette M: HIV-1 biological phenotype in long-term infected individuals, evaluated with an MT-2 cocultivation assay. AIDS 1992;6:49–54.

37 Dimitrov DS: How do viruses enter cells? The HIV coreceptors teach us a lesson of complexity. Cell 1997;91:721–730.

38 Cocchi F, DeVico AL, Garzino-Demo A, Cara A, Gallo RC, Lusso P: V3 domain of HIV-1 envelope glycoprotein gp120 is critical for chemokine-mediated blockade of infection. Nat Med 1996; 2:1–5.

39 Arenzana-Seisdedos F, Virelizier JL, Rousset D, Clark-Lewis I, Loetscher L, Moser B, Baggiolini M: HIV blocked by chemokine antagonist. Nature 1996;383:400.

40 Simmons G, Clapham PR, Picard L, Offord RE, Rosenkilde MM, Schwartz TW, Buser R, Wells TNC, Proudfoot AE: Potent inhibition of HIV-1 infectivity in macrophages and lymphocytes by a novel CCR5 antagonist. Science 1997;276:276–279.

41 Rucker J, Samson M, Doranz BJ, Libert F, Berson JF, Yi Y, Smyth RJ, Collman RG, Broder CC, Vassart G, Doms RW, Parmentier M: Regions in beta-chemokine receptors CCR5 and CCR2b that determine HIV-1 cofactor specificity. Cell 1996;87:437–446.

42 Dragic T, Trkola A, Lin SW, Nagashima KA, Kajumo F, Zhao L, Olson WC, Wu L, Mackay CR, Allaway GP, Sakmar TP, Moore JP, Maddon JP: Amino-terminal substitutions in the CCR5 coreceptor impair gp 120 binding and human immunodeficiency virus type 1 entry. J Virol 1998; 72:279–285.

43 Choe H, Farzan M, Sun Y, Sullivan N, Rollins B, Ponath PD, Wu L, Mackay CR, LaRosa G, Newman W, Gerard N, Gerard C, Sodroski J: The β-chemokine receptors CCR3 and CCR5 facilitate infection by primary HIV isolates. Cell 1996;85:1135–1148.

44 Deng HR, Liu R, Eilmeler W, Choe S, Unutmaz D, Burkhart M, Di Marzio P, Marmon S, Sutton RE, Hill CM, Davis CB, Pelper SC, Schall TJ, Littman DR, Landau NR: Identification of a major co-receptor for primary isolates of HIV-1. Nature 1996;381:661–666.

45 Doranz BJ, Rucker J, Yi Y, Smyth RJ, Samson M, Peiper SC, Parmentier M, Collman RC, Dooms RW: A dual-tropic primary HIV-1 isolate that uses fusin and the β-chemokine receptors CKR-5, CKR-3, and CKR-2b as fusion cofactors. Cell 1996;85:149–1158.

46 Jinno A, Shimizu N, Soda Y, Haraguchi Y, Kitamura T, Hoshino H: Identification of the chemokine receptor TER1/CCR8 expressed in brain-derived cells and T cells as a new coreceptor for HIV-1 infection. Biochem Biophys Res Commun 1998;243:497–502.

47 Tscherning C, Alaeus A, Fredriksson R, Bjorndal A, Deng H, Littman DR, Fenyo EM, Albert J: Differences in chemokine coreceptor usage between genetic subtypes of HIV-1. Virology 1998;241: 181–185.

48 Schools D, Proost P, Van Damme J, De Clercq E: RANTES and MCP-3 inhibit the replication of T-cell-tropic human immunodeficiency virus type 1 strains (SF-2, MN, and HE). J Virol 1997;71: 7300–7304.

49 Berger EA, Doms RW, Fenyo EM, Korber BT, Littman DR, Moore JP, Sattentau QJ, Schuitemaker H, Sodroski J, Weiss RA: A new classification for HIV-1. Nature 1998;391:240.

50 Connor RI, Sheridan KE, Ceradini D, Choe S, Landau NR: Change in coreceptor use correlates with disease progression in HIV-1 infected individuals. J Exp Med 1997;185:621–628.

51 Scarlatti G, Tresoldi E, Bjorndal A, Fredriksson R, Colognesi C, Deng HK, Malnati MS, Plebani A, Siccard AG, Littman DR, Fenyo EM, Lusso P: In vivo evolution of HIV-1 co-receptor usage and sensitivity to chemokine-mediated suppression. Nature Med 1997;3:1259–1265.
52 Zaitseva M, Blauvelt A, Lee S, Lapham CK, Klaus-Kovtun V, Mostowski H, Manischewitz J, Golding H: Expression and function of CCR5 and CXCR4 on human Langerhans' cells and macrophages: Implications for HIV primary infection. Nat Med 1997;3:1369–1375.
53 Gong W, Howard OM, Turpin JA, Grimm MC, Ueda H, Gray PW, Raport CJ, Oppenheim JJ, Wang JM: Monocyte chemotactic protein-2 activates CCR5 and blocks CD4/CCR5-mediated HIV entry/replication. J Biol Chem 1998;273:4289–4292.
54 Frade JMR, Llorente M, Mellado M, Alcami J, Gutierrez-Ramos JC, Zaballos A, Del Real G, Martinez AC: The amino-terminal domain of the CCR2 chemokine receptor acts as a coreceptor for HIV-1 infection. J Clin Invest 1997;100;497–502.
55 Horuk R, Hesselgesser J, Zhou Y, Faulds D, Halks-Miller M, Harvey S, Taub D, Samson M, Parmentier M, Rucker J, Doranz BJ, Doms RW: The CC chemokine I-309 inhibits CCR8-dependent infection by diverse HIV-1 strains. J Biol Chem 1998;273:386–391.
56 He J, Chen Y, Farzan M, Choe H, Ohagen A, Busciglio J, Yang X, Hofmann W, Newman W, Mackay CR, Sodroski J, Gabuzda D: CCR3 and CCR5 are co-receptors for HIV infection of microglia. Nature 1997;385:645–649.
57 Conant K, Garzino-Demo A, Nath A, McArthur JC, Halliday W, Power C, Gallo RC, Major EO: Induction of monocyte chemoattractant protein-1 in HIV-1 tat-stimulated astrocytes and elevation in aids dementia. Proc Natl Acad Sci USA 1988;95:3117–3121.
58 Cinque P, Vago L, Mengozzi M, Torri V, Cerasa D, Vincenzi E, Transidico P, Vagani A, Sozzani S, Mantovani A, Lazzarin A, Poli G: Elevated cerebrospinal fluid levels of monocyte chemotactic protein-1 are a correlate of human immunodeficiency virsus type 1 encephalitis and local viral replication. AIDS 1998;12:1327–1332.
59 Canque B, Rosenzwajg M, Gey A, Tartour E, Fridman WH, Gluckman JC: Macrophage inflammatory protein-1-alpha is induced by human immunodeficiency virus infection of monocyte-derived macrophages. Blood 1996;87:2011–2019.
60 Schmidtmayerova H, Nottet HS, Nuovo G, Raabe T, Flanagan CR, Dubrovsky L, Gendelman HE, Cerami A, Bukrinsky M, Sherry B: Human immunodeficiency virus type 1 infection alters chemokine beta peptide expression in human monocytes: Implications for recruitment of leukocytes into brain and lymph nodes. Proc Natl Acad Sci USA 1996;93:700–704.
61 Bernasconi S, Cinque P, Peri G, Sozzani S, Crociati A, Torri V, Vicenzi E, Vago L, Lazzarin A, Poli G, Mantovani A: Selective elevation of monocyte chemotactic protein-1 (MCP)-1 in the cerebrospinal fluid of AIDS patients with cytomegalovirus encephalitis. J Infect Dis 1996;174:1098–1101.
62 Pleskoff O, Treboute C, Brelot A, Heveker N, Seman M, Alizon M: Identification of a chemokine receptor encoded by human cytomegalovirus as a cofactor for HIV-1 entry. Science 1997;276:1874–1878.
63 Godiska R, Chantry D, Raport CJ, Sozzani S, Allavena P, Leviten D, Mantovani A, Gray PW: Human macrophage-derived chemokine (MDC), a novel chemoattractant for monocytes, monocyte-derived dendritic cells, and natural killer cells. J Exp Med 1997;185:1595–1604.
64 Imai T, Chantry D, Raport CJ, Wood CL, Nishimura M, Godiska R, Yoshie O, Gray PW: Macrophage-derived chemokine is a functional ligand for the CC chemokine receptor 4. J Biol Chem 1998;273:1764–1768.
65 Pal R, Garzino-Demo A, Markham PD, Burns J, Brown M, Gallo RC, DeVico AL: Inhibition of HIV-1 infection by the β-chemokine MDC. Science 1997;278:695–698.
66 Struyf S, Proost P, Sozzani S, Mantovani A, Wuyts A, De Clerq E, Schols D, Van Damme J: Cutting edge: Enhanced anti-HIV activity and altered chemotactic potency of NH_2-terminally processed macrophage-derived chemokine imply an additional MDC receptor. J Immunol 1998; 161:2672–2675.
67 Lee B, Rucker L, Doms RW, Tsang M, Hu X, Dietz M, Bailer R, Montaner LJ, Gerard C, Sullivan N, Sodroski J, Stantchev TS, Border CC: β-Chemokine MDC and HIV-1 infection (abstract). Science 1998;281:487.
68 Arenzana-Seisdedos F, Amara A, Thomas D, Virelizier J: β-Chemokine MDC and HIV-1 infection. Science 1998;281:487.

69 Weissman D, Rabin RL, Arthos J, Rubbert A, Dybul M, Swofford R, Venkatesan S, Farber JM, Fauci AS: Macrophage-tropic HIV and SIV envelope proteins induce a signal through the CCR5 chemokine receptor. Nature 1997;389:981–985.
70 Davis CB, Dikic I, Unutmaz D, Hill CM, Arthos J, Siani MA, Thompson DA, Schlessinger J, Littman DR: Signal transduction due to HIV-1 envelope interactions with chemokine receptors CXCR4 or CCR5. J Exp Med 1997;186:1793–1798.
71 Mack M, Luckow B, Nelson PJ, Cihak J, Simmons G, Clapham PR, Signoret N, Marsh M, Stangassinger M, Borlat F, Wells TN, Schlondorff D, Proudfoot AE: Aminooxypentane-RANTES induces CCR5 internalization but inhibits recycling: A novel inhibitory mechanism of HIV infectivity. J Exp Med 1998;187:1215–1224.
72 Amara A, Gall SL, Schwartz O, Salamero J, Montes M, Loetscher P, Baggiolini M, Virelizier JL, Arenzana-Seisdedos F: HIV coreceptor downregulation as antiviral principle: SDF-1-alpha-dependent internalization of the chemokine receptor CXCR4 contributes to inhibition of HIV replication. J Exp Med 1997;186:139–146.
73 Kinter AL, Catanzaro A, Monaco JA, Ruiz M, Justement J, Moir S, Arthos J, Oliva A, Ehler L, Mizell S, Jackson R, Ostrowski M, Hoxie J, Offord R, Fauci AS: C-C chemokines enhance the replication of T-tropic strains of HIV-1 in CD4+ T cells: Role of signal transduction. Proc Natl Acad Sci USA 1998;95:11880–11885.
74 Schmidtmayerova H, Sherry B, Bukrinsky M: Chemokines and HIV replication. Nature 1996;382:767.
75 Kelly MD, Naif NM, Adams SL, Cunningham AL, Lloyd AR: Cutting edge: Dichotomous effects of β-chemokines on HIV replication in monocytes and monocyte-derived macrophages. J Immunol 1998;160:3091–3095.
76 Dolei A, Biolchini A, Serra C, Curreli S, Gomes E, Dianzani F: Increased replication of T-cell-tropic HIV strains and CXC-chemokine receptor-4 induction in T cells treated with macrophage inflammatory protein (MIP)-1-alpha, MIP–1-beta and RANTES beta-chemokines. AIDS 1998;12:183–190.
77 Dean M, Carrington M, Winkler C, Huttley GA, Smith MW, Allikmets R, Goedert JJ, Buchbinder SP, Vittinghoff E, Gomperts E, Donfield S, Vlahov D, Kaslow R, Saah A, Rinaldo C, Detels R, O'Brien SJ: Genetic restriction of HIV-1 infection and progression to AIDS by a deletion allele of the CKR5 structural gene. Hemophilia Growth and Development Study, Multicenter AIDS Cohort Study, Multicenter Hemophilia Cohort Study, San Francisco City Cohort, ALIVE Study. Science 1996;273:1856–1862.
78 Huang Y, Paxton WA, Wolinsky SM, Neumann AU, Zhang L, He T, Kang S, Ceradini D, Jin Z, Yazdanbakhsh K, Kunstman K, Erickson D, Dragon E, Landau NR, Phair J, Ho DD, Koup RA: The role of a mutant CCR5 allele in HIV-1 transmission and disease progression. Nat Med 1996; 2:1240–1243.
79 Morawetz R, Rizzardi GP, Glauser D, Rutschmann O, Hirschel B, Perrin L, Opravil M, Flepp M, von Overbeck J, Glauser MP, Ghezzi S, Vicenzi E, Poli G, Lazzarin A, Pantaleo G for the Swiss HIV Cohort: The heterozygous (CCR5/Δccr5) genotype is neither essential nor sufficient for protection against disease progression.. Eur J Immunol 1997;27:3233–3227.
80 Benkirane M, Jin DY, Chun RF, Koup RA, Jeang KT: Mechanism of transdominant inhibition of CCR5-mediated HIV-1 infection by ccr5delta32. J Biol Chem 1997;272:30603–30606.
81 Biti R, French R, Young J, Bennetts B, Stewart G, Liang T: HIV-1 infection in an individual homozygous for the CCR5 deletion allele. Nat Med 1997;3:252–253.
82 Smith MW, Dean M, Carrington M, Winkler C, Huttley GA, Lomb DA, Goedert JJ, O'Brien TR, Jacobson LP, Kaslow R, Buchbinder S, Vittinghoff E, Vlahov D, Hoots K, Hilgartner MW, O'Brien SJ: Contrasting genetic influence of CCR2 and CCR5 variants on HIV-1 infection and disease progression. Hemophilia Growth and Development Study (HGDS), Multicenter AIDS Cohort Study (MACS), Multicenter Hemophilia Cohort Study (MHCS), San Francisco City Cohort (SFCC), ALIVE Study. Science 1997;277:959–965.
83 Kostrikis LG, Huang Y, Moore JP, Wolinsky SM, Zhang L, Guo Y, Deutsch L, Phair J, Neumann AU, Ho DD: A chemokine receptor CCR2 allele delays HIV-1 disease progression and is associated with CCR5 promotor mutation. Nat Med 1998;4:350–353.
84 Rizzardi GP, Morawetz RA, Vicenzi E, Ghezzi S, Poli G, Lazzarin A, Pantaleo G for the Swiss HIV Cohort: CCR2 polymorphism in HIV disease. Nat Med 1998;4:252–253.

85 Michael NL, Louie LG, Rohrbaugh AL, Schultz KA, Dayhoff DE, Wang CE, Sheppard HW: The role of CCR5 and CCR2 polymorphisms in HIV-1 transmission and disease progression. Nat Med 1997;3:1160–1162.

86 Winkler C, Modi W, Smith MW, Nelson GW, Wu X, Carrington M, Dean M, Honjo T, Tashiro K, Yabe D, Buchbinder S, Vittinghoff E, Goedert JJ, O'Brien TR, Jacobson LP, Detels R, Donfield S, Willoughby A, Gomperts E, Vlahov D, Phair J, O'Brien SJ: Genetic restriction of AIDS pathogenesis by an SDF-1 chemokine gene variant. ALIVE study, Hemophilia Growth and Development Study (HGDS), San Francisco City Cohort (SFCC). Science 1998;279:389–393.

87 Endres MJ, Clapham PR, Marsh M, Ahuja M, Turner JD, McKnight A, Thomas JF, Stoebenau-Haggarty B, Choe S, Vance PJ, Wells TN, Power CA, Sutterwala SS, Doms RW, Landau NR, Hoxie JA: CD4-independent infection by HIV-2 is mediated by fusin/CXCR4. Cell 1996;87:745–756.

88 Littman DR: Chemokine receptors – Keys to AIDS pathogenesis. Cell 1998 93:677–680.

89 Oravecz T, Pall M, Wang J, Roderiquez G, Ditto M, Norcross MA: Regulation of anti-HIV-1 activity of RANTES by heparan sulfate proteoglycans. J Immunol 1997;59:4587–4592.

90 Quillent C, Oberlin E, Braun J, Rousset D, Gonzalez-Canali G, Metais P Montagnier L, Virelizier JL, Arenzana-Seisdedos F, Beretta A: HIV-1-resistance phenotype conferred by combination of two separate inherited mutations of CCR5 gene. Lancet 1998;351:14–18.

91 Carrington M, Kissner T, Gerrard B, Ivanov S, O'Brien SJ, Dean M: Novel alleles of the chemokine-receptor gene CCR5. Am J Hum. Genet 1997;61:1261–1267

92 Schols D, Struyf S, Van Damme J, Este JA, Henson G, De Clercq E: Inhibition of T-tropic HIV strains by selective antagonization of the chemokine receptor CXCR4. J Exp Med 1997;186: 1383–1388.

93 Donzella GA, Schols D, Lin SW, Este JA, Nagashima KA, Maddon PJ, Allaway GP, Sakmar TP, Henson G, De Clercq E, Moore JP: AMD3100, a small molecule inhibitor of HIV-1 entry via the CXCR4 co-receptor. Nat Med 1998;4:72–77.

94 Doranz BJ, Grovit-Ferbas K, Sharrron MP, Mao SH, Goetz MB, Daar ES, Doms RW, O'Brien WA: A small-molecule inhibitor directed against the chemokine receptor CXCR4 prevents its use as an HIV-1 coreceptor. J Exp Med 1997;186:1395–1400.

95 Murakami T, Nakajima T, Koyanagi Y, Tachibana K, Fujii N, Tamamura H, Yoshida N, Waki M, Matsumoto A, Yoshie O, Kishimoto T, Yamamoto N, Nagasawa T: A small molecule CXCR4 inhibitor that blocks T cell line-tropic HIV-1 infection. J Exp Med 1997;186:1389–1393.

96 Oravecz T, Pall M, Roderiquez G, Gorrell MD, Ditto M, Nguyen NY, Boykins R, Unsworth E, Norcross MA: Regulation of the receptor specificity and function of the chemokine RANTES (regulated on activation, normal T-cell expressed and secreted) by dipeptidyl peptidase IV (CD26)-mediated cleavage. J Exp Med 1997;186:1865–1872.

97 Proost P, De Meester I, Schols D, Struyf S, Lambeir AM, Wuyts A, Opdenakker G, De Clercq E, Scharpe S, Van Damme J: Amino-teminal truncation of chemokines by CD26/dipeptidyl-peptidase IV. Conversion of RANTES into a potent inhibitor of monocyte chemotaxis and HIV-1 infection. J Biol Chem 1998;273:7222–7227.

98 Bieniasz PD, Fridell RA, Aramori I, Ferguson SS, Caron MG, Cullen BR: HIV-1-induced cell fusion is mediated by multiple regions within both the viral envelope and the CCR-5 co-receptor. EMBO J 1997;16:2599–2609.

99 Chen JD, Bai X, Yang AG, Cong Y, Chen SY: Inactivation of HIV-1 chemokine co-receptor CXCR-4 by a novel intrakine strategy. Nat Med 1997;3:1110–1116.

100 Yang AG, Bai X, Huang XF, Yao C, Chen S: Phenotypic knockout of HIV type 1 chemokine coreceptor CCR-5 by intrakines as potential therapeutic approach for HIV-1 infection. Proc Natl Acad Sci USA 1997;94:11567–11572.

101 Paxton WA, Martin SR, Tse D, O'Brien J, Skurnick J, Van Devanter NL, Padain N, Braun JF, Kotler SM, Wolinsky SM, Koup RA: Relative resistance to HIV-1 infection of CD4 lymphocytes from persons who remain uninfected despite multiple high-risk sexual exposures. Nat Med 1996; 2:412–417.

102 Zagury D, Lachgar A, Chams V, Fall LS, Bernard J, Zagury JF, Bizzini B, Gringeri A, Santagostino E, Rappaport J, Feldman M, O'Brien SJ, Burny A, Gallo RC; C-C chemokines, pivotal in protection against HIV type 1 infection. Proc Natl Acad Sci USA 1998;95:3857–3861.

103 Furci L, Scarlatti G, Burastero S, Tambussi G, Colognesi C, Quillent C, Longhi R, Loverro P, Borgonovo B, Gaffi D, Carrow E, Malnati M, Lusso P, Siccardi AG, Lazzarin A, Beretta A: Antigen-driven C-C chemokine-mediated HIV-1 suppression by CD4(+) T cells from exposed uninfected individuals expressing the wild-type CCR-5 allele. J Exp Med 1997;186:455–460.
104 Verani A, Scarlatti G, Comar M, Tresoldi E, Polo S, Giacca M, Lusso P, Siccardi AG, Vercelli D: C-C chemokines released by lipopolysaccharide-stimulated human macrophages suppress HIV-1 infection in both macrophages and T cells. J Exp Med 1997;185:805–816.
105 Kornbluth RS, Kee K, Richman DD: CD40 ligand (CD154) stimulation of macrophages to produce HIV-1-suppressive β-chemokines. Proc Natl Acad Sci USA 1998;95:5205–5210.
106 Lehner T, Wang Y, Cranage M, Bergmeier LA, Mitchell E, Tao L, Hall G, Dennis M, Cook N, Brookes R, Klavinskis L, Jones I, Doyle C, Ward R: Protective mucosal immunity elicited by targeted iliac lymph node immunization with a subunit SIV envelope and core vaccine in macaque. Nat Med 1996;2:767–775.
107 Sozzani S, Ghezzi S, Iannolo G, Luini W, Borsatti A, Polentarutti N, Sica A, Locati M, Mackay C, Wells TNC, Biswas P, Vicenzi E, Poli G, Mantovani A: IL-10 increases CCR5 expression and HIV infection in human monocytes. J Exp Med 1998;187:439–444.
108 Jourdan P, Abbal C, Nora N, Hori T, Uchiyama T, Vendrell JP, Bousquet J, Taylor N, Pène J, Yssel H: Cutting edge: IL-4 induces functional cell-surface expression of CXCR4 on human T cells. J Immunol 1998;160:4153–4157.
109 Valentin A, Lu W, Rosati M, Schneider R, Albert J, Karlsson A, Pavlakis GN: Dual effect of interleukin-4 on HIV-1 expression: Implications for viral phenotypic switch and disease progression. Proc Natl Acad Sci USA 1998;95:8886–8891.
110 Biswas P, Mengozzi M, Mantelli B, Delfanti F, Brambilla A, Vicenzi E, Poli G: 1,25-Dihydroxyvitamin D_3 upregulates functional CXCR4 human immunodeficiency virus type-1 coreceptors in U937 minus clones. NF-κB independent enhancement of viral replication. J Virol 1998;72:8380–8383.
111 Emery S, Lane HC: Immune reconstitution in HIV infection. Curr Opin Immunol 1997;9:568–572.
112 Deng HK, Unutmaz D, Kewal-Ramani VN, Littman DR: Expression cloning of new receptors used by simian and human immunodeficiency viruses. Nature 1997;388:296–300.
113 Mengozzi M, De Filippi C, Transidico P, Biswas P, Cota M, Ghezzi S, Vicenzi E, Mantovani A, Sozzani S, Poli G: Human immunodeficiency virus replication induces monocyte chemotactic protein-1 in human macrophages and U937 promonocytic cells. Blood 1999;93:1851–1857.
114 Galli G, Annunziato F, Mavilia C, Romagnani P, Cosmi L, Manetti R, Pupilli C, Maggi E, Romagnani S: Enhanced HIV expression during Th2-oriented responses explained by the opposite regulatory effect of IL-4 and IFN-gamma of fusin/CXCR4. Eur J Immunol 1998;28:3280–3290.

Guido Poli, P2-P3 Laboratories, DiBiT, Via Olgettina n. 58, I–20132 Milano (Italy)
Tel. +39 02 2643 4909, Fax +39 02 2643 4905, E-Mail poli.guido@hsr.it

Mantovani A (ed): Chemokines.
Chem Immunol. Basel, Karger, 1999, vol 72, pp 141–160

Inhibition of the Expression and Function of Chemokine Receptors on Human CD4+ Leukocytes by HIV-1 Envelope Protein gp120

Shao Bo Su[a], *Hirotsugu Ueda*[a], *O.M. Zack Howard*[c], *Michael C. Grimm*[a], *Wanghua Gong*[c], *Francis W. Ruscetti*[b], *Joost J. Oppenheim*[a], *Ji Ming Wang*[a]

[a] The Laboratory of Molecular Immunoregulation and
[b] The Laboratory of Leukocyte Biology, Division of Basic Sciences and
[c] Intramural Research Support Program, SAIC, Frederick, National Cancer Institute, Frederick Cancer Research and Development Center, Frederick, Md., USA

HIV-1 infection is initiated by high-affinity binding of the virus envelope glycoprotein, gp120, to CD4 which was identified as the primary receptor for HIV-1 infection over a decade ago [1, 2]. Members of the 7TM chemokine receptor superfamily have been identified as coreceptors for HIV-1 infection [3–12]. HIV-1 cell-type tropism is dictated by chemokine receptor usage, since T-cell-tropic viruses use CXCR4, while monocyte tropic viruses primarily use CCR5 as fusion coreceptors. A minority of HIV-1 strains may also use other C-C chemokine receptors such as CCR2b and CCR3 as their fusion cofactors [3, 11, 12]. Dual tropic HIV-1 strains interact with either type of chemokine receptor or a newly described cofactor STRL33 [13] for cell entry. Purified gp120 from monocyte tropic virus has been shown to competitively inhibit MIP-1β binding to CCR5 transfected cells or T cells in the presence of CD4 [14, 15]. In contrast, gp120 from T-cell-line adapted viruses downregulates

CXCR4 on T cells [16], in agreement with HIV-1 tropism studies. In addition, purified gp120 from laboratory-adapted HIV-1 was previously shown to induce Ca^{2+} mobilization and chemotaxis of CD4 T lymphocytes [17] and recently it was reported that envelope protein of the monocyte tropic strain also mobilized Ca^{2+} and chemoattracted CD4 T lymphocytes through CCR5 [18]. Consequently, there is considerable evidence that gp120 from various strains of HIV-1 utilizes chemokine receptors to activate T cells.

Although CD4+ T lymphocyte depletion is a central feature of the immunosuppression in AIDS patients, monocyte-macrophages are also targets of HIV-1 infection. Earlier studies demonstrated that monocytes from AIDS patients exhibited a significantly compromised capacity to migrate in response to several chemotactic factors including activated complement component C5a, the bacterial peptide fMLP and undefined lymphocyte-derived chemotactic factors [19]. Incubation of monocytes with soluble gp120 has been reported to suppress the expression of receptors for C5a and fMLP [20]. Since chemokines are important mediators of host defense, we postulated that shed gp120, which can be present in copious quantities in AIDS patients [21], may also inhibit the monocyte response to chemokines thus contributing to the anti-inflammatory and immunosuppressive effects of HIV-1. Our study shows that preincubation with gp120 from various strains of HIV-1 can suppress monocyte responses to a variety of chemokines as well as to fMLP in association with CD4 signal-dependent downregulation of chemokine receptors. In addition, gp120 downregulates the expression and function of CXCR4 on CD4+ T lymphocytes, and this downregulation requires the activation of tyrosine kinase activation by gp120.

gp120 Inhibits Monocyte Activation by Chemokines

Since the chemotactic response of monocytes from AIDS patients have been reported to be defective [19] and soluble gp120 suppresses the expression of receptors for C5a and the bacterial chemotactic peptide fMLP on normal monocytes [20], we initially investigated the effect of gp120 on the capacity of monocytes to respond to chemokines as well as to fMLP. We confirmed a previous report [22] that both native [23] and recombinant gp120 were also weakly chemotactic for human monocytes. However, gp120 was not chemotac-

Abbreviations: CCR, C-C chemokine receptor; CXCR, CXC chemokine receptor; HIV-1, human immunodeficiency virus type 1; MCP, monocyte chemotactic protein; MIP, macrophage inflammatory protein; SDF-1, stromal cell-derived factor; 7TM, seven transmembrane; HA herbimycin A.

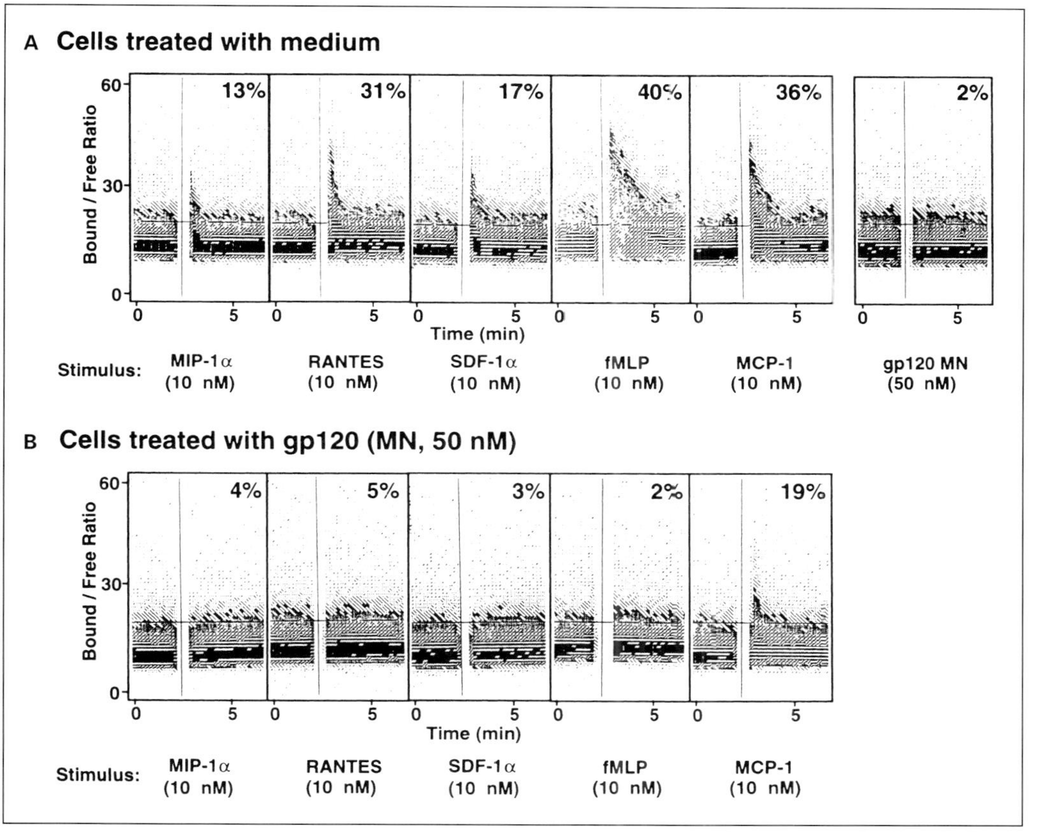

Fig. 1. Intracellular Ca^{2+} mobilization in monocytes induced by chemokines and fMLP. Monocytes loaded with Indo-1 were preincubated in the absence (*A*) or in the presence (*B*) of gp120 (MN, 50 n*M*) for 1 h at 37 °C. The Ca^{2+} mobilization stimulated by gp120, chemokines and fMLP was monitored by FACS analysis. The % values given in the figure denote the estimated percentage of responding cells in this experiment.

tic for HEK293 cells transfected with CCR5 or CXCR4 which did show significant migration in response to the chemokines SDF-1α and MIP-1β, suggesting that gp120 can only induce CD4 expressing cells to migrate. The recombinant gp120 of the MN strain did not induce significant Ca^{2+} mobilization in monocytes (fig. 1A). This gp120 also did not desensitize subsequent (within 100 s) monocyte response to chemokines or fMLP, suggesting that the gp120 used in the assay did not activate the receptors for fMLP or for the chemokines tested. However, preincubation of monocytes with increasing con-

Table 1. Effect of soluble CD4 (sCD4) on the inhibition by rgp120 (MN) of monocyte chemotaxis in response to C-C chemokines, SDF-1 and fMLP[a]

Chemoattractants	CI and (% inhibition of migration by preincubation with)		
	medium	rgp120	rgp120 + sCD4
MIP-1α	3.51	1.0 (100)[b]	3.23 (11)
MIP-1β	2.42	0.96 (100)[b]	2.50 (0)
RANTES	3.13	1.0 (100)[b]	2.70 (20)
MCP-1	4.60	3.0 (45)[b]	3.92 (19)
MCP-2	3.62	2.57 (40)[b]	3.62 (0)
fMLP	11.02	4.51 (65)[b]	11.20 (0)
SDF-1α	6.43	1.54 (90)[b]	6.51 (0)

[a] Recombinant gp120 at 25 n*M* was preincubated in the presence or absence of sCD4 for 30 min at 37 °C, then was further incubated with monocytes for 60 min at 37 °C. After washing, the cell migration in response to C-C chemokines (10 n*M*) SDF-1α (100 n*M*) or fMLP (10 n*M*) was determined. The results represent a summary of five experiments performed.

[b] $p < 0.05$ (Student's t test) compared to the migration of monocytes preincubated with medium alone.

centration of gp120 for 1 h at 37 °C significantly reduced monocyte response to a number of chemokines and the bacterial chemotactic peptide fMLP. Figure 1 shows that at 50 n*M* concentration, gp120 of the MN strain almost completely abolished the Ca^{2+} mobilization induced by MIP-1α, RANTES, SDF-1α (12 n*M*) as well as fMLP (10 n*M*) (fig. 1B). The Ca^{2+} mobilization induced by MCP-1 (12 n*M*) was also significantly reduced by preincubation of monocytes with gp120 (fig. 1B).

The effect of gp120 on the capacity of monocytes to migrate in response to chemoattractants was then examined. As observed for Ca^{2+} mobilization assays, gp120 preincubation of monocytes with gp120, also in a dose-dependent manner, inhibited the cell migration in response to a number of chemoattractants, including C-C chemokines as well as CXC chemokine SDF-1α, the ligand for CXCR4/Fusin (table 1). The inhibition of monocyte migration by gp120 could also be demonstrated for fMLP (table 1), which utilizes a 7TM receptor structurally related to chemokine receptors. Since gp120 had previously been considered to be a ligand for CD4, the contribution of CD4 to these 'desensitizing' effects of gp120 was evaluated. gp120 failed to inhibit directional migration of chemokine receptor transfected HEK293 cells lacking CD4 in response to their respective chemokines. In addition, as shown in table 1, preincubation of gp120 with soluble CD4 completely abolished the inhibitory effect of gp120 on monocyte migration induced by chemokines and fMLP, suggesting a critical role of cell membrane CD4 molecules in mediating this suppressive activity of gp120. The inhibitory effect of gp120 on monocyte migration was totally eliminated by preincubation with a monoclonal anti-gp120 antibody (data not shown). gp120 did not affect the chemotactic response of neutrophils to fMLP or IL-8 (data not shown), further supporting a requirement for cell surface CD4 for the gp120 effect.

gp120 Inhibits Monocyte Expression of Chemokine Binding Sites

To test whether gp120 might compete with chemokines for binding sites on monocytes, soluble recombinant or purified natural gp120 (MN) [23] and radiolabeled chemokines were added simultaneously to human peripheral blood monocytes [24]. While all unlabeled chemokines (60–120 n*M*) showed the expected competition for binding by radiolabeled ligands (fig. 2, horizontal lines), gp120 showed little or no direct competition with radiolabeled chemokines for binding sites on monocytes or neutrophils (fig. 2, hatched columns).

We then examined the possibility that more prolonged incubation with gp120 might downregulate monocyte expression of chemokine receptors. Preincubation of monocytes with soluble gp120 at 37 °C for 60 min resulted in a marked dose-dependent inhibition of the capacity of monocytes to bind C-C chemokines (fig. 2A–E, shaded columns). The IC_{50} for gp120 inhibition of monocyte binding of chemokines (0.1, 1.0 and 5.0 n*M* for MIP-1α, MIP-1β and RANTES, respectively) was similar to the IC_{50} obtained by the direct competitive effect of the native ligands (0.3, 0.6 and 1.0 n*M* for MIP-1α, MIP-1β and RANTES, respectively). Consequently, preincubation of monocytes with gp120 not only inhibited their capacity to bind MIP-1β, which utilizes exclusively CCR5 [25, 26], but also inhibited their binding of MIP-1α and RANTES which in addition use CCR1 [27, 28] and other C-C chemokine receptors [3, 25]. Furthermore, the capacity of monocytes to bind ^{125}I-MCP-1 and ^{125}I-MCP-2 was inhibited up to 50% by preincubation of the cells with gp120 (fig. 2D, E), even though these chemokines have been reported to predominantly use CCR2b [3, 25] and/or CCR1 [29], respectively. Preincubation with gp120 also significantly inhibited the monocyte expression of the binding sites for SDF-1α, the only known ligand for the T-tropic HIV-1 fusion cofactor CXCR4. The suppressive effect on monocyte expression of chemokine binding sites was not limited to purified gp120 of the MN strain. Preincubation with other native and recombinant gp120 from T-cell-line adapted virus such as IIIB, as well as a recombinant gp120 from a monocyte tropic strain, CM, all

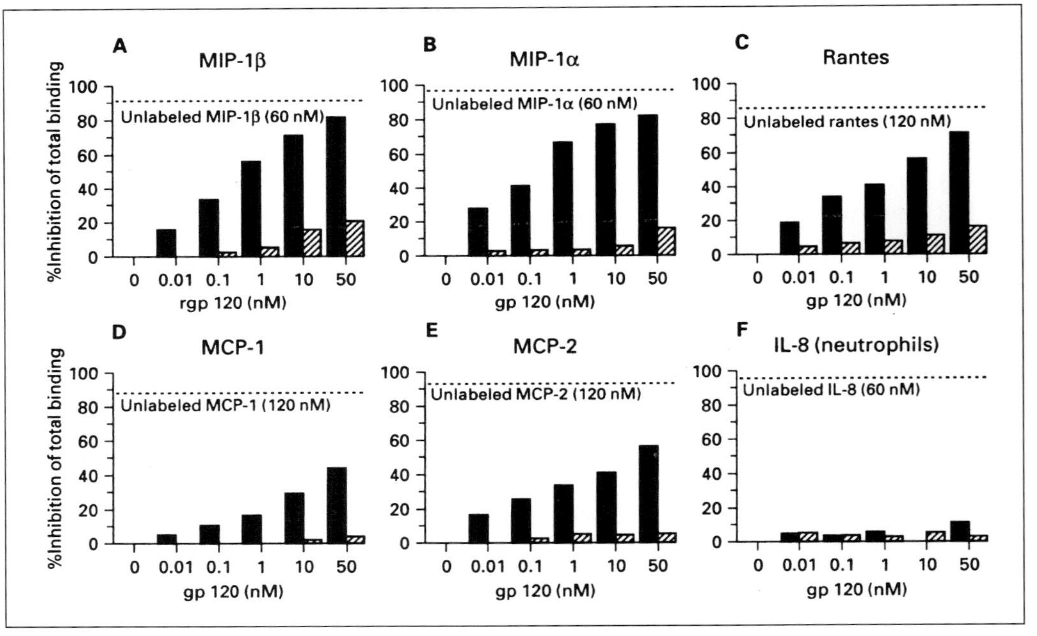

Fig. 2. gp120 inhibits the capacity of monocytes to bind chemokines. Monocytes were preincubated in duplicate with medium alone or different concentrations of purified gp120 (MN) for 60 min at 37 °C. ^{125}I-labeled chemokines were added and the cultures were continued for 40 min at room temperature. The cells were then centrifuged through a sucrose cushion and measured for radioactivity. Direct competition experiments were performed in parallel by adding different concentrations of gp120 simultaneously with ^{125}-I-labeled chemokines to duplicate monocyte samples (shown as hatched columns). Unlabeled chemokines were used as control competitors (60 n*M* for MIP-1α and MIP-1β, 120 n*M* for RANTES, MCP-1, MCP-2 and IL-8). The cells were incubated at room temperature for 40 min and harvested. Shaded columns represent the percent reduction of monocyte binding for chemokines. Hatched columns indicate the levels of direct competition with chemokines for binding by gp120. Horizontal lines depict the maximal level of direct competition of chemokine binding by unlabeled native ligands (60–120 n*M*). *A–E* Reduction of ^{125}I-labeled C-C chemokine binding to monocytes pretreated with gp120 (shaded columns) and competition by gp120 of chemokine binding to monocytes (hatched columns). *F* Effect of gp120 on neutrophil binding for ^{125}I-IL-8.

significantly interfered with the capacity of monocytes to bind chemokines. In contrast, gp120 did not inhibit the neutrophil binding of the CXC chemokine, IL-8, a potent chemotactic factor for neutrophils rather than monocytes (fig. 2F). These results showed that the reduction in chemokine binding to monocytes preincubated with soluble gp120 is more generalized than the

Table 2. Effect of preincubation with recombinant gp120 on the expression of chemokine binding sites by monocytes[a]

^{125}I-chemokine	Cells preincubated with					
	medium		gp120 (MN, 10 n*M*)		gp120 (MN) & sCD4[b]	
	Kd (n*M*)	sites/cell	Kd (n*M*)	sites/cell (% reduction)	Kd (n*M*)	sites/cell
MIP-1α	0.20	1,500	0.30	600 (60)[c]	0.31	1,200
MIP-1β	0.62	4,500	1.33	1,300 (71)[c]	0.84	3,900
RANTES	0.35	4,650	1.22	1,100 (76)[c]	0.55	4,050
MCP-1	2.10	6,700	3.22	4,500 (32)[c]	2.50	5,900
MCP-2	1.80	8,100	2.46	5,300 (34)[c]	2.00	7,500
SDF-1α	2.50	4,680	5.32	1,240 (74)[c]	2.43	4,440

[a] Monocytes were preincubated with medium alone or gp120 (MN, 10 n*M*) w/wo sCD4 for 60 min at 37 °C, and their capacity to bind C-C chemokines assessed. The binding data were analyzed using the Macintosh program LIGAND, and the results shown are representative of three experiments performed.

[b] rgp120 was preincubated with molar concentrations of sCD4 at a ratio of 1:25 for 30 min and the mixture was then added to the monocyte cultures.

[c] $p<0.05$ (Student's t test) compared to cells incubated with medium alone.

reported capacity of chemokines to competitively inhibit HIV-1 entry and envelope-mediated cell fusion [30, 31].

Downregulation of Chemokine Binding Sites on Monocytes by gp120 Requires CD4

We examined whether the downregulation by gp120 of chemokine binding sites on monocytes also required the presence of CD4 as manifested in chemotaxis experiments. Preincubation of HEK293 cells expressing functional CCR5, CCR1 or CXCR4 with gp120 from MN, IIIB or CM strains did not reduce their ability to bind chemokines (data not shown), indicating these chemokine receptors did not directly interact with the gp120 tested. On the other hand, the inhibitory effect of gp120 on monocyte binding of C-C chemokines was blocked by pretreatment of gp120 with soluble CD4 (table 2), in correlation with the observation in cell migration (table 1). This suggests that soluble CD4 sequesters gp120 and prevents its binding to cell membrane anchored CD4 and the consequent downregulation of chemokine receptors. In order to examine whether the suppressive effect on monocyte expression of chemokine

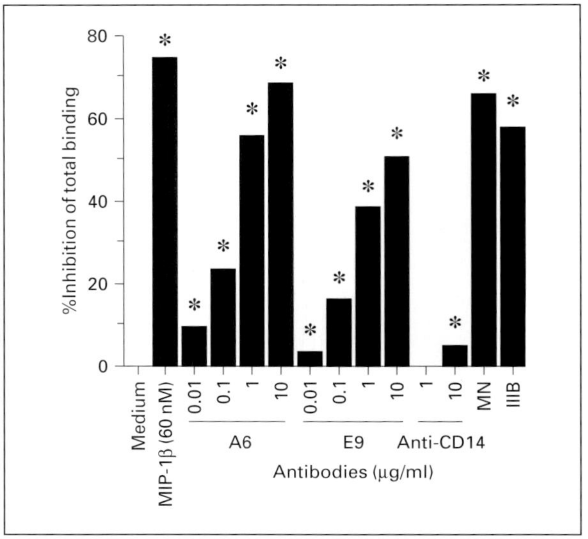

Fig. 3. Monoclonal anti-CD4 antibodies inhibit monocyte binding for MIP-1β. Monocytes were preincubated with recombinant gp120 (MN and IIIB) or different concentrations of monoclonal anti-CD4 antibodies for 60 min at 37 °C. ^{125}I-MIP-1β was added to the cells at room temperature for 40 min. The cells were then pelleted through sucrose cushion and the cell-associated radioactivity was determined. Antibodies from both clones A6 and E9 stained CD4+ cells, but only clone E9 blocked HIV binding by HIV-1 (as per Biogenics, Poole, UK). Unlabeled MIP-1β was used to define the level of maximal direct competition by native ligand. * $p < 0.05$ in comparison to MIP-1β binding to cells incubated with medium.

binding sites was exclusive for gp120 or whether other activators of CD4 have similar effect, we utilized monoclonal anti-CD4 antibodies. Preincubation with monoclonal anti-CD4 antibodies reproduced the effect of gp120 in inhibiting monocyte binding of MIP-1β, whereas monoclonal anti-CD14 antibody had no effect (fig. 3). The anti-CD4 antibodies also reduced the capacity of monocytes to bind other chemokines such as SDF1, MCP-1 and MCP-2.

These observations led us to use confocal microscopy to visualize the effect of gp120 as well as anti-CD antibody on chemokine receptor localization. Confocal microscopy indicated that preincubation with gp120 or anti-CD4 monoclonal antibody caused marked time-dependent internalization of CXCR4/Fusin (fig. 4) in HEK293 cells transfected to express both CD4 and CXCR4/Fusin, but not in cells expressing CXCR4/Fusin alone. The apparent requirement for initial interaction of gp120 with CD4 is in agreement with the recent report that preincubation of CD4+/Fusin (CXCR4)$^{+}$ T cells with gp120 resulted in the formation of a gp120/CD4/Fusin complex which could

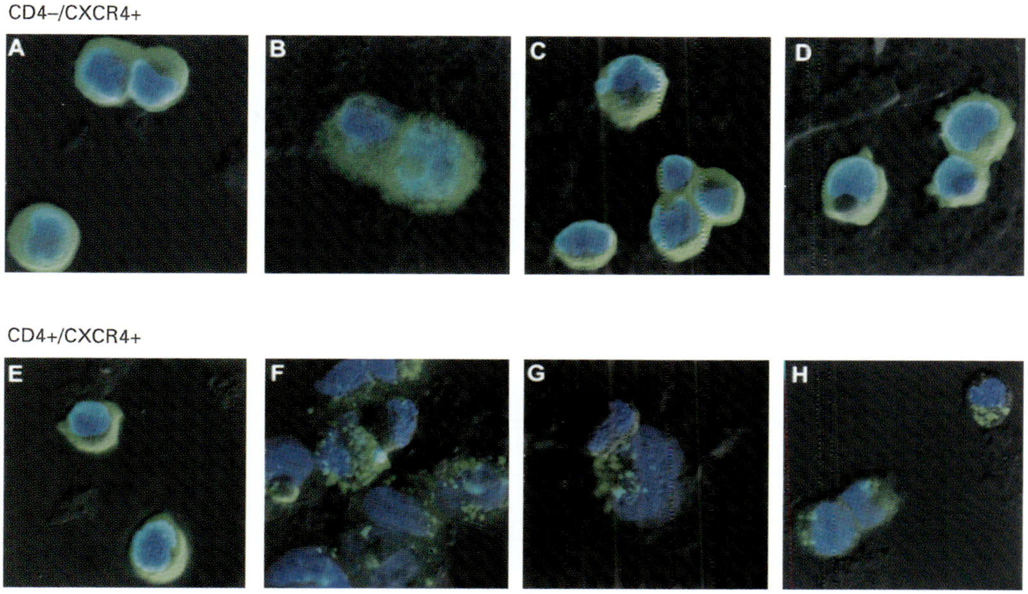

Fig. 4. Internalization of CXCR4/Fusin by pretreatment of CD4+/CXCR4+ HEK293 cells with gp120 and anti-CD4 antibody. FITC staining shows CXCR4/Fusin localized to the cell surface in medium-treated (control) cells (*A, E*), but internalized into the perinuclear cytoplasma in response to the native ligand of CXCR4, SDF-1α (1 µg/ml), in both CD4– (*B*) and CD4+ (*F*) cells. gp120 (IIIB, 25 n*M*) and anti-CD4 (5 µg/ml) resulted in internalization of CXCR4/Fusin in cells coexpressing CD4 (*G, H*), but not in CD4– cells (*C, D*).

be coprecipitated with antibodies against any one of these three molecules [32]. Our results also indicate that ligation of CD4 with anti-CD4 is sufficient to internalize chemokine receptors with the resultant inhibition of the ability of CD4+ cells to bind chemokines. Although in figure 4, only the results obtained with gp120 IIIB and CXCR4/CD4/293 cells after 3 h treatment are presented, the internalization was already significant at 1 h incubation and similar internalizing effects were obtained with gp120 of the MN and CM strains. In addition, CCR5 was also markedly internalized by gp120 in 293 cells provided they were also transfected to express CD4.

Signaling Is Involved in the Inhibition of Chemokine Receptors on Monocytes by gp120

The interaction of HIV-1 with CD4 and the coreceptors and the resultant HIV-1 cell fusion was reported to be resistant to pertussis toxin suggesting

Table 3. Staurosporine reverses the inhibitory effect of gp120 on monocyte expression of MIP-1β binding sites[a]

Cell treatment						
medium			rgp120 (MN, 25 n*M*)		staurosporine followed by gp120[b]	
n	sites/cell	Kd (n*M*)	sites/cell	Kd (n*M*)	sites/cell	Kd (n*M*)
1	1,520	0.2	750[c]	0.3	1,560	0.4
2	1,460	0.3	780[c]	0.4	1,370	0.5
3	1,500	0.2	690[c]	0.5	1,450	0.3
4	2,000	0.4	990[c]	0.4	1,950	0.5
5	3,500	0.5	1,350[c]	0.6	3,180	0.7
6	2,430	0.5	1,100[c]	0.6	2,240	0.5

[a] Monocytes were incubated with medium alone or recombinant gp120 (MN, 25 n*M*) for 60 min at 37 °C. After washing, duplicate aliquots of the cells were incubated with 0.12 n*M* radioiodinated MIP-1β in the presence of increasing concentrations of unlabeled ligand. The samples were cultured at room temperature for 40 min then were harvested and measured for radioactivity. The data was analyzed with LIGAND program. Results obtained with cells from 6 donors are shown.

[b] Cells were first preincubated with staurosporine (1 ng/ml) for 15 min at 37 °C followed by treatment with gp120.

[c] Significant reduction of MIP-1β binding sites on monocytes treated with gp120 ($p<0.05$, Student's t test).

that the virus competes for chemokine receptor occupancy, resulting in fusion without requiring G-protein signaling in target cells [31, 33]. However, interaction of gp120 with CD4 and coreceptors has been reported to induce G-protein activation [18] and tyrosine kinase signaling events in T cells or transfected cells [34]. In our study, the need to preincubate monocytes at 37 °C for 1 h with gp120 to downregulate chemokine binding sites suggested that binding of CD4 by gp120 may transduce signals. It has been observed previously that gp120 triggers intracellular signals, such as translocation of PKC and the production of metabolites of arachidonic acid in monocytes [35, 36]. It has also been reported that PMA, a PKC activator, downregulated an HIV-1 fusion cofactor, later identified as CXCR4/Fusin [32] and inhibited T-cell viral entry [37]. We therefore investigated whether the suppressive effect of gp120 on chemoattractant receptors requires CD4-dependent protein kinase activation. We confirmed that gp120 as well as anti-CD4 antibody enhanced the PKC activation in monocytes and pretreatment of monocytes with the protein kinase inhibitor, staurosporine, prevented the downregulation of MIP-1β binding sites on monocytes by gp120 (table 3). The ability of monocytes to bind

Table 4. Preincubation with gp120 of CCR5 HEK293 cells expressing intact CD4 downregulates the cell binding for ^{125}I-MIP-1β[a]

Cell type	cpm (% inhibition of binding)			
	preincubation of cells with			
	medium (binding in the absence of cold MIP-1β)	medium[b] (binding in the presence of cold MIP-1β)	gp120 (MN, 25 n*M*)	anti-CD4 (A6)
CCR5/293	4,435	1,101 (75)[c]	4,306 (3)	4,634 (0)
Control vaccinia vector	5,927	1,372 (74)[c]	5,671 (4)	5,452 (8)
VCB2 (tailless CD4)	4,203	1,449 (56)[c]	3,882 (8)	3,981 (5)
VCB7 (intact CD4)	4,217	1,027 (76)[c]	1,796 (57)[c]	1,991 (53)[c]

[a] CCR5/293 cells were infected with control vaccinia virus, or recombinant vaccinia virus encoding tailless CD4 (VCB2) or intact CD4 (VCB7) at 37 °C for 1 h, at multiplicity of infection of 5 in DMEM containing 2% FCS and antibiotics. The cells were washed and cultured for 10 h at 37 °C in DMEM containing 400 μg/ml, 10% FCS and antibiotics. The cells were then gently detached with trypsin/EDTA, resuspended in binding medium, aliquoted, and incubated for 10 h in the presence or absence of gp120 or anti-CD4 mAb. Binding assays utilizing ^{125}I-MIP-1β were performed at room temperature for 40 min. Both VCB2 and VCB7 infected CCR5/293 cells were more than 90% CD4+ as assessed by FACS analysis (not shown).

[b] Cells were preincubated with medium and bindings were performed in the presence of 120 n*M* unlabeled MIP-1β.

[c] Significant inhibition of ^{125}I-MIP-1β binding compared to cells preincubated with medium alone ($p < 0.05$). Preincubation of gp120 with soluble CD4 reversed the inhibitory effect of gp120 on cell binding for MIP-1β.

other CC chemokines and SDF-1α could also be protected by pretreatment with staurosporine before the addition of gp120. A more specific PKC inhibitor, Calphostin C, could mimic the protective effect of staurosporine. These observations suggest that binding of gp120 to CD4 on monocytes activates intracellular protein kinase activity which in turn downregulates chemoattractant receptor expression and function. This was further investigated by comparing the response to gp120 of HEK293 cells transfected with tailless or intact CD4. The ability of HEK293 cells to bind MIP-1β could not be inhibited by preincubation of the cells with gp120 or anti-CD4 antibody if the cells expressed CCR5 and a CD4 lacking its cytoplasmic tail, whereas the binding capacity of the CCR5/293 cells transfected with intact CD4 was inhibited by gp120 or anti-CD4 antibody (table 4), again suggesting that CD4 is an active rather than passive participant in the downregulation of chemoattractant receptor expression by gp120.

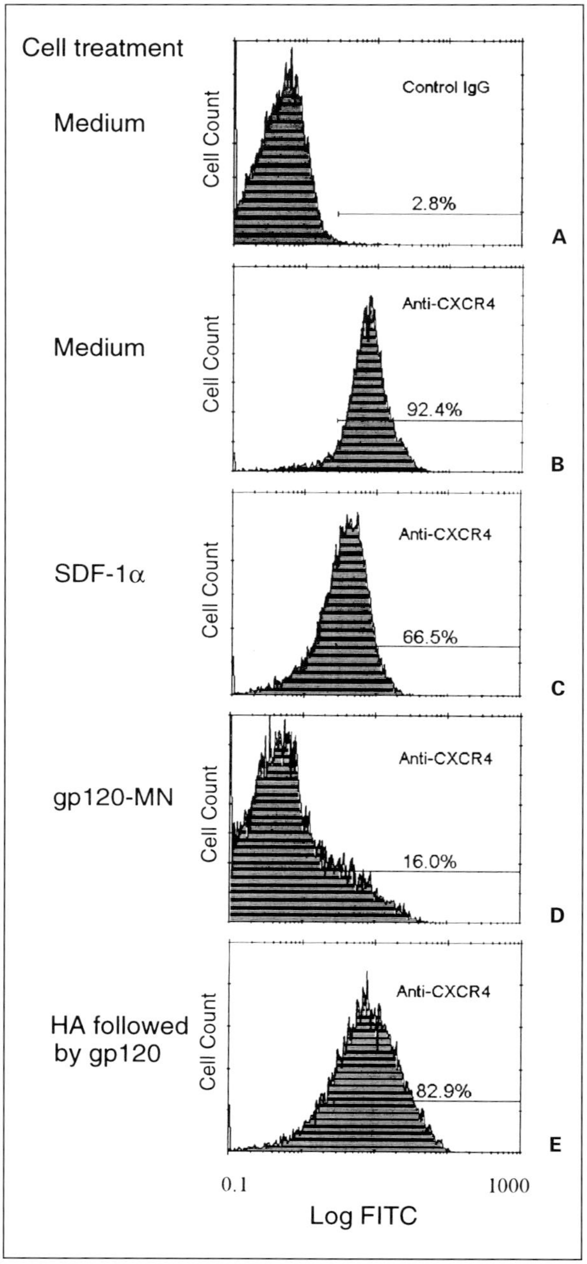

Fig. 5. FACS analysis of CXCR4 expression on CD4+ lymphocytes pretreated with gp120 MN. Peripheral blood CD4+ lymphocytes were treated with HA (2 μ*M*) or medium

CXCR4 Downregulation by gp120 on CD4+ T Lymphocytes Requires the Activation of Protein Tyrosine Kinase(s)

We further observed that gp120 downregulated the expression and function of CXCR4 in CD4+ but not CD8+ lymphocytes. Since as in monocytes, gp120 did not directly compete with CXCR4 ligand SDF-1α for binding, we postulated that a metabolic process might be required for gp120 to downregulate CXCR4. We examined this possibility by using FACS with a monoclonal anti-CXCR4 antibody (clone 12G5). Normal CD4+ T cells express a substantial level of CXCR4 on cell surface (fig. 5A, B), which as expected is substantially downregulated by incubation of the cells with SDF-1α (fig. 5C). Preincubation of T cells with gp120 at 37 °C for 1 h also markedly reduced CXCR4 expression on the cell surface (fig. 5D) and the T cells pretreated with tyrosine kinase inhibitor HA, but not PKC inhibitors, became very resistant to the downregulating effect of gp120 (fig. 5E). These observations indicate that unlike in monocytes in which the inhibitory effect of gp120 on chemokine receptors requires the participation of PKC, downregulation of CXCR4 in CD4+ T lymphocytes by gp120 is mediated primarily by tyrosine kinase activation. Indeed, the src-like tyrosine kinase $p58^{lck}$ is rapidly phosphorylated by gp120 (fig. 6), and treatment of the cells with HA abolished the phosphorylation induced by gp120, in agreement with the effects seen on the expression of cell surface CXCR4. Furthermore, anti-CD4 antibody is also able to induce tyrosine phosphorylation of $p58^{lck}$ in association with the downregulation of CXCR4 from the cell surface. Therefore the activation of CD4 plays an essential role in the modulation of CXCR4 expression in CD4+ T cells.

CD4-Dependent Cell Activation Plays an Important Role in the Modulation of Immune System

Much attention has been focused on how the gp120 envelop protein may interact with chemokine receptors and considerable information has been generated concerning the interaction of HIV-1 with CD4 and chemokine coreceptors on T cells and transfected cells. It has been suggested that after

alone at 37 °C for 18 h then were incubated with medium alone (*A, B*), SDF-1α (1 μg/ml, *C*), gp120 MN (50 n*M*, *D, E*) at 37 °C for 60 min. After washing, cells were stained with control mouse IgG (*A*) or monoclonal antibody to CXCR4 (12G5, *B–E*), followed by FITC-conjugated goat anti-mouse IgG antibody. The percentage of cells positively stained with anti-CXCR4 antibody is shown in each panel. Data shown are from one experiment out of three performed.

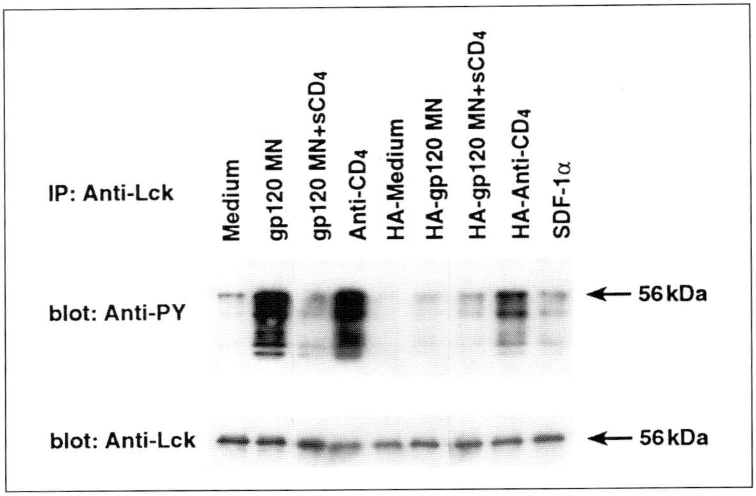

Fig. 6. Tyrosine phosphorylation of lck induced by gp120 MN. CD4+ CEM-SS cells were cultured with medium alone or HA (2 μ*M*) at 37 °C for 18 h, then were stimulated with gp120 MN (50 n*M*), gp120 NM + sCD4 (100 n*M*), anti-CD4 (E9 clone, 10 μg/ml) or SDF-1α (1 μg/ml) at 37 °C for 5 min. The cells were pelleted and lysed in lysing buffer. The tyrosine phosphorylation was examned by immunoprecipitation with anti-p56[lck] followed by immunoblotting with anti-phosphotyrosine antibodies. Representative results obtained in three experiments is shown.

binding of gp120 to CD4, a conformational change endows an epitope of gp120 (presumably the V3 loop) with the capacity to bind chemokine receptor cofactors [3, 31]. This was supported by the observation that in the presence of cell membrane CD4, gp120 competes with MIP-1β for binding to CCR5 [14, 15]. It has also been proposed that a complex of CXCR4 and CD4 may preexist and stimulation with gp120 may further promote the complex formation [32]. Studies on T cells and transfectants have shown that interaction of HIV-1 envelope proteins with CD4 and coreceptor CCR5 or CXCR4 activated these receptors causing G-protein-mediated signaling and tyrosine kinase activation [18, 34]. Although the chemotactic activity of soluble gp120 for CD4 T lymphocytes and monocytes were documented a number of years ago [17, 23], only recently Weissman et al. [18] reported that mammalian cell-derived recombinant monotropic gp160, a precursor of the gp120, was able to induce Ca^{2+} flux and migration of CD4 T lymphocytes by using CCR5. Since the signaling of gp160 in CD4+ T cells could be homologously desensitized by MIP-1β, it was concluded that this gp160 was able to directly activate CCR5. Whether this gp160 was also capable of inducing CD4+ monocyte migration or migration of CCR5 transfectants in the presence or absence of CD4 was not reported. In our study, the recombinant gp120 preparations were only weakly chemotactic for monocytes but they did not induce significant Ca^{2+} flux. There was no homologous desensitization by gp120 of Ca^{2+} mobilization in monocytes induced by a number of chemokines. Furthermore, our gp120 did not induce migration or Ca^{2+} flux in HEK293 cells transfected with CXCR4 and CCR5 alone or in combination with CD4. Therefore, in our assay systems the gp120 did not show direct activation of CCR5 or CXCR4, but rather, activation of CD4 was a prerequisite for downregulation of chemoattractant receptors.

In contrast with T cells, the nature of the interaction of gp120 with CD4 and cofactors on monocytes has not been as well characterized. CD4 on monocytes/macrophages is known to act as an HIV-1 fusion cofactor for monocyte tropic strains. In this study, we demonstrated for the first time that HIV-1 gp120 markedly inhibited monocyte responses to a variety of chemokines in association with downregulation of the receptor expression on the cell surface via a CD4-dependent pathway. This inhibition was apparently not due to a direct competition with chemokines for binding sites by gp120, but required CD4-mediated signaling events operationally resembling 'heterologous desensitization'. This was demonstrated by the facts that (1) the effect of gp120 required a period of preincubation and was observed only on CD4+ monocytes and HEK293 cells transfected to express intact CD4; (2) monoclonal anti-CD4, but not anti-CD14, antibodies emulated the inhibitory effect of gp120 on both monocytes and CD4+/HEK293 cells; (3) the effect was observed on HEK293 cells expressing only intact CD4 that retains the cytoplasmic domain but not a tailless CD4; (4) monocytes pretreated with protein kinase inhibitors such as staurosporine (fig. 5) and Calphostin C (data not shown), but not pertussis toxin, were protected from the inhibitory effect of gp120. In addition, preincubation of monocytes with gp120 at 37 °C for 1 h markedly inhibited Ca^{2+} mobilization and chemotactic migration in response to chemokines as well as fMLP. Confocal microscopy clearly demonstrated internalization of CXCR4/Fusin by gp120 in the presence of CD4. gp120 from various strains as well as anti-CD4 antibody all suppressed the expression and function of chemoattractant receptors on monocytes. The downregulation of CXCR4 and CCR5 on monocytes by gp120 of the MN or CM strain was confirmed by FACS analyses using commercially available antibodies. After 1 h incubation with 50 n*M* gp120, the CXCR4 or CCR5 staining on monocytes was reduced by more than 50% (data not shown). These observations strongly suggest that inhibition of chemoattractant receptor expression and function by gp120 is dependent on cross-talk between CD4 and 7TM receptor. This cross-talk of CD4 and CXCR4 or CCR5 could also initiate a cascade of signaling events that leads to the desensitization of the receptors for other chemoattractants and IL-2 [18, 34]. Further studies are in progress to elucidate whether chemoattractant receptors are phosphorylated by CD4-mediated kinase activation.

CD4 has been shown to play many roles that either serve to increase or suppress immune responses. CD4 was originally identified as a phenotypic marker and subsequently as a high-affinity receptor for HIV-1 envelope protein gp120 [38]. CD4 facilitates T-cell function by binding to the nonpolymorphic region of the MHC class II antigens expressed on the surface of antigen-presenting cells. However, an inhibitory role for CD4 in the activation of T lymphocytes has been suggested by reports that anti-CD4 antibodies abrogate a variety of T-lymphocyte effector functions in vitro, including IL-2 receptor γ chain expression and IL-2-induced lymphocyte proliferation, and graft rejection [38]. CD4 participates in signal transduction by its cytoplasmic domain through association with the src-like protein tyrosine kinase lck in T lymphocytes [39] and such signals may lead to downregulation of TCR as well as cytokine (IL-2) receptors. Our data suggest that signals emanating from CD4 culminate in downregulation of chemoattractant receptors in monocytes. We have also observed that downregulation of chemokine receptor CXCR4 by gp120 occurred in resting CD4+ T lymphocytes, which involves activate participation of CD4. In CD4+ but not CD8+ T cells, gp120 induced rapid tyrosine phosphorylation of the src-like kinase $p56^{lck}$, associated with downregulation of CXCR4 expression and function. Pretreatment of the CD4 T cells with tyrosine kinase inhibitor HA, but not staurosporine, completely restored the ability of CD4 T cells to express functional CXCR4. These observations suggest that although diverse signaling events are triggered by gp120 through CD4 in T cells and monocytes, each of them results in the downregulation of chemokine receptors.

We have observed that natural and recombinant gp120 from T-cell-tropic strains MN, IIIB and RF, as well as recombinant monocyte tropic CM, all exhibited similar effects on monocytes which differs from the restricted tropism exhibited during the viral fusion process. This could be due to the fact that the CD4 binding region is conserved in gp120 from primary isolates [39] and T-cell-line adapted viruses, thus enabling gp120 from different HIV-1 strains to bind and activate monocyte CD4, with consequent downregulation of chemoattractant receptor expression. Further efforts are needed to identify critical epitopes responsible for CD4 binding, and possibly signaling, on both mono- and T-tropic viral envelope proteins.

gp120 Is Accessible to Host Immune Cells in AIDS Patients

The availability of gp120 in AIDS patients has been documented in a number of reports. In the course of the HIV-1 infection, some of the gp120 detected in the sera of patients may in fact be complexed by anti-gp120. However, it is unlikely that the effects of gp120 are completely blocked by the antibodies because there are considerable variations in the specificity, amount and timing of anti-gp120 antibody production [40–42]. In most patients, serum anti-gp120 antibodies appear relatively late and were first detected only after p24 antigen and infectious-virus titer in the peripheral blood had already declined manyfold from their highest values [40]. Many of the anti-gp120 antibodies do not actually have the capacity to recognize the CD4 binding structure on gp120. This is manifested by the failure of these antibodies to compete for gp120 binding to CD4 with a neutralizing anti-gp120 human monoclonal antibody which does recognize the conformational CD4 binding structure on gp120 [42]. Such neutralizing antibody appeared later in the patients' sera than other anti-gp120 antibodies which do not block the CD4 binding structure on gp120 [41]. These observations suggest that there could be an ample opportunity for the virus-associated for 'shed' gp120 [21] to interact with CD4 on immune cells. Furthermore, the binding of gp120 to CD4 is of high affinity, which is comparable to or even better than the antibody affinities [43]. In fact, gp120 that is not associated with viral particles can be detected on the surface of explanted CD4+ T cells from patients [44]. These observations strongly argue that gp120 can have biological effects on cells of infected individuals.

Our findings suggest that gp120 can have a number of intriguing effects on the host that require further evaluation. On the one hand, gp120 may recruit and activate CD4+ cells during the course of viral infection. On the other hand, this activation of the cells by gp120 results in the internalization of a number of chemoattractant receptors including HIV-1 fusion coreceptors, which may contribute to the reported viral interference following initial infection [39] but also to the suppression of monocyte-dependent inflammatory reactions. The inhibitory effects of gp120 on chemokine and other chemoattractant receptors can be exploited to develop anti-inflammatory agents that interfere with monocyte recruitment based on the structure and mechanism of gp120 action.

Conclusion

Human peripheral blood monocytes, when preincubated with gp120 either purified from laboratory-adapted strains or as recombinant proteins, exhibited markedly reduced binding, calcium mobilization and chemotactic response to chemokines. gp12-pretreated monocytes also showed a decreased response to fMLP. This broad inhibition of monocyte activation by chemoattractants required interaction of gp120 with CD4, since the effect of gp120 was only observed in CD4+ monocytes and in HEK293 cells only if cotransfected with both chemokine receptors and an intact CD4, but not a CD4 lacking its cytoplasmic domain. Anti-CD4 monoclonal antibodies mimicked the effect of gp120 and both anti-CD4 antibody and gp120 caused internalization of CXCR4 in HEK293 cells provided they also expressed CD4. Staurosporine blocked the inhibitory effect of gp120 on monocytes, suggesting that cellular signaling was required for gp120 to inhibit the response of CD4+ cells to chemoattractants. Our study demonstrates a broad suppressive effect of gp120 on monocyte activation by chemoattractants through the downregulation of cell surface receptors. Furthermore, gp120 markedly inhibited the expression and function of CXCR4 in CD4+ T lymphocytes, a process that requires the active participation of tyrosine kinase signaling cascade. Since monocyte and T-cell response to chemokines is essential in the host defense against inflammatory stimulation, gp120 may be utilized by HIV-1 to disarm the cells leading to immune suppression.

Acknowledgments

The authors thank Dr. Patrick Gray for providing us with some of the chemokine receptor transfected HEK293 cells. The technical support by N. Dunlop, K. Bengali, L. Finch, J. Resau, C. Broder and the clerical assistance by C. Fogle are gratefully acknowledged.

References

1 Klatzmann D, Champagne E, Chamaret S, Gruest J, Guetars D, Hercend T, Gluckman JC, Montaggnier L: T-lymphocyte T4 molecule behaves as the receptor for human retrovirus LAV. Nature 1984;312:767–768.

2 Dalgleish AG, Beverley PC, Clapham PR, Crawford DH, Greaves MF, Weiss RA: The CD4 (T4) antigen is an essential component of the receptor for the AIDS retrovirus. Nature 1984;312:763–767.

3 Premack BA, Schall TJ: Chemokine receptors: Gateways to inflammation and infection. Nat Med 1996;2:1174–1178.

4 Bleul CC, Farzan M, Choe H, Parolin C, Clark-Lewis I, Sodroski J, Springer TA: The lymphocyte chemoattractant SDF-1 is a ligand for LESTR/fusin and blocks HIV-1 entry. Nature 1996;382:829–832.

5 Oberlin E, Amara A, Bachelerie F, Bessia C, Virelizier JL, Arenzana-Seisdedos F, Schwartz O, Heard JM, Clark-Lewis I, Legler DF, Loetscher M, Baggilini M, Moser B: The CXC chemokine SDF-1 is the ligand for LESTR/fusin and prevents infection by T-cell-line-adapted HIV-1. Nature 1996;382:833–835.

6 Feng Y, Broder CC, Kennedy PE, Berger EA: HIV-1 entry cofactor: Functional cDNA cloning of a seven-transmembrane, G protein-coupled receptor. Science 1996;272:872–877.

7 Deng HK, Liu R, Ellmeier W, Choe H, Unutmaz D, Burkhart M, Di Marzio P, Marmon S, Sutton RE, Hill CM, Davis C, Peiper SC, Schall TJ, Littman DR, Landau NR: Identification of major co-receptor for primary isolates of HIV-1. Nature 1996;381:661–666.

8 Dragic T, Litwin V, Allaway GP, Martin SR, Huang Y, Nagashima KA, Paxton WA: HIV-1 entry into CD4+ cells is mediated by the chemokine receptor CC-CKR-5. Nature 1996;381:667–673.

9 Alkhatib G, Combatiere C, Broder CC, Feng Y, Kennedy PE, Murphy PM, Berger EA: CC CKR5: A RANTES, MIP-1α, MLIP-1β receptor as a fusion cofactor for macrophage-tropic HIV-1. Science 1996;272:1955–1958.

10 Liu R, Paxton WA, Choe H, Ceradini D, Martin SR, Horuk R, MacDonald ME, Stuhlmann H, Koup RA, Landau NR: Homozygous defect in HIV-1 coreceptor accounts for resistance of some multiply-exposed individuals to HIV-1 infection. Cell 1996;86:367–377.
11 Choe H, Farzan M, Sun Y, Sullivan N, Rollins B, Ponath PD, Wu L, Mackay CR, LaRosa G, Newman W, Gerard N, Gerard C, Sodroski J: The β-chemokine receptors CCR3 and CCR5 facilitate infection by primary HIV-1 isolates. Cell 1996;85:1135–1148.
12 Doranz BJ, Rucker J, Yi Y, Smyth RJ, Samson M, Peiper SC, Parmentier M, Collman RG, Doms RW: A dual-tropic primary HIV-1 isolate that uses fusin and the β-chemokine receptors CKR-5, CKR-3, and CKR-2b as fusion cofactors. Cell 1996;85:1149–1158.
13 Liao F, Alkhatib G, Peden KW, Sharma G, Berger EA, Farber JM: STRL33, a novel chemokine receptor-like protein, functions as a fusion cofactor for both macrophage-tropic and T cell line-tropic HIV-1. J Exp Med 1997;185:2015–2023.
14 Trkola A, Dragic T, Arthos J, Binley JM, Olson WC, Allaway GP, Cheng-Mayer C, Robinson J, Maddon PJ, Moore JP: CD4-dependent, antibody-sensitive interactions between HIV-1 and its co-receptor CCR-5. Nature 1996;384:184–187.
15 Wu L, Gerard NP, Wyatt R, Choe H, Parolin C, Ruffing N, Borsetti A, Cardoso AA, Desjardin E, Newman W, Gerard C, Sodroski J: CD4-induced interaction of primary HIV-1 gp120 glycoproteins with the chemokine receptor CCR-5. Nature 1996;384:179–183.
16 Ugoni S, Moulard IM, Mondor I, Barois N, Demandolx D, Hoxie J, Brelot A, Alizon M, Davoust J, Sattentau QJ: HIV-1 gp120 induces an association between CD4 and the chemokine receptor CXCR4. J Immunol 1997;159:3000–3008.
17 Kornfeld H, Cruikshank WW, Pyle SW, Berman JS, Center DM: Lymphocyte activation by HIV-1 envelope glycoprotein. Nature 1988;335:445–448.
18 Weissman D, Rabin RL, Arthos J, Rubbert A, Dybul M, Swofford R, Venkatesan S, Farber JM, Fauci A: Macrophage-tropic HIV and SIV envelope proteins induce a signal through the CCR5 chemokine receptor. Nature 1997;389:982–985.
19 Smith PD, Ohura K, Masur H, Lane HC, Fauci AS, Wahl SM: Monocyte function in the acquired immune deficiency syndrome. Defective chemotaxis. J Clin Invest 1984;74:2121–2128.
20 Wahl SM, Allen JB, Gartner S, Orenstein JM, Popovic M, Chenoweth DE, Arthur LO, Farrar WL, Wahl LM: HIV-1 and its envelope glycoprotein down-regulate chemotactic ligand receptors and chemotactic function of peripheral blood monocytes. J Immunol 1989;142:3553–3559.
21 Gelderblom HR, Hausmann EHS, Ozel M, Pauli G, Koch MA: Fine structure of human immunodeficiency virus (HIV) and immunolocalization of structural proteins. Virology 1987;156:171–176.
22 Cruikshank WW, Center DM, Pyle SW, Kornfeld H: Biologic activities of HIV-1 envelope glycoprotein: The effects of crosslinking. Biomed Pharmacother 1990;44:5–11.
23 Pyle SW, Dubois GC, Robey WG, Bess JW Jr, Fischinger PJ, Arthur LO: Purification and characterization of the external envelope glycoprotein from two human immunodeficiency virus type 1 variants, HTLV-IIIB and HTLV-IIIRF. J Virol 1988;62:2258–2264.
24 Xu LL, McVicar DW, Ben-Baruch A, Kuhns DB, Johnston J, Oppenheim JJ, Wang JM: Monocyte chemotactic protein-3 (MCP3) interacts with multiple leukocyte receptors: Binding and signaling of MCP3 through shared as well as unique receptors on monocytes and neutrophils. Eur J Immunol 1995;25:2616–2617.
25 Murphy PM: Chemokine receptors: Structure, function and role in microbial pathogenesis. Cytokine Growth Factor Rev 1996;7:47–64.
26 Combadiere C, Ahuja SK, Tiffany HL, Murphy PM: cloning and functional expression of CC CKR5, a human monocyte CC chemokine receptor selective for MIP-1α, MIP-1β and RANTES. J Leukoc Biol 1996;60:147–152.
27 Neote K, DiGregorio D, Ma JY, Horuk R, Schall TJ: Molecular cloning, functional expression, and signaling characteristics of a C-C chemokine receptor. Cell 1993;72:415–425.
28 Gao JL, Kuhns DB, Tiffany HL, McDermot D, Li X, Francke U, Murphy PM: Structure and functional expression of the human macrophage inflammatory protein 1α/RANTES receptor. J Exp Med 1993;177:1421–1427.
29 Gong X, Gong W, Kuhns DB, Ben-Baruch A, Howard OMZ, Wang JM: Monocyte chemotactic protein-2 (MCP-2) uses CCR1 and CCR2B as its functional receptors. J Biol Chem 1997;272:11682–11685.

30 Cocchi F, DeVico AL, Garzino-Demo A, Arya SK, Gallo RC, Lusso P: Identification of RANTES MIP-1α, MIP-1β as the major HIV-suppressive factors produced by CD8+ T cells. Science 1995 270:1811–1815.

31 Cocchi F, DeVico AL, Garzino-Demo A, Gallo RC, Lusso P: The V3 domain of the HIV-1 gp120 envelope glycoprotein is critical for chemokine-mediated blockade of infection. Nat Med 1996;2 1244–1247.

32 Lapham CK, Ouyang J, Chandrasekhar B, Nguyen NY, Dimitrov DS, Golding H: Evidence for cell-surface association between fusin and the CD4– gp120 complex in human cell lines. Science 1996;274:602–605.

33 Oravecz T, Pall M, Norcross A: β-Chemokine inhibition of monocytrotropic HIV-1 infection. J Immunol 1996;157:1329–1332.

34 Davis CB, Dikic I, Unutmaz D, Hill CM, Arthos J, Siani MA, Thompson DA, Schlessinger J, Littman DR: Signal transduction due to HIV-1 envelope interaction with chemokine receptors CXCR4 or CCR5. J Exp Med 1997;186:1793–1798.

35 Parada NA, Cruikshank WW, Danis HL, Ryan TC, Center DM: IL-16- and other CD4 ligand-induced migration is dependent upon protein kinase C. Cell Immunol 1996;168:100–106.

36 Wahl LM, Corcoran ML, Pyle SW, Arthur LO, Harel-Bellan A, Farrar WL: Human immunodeficiency virus glycoprotein (gp120) induction of monocyte arachidonic acid metabolites and interleukin-1. Proc Natl Acad Sci USA 1989;86:621–625.

37 Golding H, Manischewitz J, Vujcic L, Blumenthal R, Dimitrov DS: The phorbol ester phorbol myristate acetate inhibits human immunodeficiency virus type 1 envelope-mediated fusion by modulating an accessory component(s) in CD4-expressing cells. J Virol 1994;68:1962–1969.

38 Ravichandran KS, Collins TL, Burakoff SJ: CD4 and signal transduction. Curr Top Microbiol Immunol 1996;205:47–62.

39 Volsky DJ, Simm M, Shahabuddin M, Chao W, Potash MJ: Interference to human immunodeficiency virus type 1 infection in the absence of down-modulation of the principal virus receptor, CD4. J Virol 1996;6:3823–3833.

40 Moore JP, Cao Y, Ho DD, Koup RA: Development of the anti-gp120 antibody response during seroconversion to human immunodeficiency virus type 1. J Virol 1994;68:5142–5155.

41 Moore JP, Jarrett RF: Sensitive ELISA for the gp120 and gp160 surface glycoproteins of HIV-1. AIDS Res Hum Retroviruses 1988;4:369–379.

42 Ho DD, McKeating JA, Li XL, Moudgil T, Daar ES, Sun NC, Bobinson JE: Conformational epitope on gp120 important in CD4 binding and human immunodeficiency virus type 1 neutralization identified by a human monoclonal antibody. J Virol 1991;65:489–493.

43 Nara PL, Garrity RR, Goudsmit J: Neutralization of HIV: A paradox of humoral proportions. FASEB J 1991;5:2437–2455.

44 Sunila I, Vaccarezza M, Pantaleo G, Fauci AS, Orenstein JM: gp120 is present on the plasma membrane of apoptotic CD4 cells prepared from lymph nodes of HIV-1-infected individuals: An immunoelectron microscopic study. AIDS 1997;11:27–32.

Ji Ming Wang, LMI, DBS, NCI-FCRDC, Building 560, Room 31-40,
Frederick, MD 21702-1201 (USA)
Tel. +1 301 846 1347, Fax +1 301 846 7042, E-Mail wangji@mail.ncifcrf.gov

Mantovani A (ed): Chemokines.
Chem Immunol. Basel, Karger, 1999, vol 72, pp 161–180

Virally Encoded Chemokines and Chemokine Receptors: Genetic Embezzlement of Host DNA

Johnny T. Stine, David Chantry, Patrick Gray

ICOS Corporation, Bothell, Wash., USA

From a historical perspective, RNA tumor viruses were among the first viruses to give us clues to normal cellular gene function by their acquisition of host DNA. Homologues of cellular genes encoded by retroviruses enable viral propagation by subverting host cell cycle control mechanisms. Studying these genes has led to an understanding of the roles which they play in the pathobiology of the virus; however, more importantly, it has led to the elucidation of the biological function of oncogenes, their respective cellular counterparts [1].

Through selective pressures incited by coevolution with the host's immune system, DNA viruses have acquired a wide range of strategies to circumvent prevailing immune responses [2]. In order to discover novel viral genes which may be involved in the underlying mechanisms of viral pathogenesis, investigators have resorted to sequencing entire genomes of herpesviruses and poxviruses – two genre of viruses notorious for their ability to subvert host immunity. As a result, various novel open reading frames have been identified and compared 'in silico' to the current, expansive genetic data base of mammalian genes. Similar to the retrovirology field, several of the open reading frames identified have been found to share significant homology with cellular genes. As predicted from the activities of their cellular counterparts, many of these genes have subsequently been shown to be involved in cellular processes such as cell cycle control, growth factor signal transduction, apoptosis and immunomodulation [3].

To date, herpesviruses and poxviruses are the only viruses known to contain cellular homologues of chemokines and chemokine-binding proteins

[4–6]. Viral embezzlement of host chemokine components along with their role in HIV infection has generated increased interest in these immunomodulatory molecules. Just as retroviruses taught us lessons in tumorigenesis, signaling and cell cycle control mechanisms, studying viral chemokine, chemokine-binding proteins and receptors has already begun to create a greater understanding of cellular chemokine biological properties.

Recent characterization of virally encoded chemokine components has provided additional insight concerning host/virus relationships and pathogenic mechanisms. This chapter will review the rapidly growing field of virally encoded chemokines and chemokine receptors and, where applicable, discuss their potential role in viral pathogenicity.

Cellular Chemokines and Chemokine Receptors

Chemokines are small, secreted proteins approximately 80 amino acids in length and display a conserved arrangement of cysteine residues [7]. The chemokine family has been subdivided into the CXC class in which there is an intervening nonconserved amino acid separating the first and second cysteine, and the CC class where the two cysteines are juxtaposed. Other classes of chemokines have recently emerged with the discovery of fractalkine, a CX_3C chemokine, and a C chemokine, lymphotactin. CXC chemokines act principally on neutrophils, whereas the CC chemokines are mainly chemotactic for lymphocytes and monocytes.

Chemokines elicit their biological responses through seven transmembrane G-protein-coupled receptors (GPCR). Chemokine receptors are classified based on the category of chemokine it binds. With regard to human chemokine receptors, ten CC, five CXC and one CX_3C chemokine receptor have been characterized to date. In addition, the Duffy blood group antigen is a promiscuous chemokine receptor which binds both CC and CXC categories. Beyond chemokine binding, several of these receptors have recently been demonstrated to act as HIV coreceptors [12].

Chemokines selectively chemoattract specific subsets of leukocytes to initiate various immunomodulatory functions. Besides inflammation, chemokines have been demonstrataed to be involved in lymphocyte homing, T-cell polarization/activation, and hematopoiesis [8–10, R. Bonecchi, in press]. Additionally, they have been shown to be expressed in areas of the central nervous system suggesting their involvement in various neurological processes [11].

Herpesviruses

Herpesviruses are subdivided into three groups (α, β, γ) based on their in vitro and in vivo properties. These classifications were subsequently confirmed by sequence analysis of these viral genomes. The α-herpesviruses, which consist of herpes simplex-1, -2 and varicella zoster virus, are characterized by their ability to efficiently establish latent infections primarily in sensory ganglia. This subfamily contains no cellular homologues of chemokines or chemokine receptors.

The β-herpesviruses, which consist of human herpesvirus-6, -7 (HHV6 and HHV7), and human and murine cytomegalovirus (HCMV and MCMV), each contain chemokine and/or receptor homologues. These viruses have a long reproductive life cycle and can maintain a latent state in secretory glands, leukocytes, and in kidney. The characteristic pathology of these viruses is cellular enlargement (cytomegalia).

γ-Herpesviruses consist of viruses which show tropism for lymphoid as well as epithelial tissues and are associated with various lymphoproliferative disorders. These viruses, which include Kaposi's sarcoma-associated herpesvirus (KSHV, also known as HHV8), herpesvirus saimiri (HVS), murine γ-herpesvirus-68 (MHV-68), and equine herpesvirus-2 (EHV-2), all encode cellular homologues of chemokines and chemokine receptors. In contrast, Epstein-Barr virus (EBV), also a γ-herpesvirus, does not encode chemokines or chemokine receptors, but induces the expression of these elements upon cellular infection [13].

KSHV-encoded chemokine components have had the greatest degree of characterization, and thus will be described first. The possible role of these chemokine/chemokine receptor homologues in the virus life cycle will be discussed.

γ-Herpesviruses

Kaposi's Sarcoma-Associated Herpesvirus

KSHV. Using representational difference analysis of Kaposi's sarcoma (KS) tissue, novel DNA sequences unique to KS tissue and homologous to herpesviruses were isolated [14]. Subsequent isolation and sequencing of the viral genome demonstrated that the novel sequences belonged to a member of the γ-herpesvirus subgroup. In addition to the angioproliferative disease KS, KSHV sequences were found to be associated with various lymphoproliferative disorders such as multicentric Castleman's disease (MCD) and primary effusion lymphoma (PEL – also known as B-cell cavity lymphoma) [15, 16].

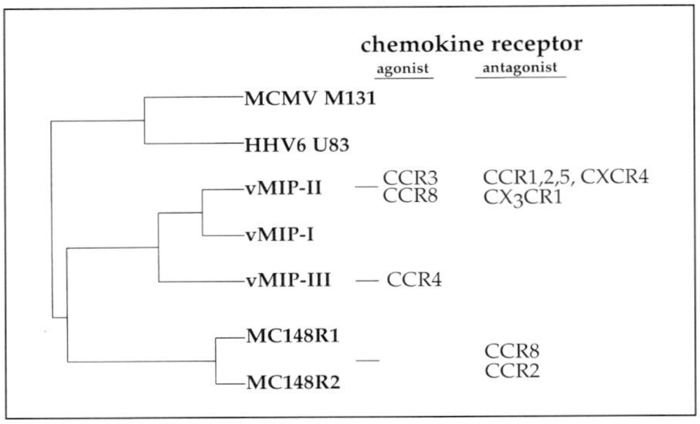

Fig. 1. Dendrogram showing the phylogenetic relationship of virally encoded chemokines. Chemokine receptors which have been shown to specifically bind these chemokines are listed and grouped based on the nature of the functional response. References for this information are listed in the text.

Although classified by the colinear conservation of open reading frames, herpesviruses of the same subgroup contain regions of genetic divergence which usually comprise clusters of unique genes present at analogous loci. These loci frequently include virus-specific cellular homologues which are predicted to confer characteristics unique to the pathobiology of the virus. Positioned within the KSHV long unique region are three homologues of cellular CC chemokines and one homologue of a chemokine receptor [17]. Recent characterization of these chemokine components has led to intriguing proposals involving KSHV subversion of host immunity and viral pathogenesis.

Chemokine Homologues. Until the identification of a chemokine homologue in the genome of rhesus γ_2-herpesvirus [S.W. Wong, pers. commun.], KSHV was the only γ-herpesvirus to encode chemokine homologues. Open reading frames K4, K4.1 and K6 encode viral CC chemokines vMIP-II, vMIP-III and vMIP-1, respectively. Each is unspliced suggesting acquisition from the infected host cell via an mRNA intermediate. Phylogenetic analysis revealed vMIP-I and -II are more similar to each other than to their more closely related cellular homologues MIP-1α and RANTES, suggesting that they may have evolved by a gene duplication event within the virus genome rather than through a separate acquisition from the host genome (fig. 1). In contrast, vMIP-III is more distantly related and thus may have been acquired independent of vMIP-I and -II.

vMIP-I. Initial attempts to understand the role of vMIPs in KSHV pathogenesis centered around HIV infection in part because of HIV's utility of chemokine receptors as coreceptors for infection and the prevalence of KS in HIV-infected individuals [12]. vMIP-1, which shares 43% sequence identity to

MIP-1α, was demonstrated to inhibit HIV infection through CCR5 suggesting a productive interaction with this receptor [13]. However, depending on the assay system used, the ability to inhibit CCR5-utilizing strains produced variable results [18].

Also in these studies, vMIP-I could not induce calcium mobilization in human neutrophils or human eosinophils, nor could it act as an agonist or antagonist in chemotaxis assays. Although vMIP-I showed inhibition of HIV/CCR5 binding, high chemokine concentrations were required. A high affinity receptor for vMIP-I remains to be identified. Nonetheless, a positive effect of vMIP-I on angiogenesis has been reported in the chick chorioallantoic assay [18].

vMIP-II. Because of high similarity to vMIP-1 (60% identity) and MIP-1α (52% identity), vMIP-II was tested for its ability to inhibit HIV infection. In contrast, vMIP-II was shown by Boshoff et al. [18] to be a potent inhibitor of HIV infection through CCR3 (95% inhibition at 200 n*M* vMIP-II), while showing only modest inhibition in cells expressing CCR5 or CXCR4. These findings suggest that vMIP-II is a ligand for CCR3. Consistent with this, vMIP-II was demonstrated to mobilize calcium in human eosinophils where CCR3 is predominantly expressed [19] and to act as an agonist in eosinophil chemotaxis assays.

Further indication of vMIP-II's role as an agonist comes from the observation that it induces chemotaxis of primary cell types as well as certain polarized T cells [Sozzani et al., in press]. Human monocytes and T cells of the Th2 phenotype (that is type II T cells secreting Th2 cytokines) were demonstrated to selectively migrate in response to vMIP-II. Th1 cells, dendritic cells, and natural killer cells, however, showed no chemotactic response. Additionally, vMIP-II induced chemotaxis of Jurkat cells stably expressing the chemokine receptor CCR8, a receptor which has been demonstrated to be selectively expressed on CD4+ and CD8+ T cells with a Th2 cytokine profile [Sozzani et al., in press].

In contrast to the preceding findings, Kledal et al. [20] have shown vMIP-II is an antagonist for a number of chemokine receptors including CCR1, -2, -3, -5 and CXCR4. Moreover, vMIP-II was subsequently shown to inhibit RANTES-, MIP-1α- and MIP-1β-induced chemotaxis of human monocytes, suggesting that vMIP-II may be a broad-spectrum chemokine antagonist. Consistent with this, recent studies indicate vMIP-II is also an antagonist of CX_3CR1 [21], the receptor for fractalkine, and effectively attenuates chemokine-mediated leukocyte trafficking in vivo [21].

Using synthetic vMIP-II corresponding to the previously described short and long forms, we have recently shown that both forms of vMIP-II are functional agonists for CCR3 based on chemotaxis of mouse pre-B cells stably expressing CCR3. The shorter form, which was shown to be the actual sequence of mature of vMIP-II [20], proved to be the more potent agonist for CCR3 which is consistent with the competition binding profiles. Thus under these circumstances, both forms of vMIP-II are capable of acting as agonists for CCR3.

vMIP-III. Of the three viral chemokines, vMIP-III is more distantly related to cellular chemokines (the highest identity is 25%) as well as to the other KSHV vMIPs (30% identity). While vMIP-1 and -II have a molecular mass of approximately 8 kDa, vMIP-III is larger at 9.7 kDa. In addition to containing two additional cysteine residues, vMIP-III diverges from vMIP-I and -II toward the COOH-terminus beginning with the loss of a conserved tryptophan-valine motif distal to the last conserved cysteine [4]. In contrast to vMIP-I and vMIP-II, vMIP-III showed no demonstrable inhibition of HIV infection [C. Boshoff, pers. commun.].

Chemokine competition binding experiments have identified CCR4 as a preferred receptor for vMIP-III [Stine et al., submitted]. Subsequent chemotaxis experiments using cells stably expressing CCR4 demonstrate vMIP-III's role as an agonist for this receptor. This chemotactic response appears to be more robust than that induced by the natural ligands for CCR4, MDC and TARC, but requires a higher dose of chemokine [J.T. Stine et al., submitted].

Within the T-cell compartment, CCR4 has been shown to be selectively expressed on T cells of the Th2 phenotype [8, 9]. Consistent with its role as an agonist for CCR4-bearing cells, vMIP-III induces chemotaxis of Th2 cells, whereas Th1 cells are virtually unresponsive [J.T. Stine et al., submitted].

Possible Role in KSHV Malignancy. While vMIP-I has yet to be fully characterized with regard to its chemokine properties, vMIP-II and -III have been shown to functionally interact with chemokine receptors which are selectively expressed on T cells of the Th2 phenotype [Sozzani et al., in press; J.T. Stine et al., submitted]. Recent analysis of the cellular infiltrate in the KS lesion has shown that the infiltrating T cells are predominantly CD4+/CD8+ T cells with a Th2 cytokine profile [Sozzani et al., in press]. A well-documented action of Th2 cytokines is the suppression of Th1 cytokine activity, which includes the cell-mediated, antiviral immune response [22, 23]. As a mechanism of subverting host immunity, measles viruses have been shown to inhibit the establishment of a Th1-type immune response by downregulating IL-12, a Th1-inducing cytokine [24]. Consistent with this, there is evidence that activation of a Th2 response can lead to delayed viral clearance [25]. Therefore, it is likely that KSHV may utilize vMIP-II and vMIP-III to subvert host immunity by changing the microenvironment of the KS lesion from an antiviral Th1 to a Th2 phenotype. Once IL-4- and IL-13-secreting Th2 cells have migrated to

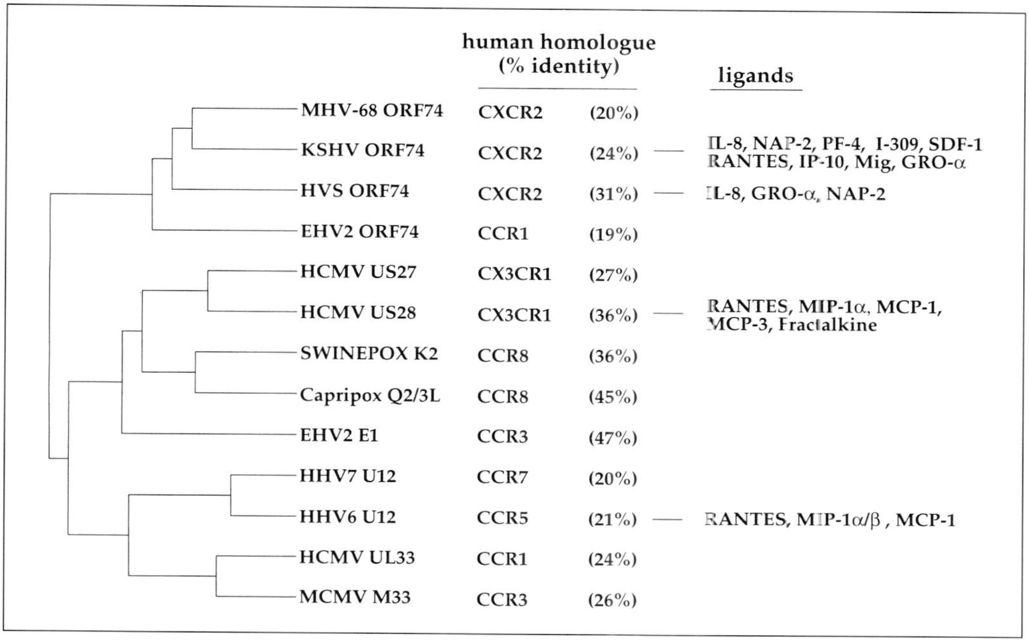

Fig. 2. Dendrogram showing the phylogenetic relationship of virally encoded chemokine receptors. Human homologues with percent identity are listed along with ligands known to bind these receptors. References for this information are listed in the text.

the lesion, they may amplify Th2 chemoattraction since these two cytokines have been shown to upregulate expression of MDC, the natural ligand for CCR4 [Bonecchi et al., 1998, in press].

With the diverse properties of vMIP-II in mind, it is tempting to speculate that vMIP-II may effectively limit a localized host antiviral response by acting as a selective agonist for those chemokine receptors expressed by Th2 cells (CCR3 and CCR8) while acting as an antagonist of those receptors expressed more broadly in the immune system or in Th1 cells [20].

An additional role for vMIP-I and -II in KS may be induction of angiogenesis. KS is classified as an angioproliferative disorder and vMIP-1 and vMIP-II have been shown to induce angiogenesis in a chick chorioallantoic assay [18].

Chemokine Receptor Homologue. The KSHV genome contains an open reading frame, with significant sequence conservation with G-protein-coupled receptors. This sequence is colinear with ORF 74 of HVS and is most similar to the human IL-8 receptor [26] (fig. 2). This gene, ORF 74 (also known as KSHV-GPCR), was demonstrated to be expressed in primary effusion lymphomas as well as in KS lesions [26, 27].

Initial characterization indicated this receptor signaled in a constitutive, agonist-independent manner and could activate cell proliferation in normal rat kidney fibroblasts [28]. As predicted by homology with the chemokine receptors CXCR1 and -2, ORF 74 binds IL-8 as well as other CXC chemokines such as NAP-2, PF-4, and GRO-α. Although CC chemokines are not known to bind IL-8 receptors, ORF 74 also binds I-309 (the ligand for CCR8) and RANTES (ligand for CCR5), whereas MIP-1β and MCP-1 do not bind.

CXC chemokines display interesting binding characteristics on ORF 74. IP-10 and Mig each act as agonists on the same receptor, CXCR3. Interestingly, while both bind ORF 74, they have opposing effects on ORF 74 signaling [29]. IP-10 acts as an inverse agonist and inhibits the constitutive signaling of this receptor. In contrast, Mig binds but does not inhibit the constitutive signaling activity of ORF 74. The CXC chemokine, SDF-1 [M.M. Rosenkilde et al., in press] and the KSHV-encoded CC chemokine, vMIP-II [M.C. Gershengorn, pers. commun.; M.M. Rosenkilde, submitted], have also been reported to act as inverse agonists. Structure/function experiments aimed at understanding this mechanism have shown that construction of a high-affinity zinc-switch through the introduction of two His residues at the extracellular end of transmembrane segment 5 enables Zn^{2+} to act as a prototypic, nonpeptide inverse agonist [M.M. Rosenkilde et al., in press].

Conversely, IL-8 and GRO-α, which contain the ELR (glutamate-leucine-arginine) motif associated with chemokine induction of angiogenesis, have been shown to elevate the activity of ORF 74 over constitutive levels. This finding indicates that a constitutively active GPCR can be hyperstimulated by agonist activity [M.C. Gershengorn, pers. commun.; M.M. Rosenkilde, submitted].

As with human receptors, the integrity of the ELR motif of chemokines is required for activation of ORF 74 [M.C. Gershengorn, pers. commun.]. Moreover, other residues that are required for IL-8 binding to human chemokine receptors CXCR1 and CXCR2 are also important for ORF 74 activation. Thus it appears that the ELR binding site and other key domains of ELR chemokine activation have been preserved in the viral ORF 74.

Possible Role in KSHV-Associated Malignancy. The significance of ORF 74 in the pathology of KSHV is highlighted by the fact that ORF 74, when transfected into nontransformed cells, stimulates cellular proliferation [28]. This effect is attributed to its constitutive signaling activity since the chemokine IP-10, which effectively inhibits ORF 74 signaling, also inhibits ORF 74-induced cell proliferation [29]. ORF 74 signaling has also been shown to be oncogenic as it leads to cell transformation and tumorigenicity [30]. Additionally, signaling through ORF 74 induces a switch to an angiogenic phenotype through the upregulation of vascular endothelial growth factor (VEG-F), an angiogenesis and Kaposi's spindle cell growth factor.

Taken together, it appears that ORF 74 may be partly responsible for the transformed phenotype of KSHV-infected cells in KS lesions and B-cell cavity lymphomas. Additionally, ORF 74 has been optimized for agonist and inverse agonist modulation by respective endogenous angiogenic, ELR-containing GRO-α/IL-8 and angiostatic, non-ELR-containing IP-10/SDF-1 chemokines. These properties along with its ability to upregulate VEG-F, strongly suggests a role for ORF 74 in neovascularization seen in KS lesions.

Herpesvirus Saimiri

HVS. This T-lymphotropic γ-herpesvirus establishes an asymptomatic infection in its natural host, the squirrel monkey, but causes acute fulminate lymphoproliferative disease in New World primates [31]. Human T cells can be immortalized by HVS such that they become independent of antigen and accessory cells while retaining many functions of primary activated T cells; however, no infectious virus is secreted from these infected cells [31, 32].

Chemokine Receptor Homologue. The first viral seven-transmembrane receptor to be functionally characterized was identified during sequencing studies of HVS [33]. This gene, termed ECRF3, shares both sequence and colinear conservation with other ORF 74 found in other γ-herpesviruses [31] (fig. 2). ECRF3 is homologous to CXCR2 and binds the same ligands, IL-8, Gro-α, and NAP-2 [34]. In contrast to the KSHV-related ORF 74, no constitutive signaling was detected [35].

HVS does not encode chemokine homologues in contrast to the closely related KSHV. However, HVS encodes vIL-17, a cellular homologue of IL-17 which has been shown to induce the expression of chemokines [36]. Assuming vIL-17 functions like cellular IL-17, this may provide a mechanism for gaining access to chemokines which may be necessary for the viral life cycle.

Epstein-Barr Virus

EBV. Although EBV encodes no chemokine or chemokine receptor genes, this γ-herpesvirus upregulates expression of MIP-1α, -β and RANTES [3] as well as the chemokine receptor CCR7 [37] upon infection. CCR7 is a chemokine receptor for SLC (secondary lymphoid-tissue chemokine) and ELC (EBV-induced ligand chemokine) [38]. The interaction of CCR7 and SLC/ELC is thought to be responsible for chemoattracting activated B and T cells to secondary lymphoid organs.

While their role in EBV-mediated disease is not known, it is interesting to note that chemokine elements upregulated by EBV exist as homologues in the genome of closely related KSHV. Unlike KSHV, EBV is not associated with angioproliferative diseases; therefore, the significance of this correlation may be more appropriately represented in their respective B-cell proliferative disorders. In this context, both ORF 74 and the upregulated CCR7 may induce B-cell trafficking and increase viral dissemination.

Murine γ-Herpesvirus-68

MHV-68. Like the human γ-herpesviruses, lymphoproliferative disorders develop in mice infected with MHV-68 [39]. Moreover, MHV-68 infects multiple organs and can establish a latent or persistent infection of the spleen. Although it is likely that B cells act as the reservoirs for latent and/or persistent virus, additonal sites may exist since mice lacking mature B cells still allow the virus to establish a latent infection [40]. Sequencing of the genome of this virus shows colinear genetic alignment with those of other γ-herpesviruses and includes a putative chemokine receptor located in ORF 74. To date, no functional data are available on this receptor.

Equine Herpesvirus-2. EHV-2 is a γ-herpesvirus which is ubiquitous in the equine population; nevertheless, its pathogenic role and tissue tropism remains to be identified [41]. While no chemokine homologues are encoded by this virus, sequence analysis of the genome of this virus discloses four putative seven-transmembrane G-protein-coupled chemokine receptors – ORF E1 which is duplicated, ORF E6 and an ORF 74-like GPCR. ORF E1 shares 47% identity with CCR3 (fig. 2), but has yet to be characterized. The ORF 74-like gene shares sequence similarity and colinear conservation with ORF 74 genes from other γ-herpesviruses and, like ORF E1, has not been characterized. ORF E6 is more distantly related and thus speculation on function cannot be made.

β-Herpesviruses

Cytomegalovirus

CMV. Similar to other β-herpesviruses, CMV infection is prevalent among the adult population and has an enhanced tropism for hematopoietic cells. Although infection is generally inocuous to healthy adults, human CMV (HCMV) causes serious congenital and neonatal diseases [42]. Moreover, this virus is an opportunistic pathogen for immunocompromised individuals, such as persons with HIV infection and immunosuppressed individuals such as organ transplant patients.

Chemokine Receptor Homologues. Sequence analysis of the HCMV genome [42] demonstrated the presence of four G-protein-coupled receptors, UL33, US27, US28 and UL78 [4]. US27 and US28 are arranged in tandem suggesting an intrinsic gene duplication event, whereas UL33 is more divergent and separated by 173 kb.

Of the four GPCRs, US28 has been most extensively studied. This open reading frame has 30% sequence identity with chemokine receptors, and encodes a promiscuous calcium-mobilizing receptor for β-chemokines RANTES, MIP-1α, MCP-1 and MCP-3, but not for CXC chemokines IL-8 or IP-10 [43, 44]. Interestingly, the CC chemokines which bind US28 have a greater affinity for US28 than to their cognate receptors [4].

Among the human chemokine receptors, CX_3CR1 shares the greatest degree of homology to US28 (36% identity) (fig. 2). Fractalkine, the ligand for CX_3CR1, has been reported to bind US28 [T.W. Schwartz, pers. commun.]. While US28 binds a wide variety of CC chemokines with single digit nanomolar affinity, it is specially optimized to recognize fractalkine. None of the other host chemokines are able to compete for fractalkine binding despite their apparent high affinity for US28.

Lastly, US28 may also play a role in dissemination of HIV. US28 was shown to function as an HIV coreceptor by facilitating infection of a CD4+ human cell line by primary isolates of HIV-1 and HIV-2. Additionally, fusion of these cells with cells expressing the HIV envelope proteins or vesicular stomatitis virus-encoded G-protein could be facilitated by US28 [45, 46]. These observations suggest an attractive hypothesis describing the interplay of HIV and CMV in disease.

Although UL33 remains to be functionally characterized as a chemokine receptor, it has been demonstrated to be expressed in CMV-infected cells as well as in the region of cytoplasmic inclusions in HCMV-infected fibroblasts [47]. While UL33 is expressed in infected fibroblasts, it is not required for growth of HCMV in these cells. Moreover, UL33 has been shown to be expressed in enveloped virus particles [47].

The US27 ORF shows divergent sequences which place it further away from the chemokine receptors than US28 (fig. 2). US27 and UL78 have yet to be characterized with regard to their roles as chemokine receptors. UL78 appears to show more similarities with the fMLP (fMet-Leu-Phe) receptor [4] rather than chemokine receptors.

MCMV. Murine CMV (MCMV) genomic sequence encodes only one G-protein-coupled receptor, M33 which is conserved and colinear with UL33 in HCMV [48]. Like UL33, M33 has not been functionally characterized as a chemokine receptor; however, the importance of M33 in MCMV infection is highlighted by the fact that growth of M33-deleted MCMV was severely restricted in salivary glands of infected mice. This suggests that M33 may be important for the trafficking of infected leukocytes or transmission of virus to the salivary glands [49].

HCMV/MCMV Chemokine Homologues. Open reading frame 131 of MCMV shows homology with CC chemokines. This ORF has been demonstrated to be expressed late in the viral replication cycle suggesting that it may play a role in MCMV pathogenesis [50]. To date, ORF 131 has not been characterized.

Previous reports do not indicate the presence of chemokine homologues in HCMV. Nevertheless, an HCMV open reading frame encoding an ELR-containing CXC chemokine – designated CMV-α-1 – is currently being characterized [T.J. Schall, pers. commun.].

HHV6. The seroprevalence of human herpesvirus-6 (HHV6) in the general population is approximately 85%. Clinically, this virus has been recognized as the cause of exanthem subitum in infants [51], it has been recently implicated in multiple sclerosis [52], and is associated with bone marrow and organ transplant patients where infection results in bone marrow suppression, interstitial pneumonia and encephalitis [53]. It is most prevalent in peripheral blood lymphatic mononuclear cells, lymphatic tissues, brain-derived tissues, and is shed in the saliva [54–58]. Additionally, only during conditions of immunosuppression does the virus appear to be reactivated in the blood, as is commonly observed for other human herpesviruses.

HHV6 consists of two variants, HHV6A and HHV6B, both of which have recently been sequenced [59, 60]. DNA sequence analysis shows colinear alignment with other β-herpesviruses and includes both a chemokine and chemokine receptor homologue [58]. ORF U12 encodes a functional chemokine receptor homologue which is related by sequence to those encoded by other β-herpesviruses – HCMV UL33, MCMV M33, and HHV7 U12. U12 was demonstrated by calcium mobilization to bind RANTES, MIP-1α/β, MCP-1, but not the CXC chemokine, IL-8, suggestive of a promiscuous CC chemokine receptor [60].

HHV6 Chemokine Homologues. The open reading frame in HHV6A designated U83 encodes a gene which shares homology with CC chemokines and has yet to be characterized. While the NH_2-terminal region is conserved, the COOH-terminus greatly diverges from that of cellular CC chemokines. U83 is more closely related to MCMV 131 (fig. 1).

HHV7. HHV7 has a seroprevalence of approximately 85% in the general population with infection occurring in early childhood. Similar to HHV6, this virus is also shed as infectious virus particles in the saliva and shows a similar cellular tropism. No firm association with human disease has been made, although, like HHV6, there may be a link to exanthem subitum [61].

Sequence analysis of HHV7 [62] confirmed the placement of this virus in the β-herpesvirus family. HHV7 also encodes a G-protein-coupled receptor which is conserved colinearly with the HHV6 U12, thus named accordingly. The U12 open reading frame, although not functionally characterized, is predicted to function as the U12 ORF in HHV6. To date, no chemokine homologues have been found in HHV7.

Poxviruses

Like herpesviruses, poxviruses are large double-stranded DNA viruses that are notorious for their ability to subvert host immune responses. Many viruses within this family encode proteins which interfere with various cytokine networks, mostly by interception of receptor-ligand interactions [2, 6]. Since the eradication of smallpox, the main poxvirus that infects humans is the molluscum contagiosum virus (MCV). Clinically, this virus produces papules in the skin of young children and sexually active adults and acts as an opportunistic pathogen in immunocompromised patients, such as those with AIDS [63, 64]. Typically, infection is marked by virtually no immune response in the epidermal lesion.

Studies aimed at determining virulence factors of MCV as well as poxviruses which infect other vertebrates have led to a greater understanding of host-virus interactions and progression to disease states. Through biochemical techniques and genomic seuence analysis of various poxviruses, proteins which interfere with chemokine activity directly or indirectly have been discovered.

Molluscum contagiosum Virus

Chemokine Homologues. To date, only one poxvirus family member encodes a chemokine homologue. Sequence analysis of the genome of MCV indicates that a CC chemokine homologue exists in open reading frame MC148R [65]. Initially this gene was expressed in insect cells, purified, and characterized based on its homology with the MIP-1α/β CC chemokines. While the protein encoded by MC148R does not induce chemotaxis, it doses, however, antagonize MIP-1α-induced chemotaxis [66]. Further studies demonstrated that MC148R acts as a broad-spectrum chemokine antagonist while inhibiting the chemotactic activity of various leukocyte subsets to several CC and CXC chemokines [67]. Concomitant with MC148R's ability to inhibit MCP-1-induced chemotaxis (IC_{50} of 1.5 n*M*), it is also able to compete with ^{125}I-MCP-1 binding to CCR2B. Moreover, MC148R has been shown to inhibit I-309 binding to the chemokine receptor CCR8 also with IC_{50} of approximately 1.5 n*M* [I. Armstrong, pers. commun.].

Taken together, these observations suggest that MC148R may act as a broad-spectrum chemokine antagonist by inhibiting the activity of several chemokine receptors, thus inhibiting the leukocyte infiltrate at the site of infection. It should be noted that the antagonistic nature of MC148R may be due to the NH_2-terminal truncation of five amino acids in the mature protein as compared to other CC chemokines [66, 67]. This NH_2-terminal region of chemokines has been shown to be necessary for chemokine function [68].

Myxoma Virus

Myxoma virus is a poxvirus which induces a virulent systemic lethal disease called myxomatosis in European rabbits [69]. The severity of this disease is highlighted by the overall immunosuppression of the host's cell-mediated immune response. Myxoma virus infection of rabbits has permitted development of models to study host/virus interactions.

Using chemical crosslinking of cytokines and myxoma virus-infected cell supernatants, an open reading frame designated M-T7 was demonstrated to be a soluble, functional homologue of cellular IFN-γ receptor [70]. Using the rabbit model, M-T7 was shown to be involved in the overall reduction in cell-mediated immunity as rabbits infected with M-T7-deleted myxoma virus displayed a vigorous and effective cellular immune response to infection. Moreover, the lack of M-T7 was associated with the presence of inflammatory cells in the lesion, whereas the wild type had virtually no inflammatory cells, thus indicative of yet another role for M-T7 in viral pathogenesis.

A slight modification of the technique used to find cytokine binding proteins was adopted to find specific chemokine-binding proteins secreted from myxoma virus-infected cells. Using this method, M-T7, which was initially identified as an IFN-γ binding protein, was subsequently shown to interact with chemokines. When M-T7 was purified and assayed for chemokine interaction, it was demonstrated to bind CC and CXC chemokines as well as lymphotactin (C chemokine). Interestingly, the binding activity was localized to the heparin binding domains of the chemokines.

Using M-T7-deleted myxoma virus-infected cells, chemical crosslinking detected still another chemokine-binding protein of similar molecular weight as M-T7. This protein was purified, sequenced and found to be a product of the T1 open reading frame, thus named M-T1 [71]. M-T1 shows no sequence similarities with chemokine receptors. Additionally, a similar chemokine binding activity was observed in supernatants from cells infected with Shope fibroma virus, raccoonpox, cowpox, rabbitpox, and vaccinia virus strain Lister, but not vaccinia virus strain WR (Western Reserve). Each of these viruses was shown to encode an M-T1-like protein of approximately 35 kDa (sometimes referred to as p35) [6] (table 1).

Table 1. Poxvirus secreted chemokine-binding proteins

Virus	Open reading frame	Binding characteristics
Myxoma virus Shope fibroma virus	M-T7 S-T7	Bind heparin binding domain of C, CC, and CXC chemokines
Myxoma virus Shope fibroma virus Rabbitpox Vaccinia strain Lister Vaccinia strain Copenhagen Variola Cowpox	M-T1 S-T1 RPV, 35 kDa C23L, 35 kDa C23L, 35kDa G3R, 35 kDa ORF B, 35 kDa	~35 kDa glycoprotein binds CC chemokines more avidly than CXC chemokines

While M-T7 bound RANTES with an IC_{50} of 900 nM, M-T1 bound the same chemokine with an IC_{50} of 73 nM [71]. In addition, the rabbitpox M-T1 p35 equivalent bound MIP-1α, RANTES and eotaxin with affinities ranging from 0.1 to 0.15 nM [5]. Higher affinities were observed using the cowpox virus and variola (smallpox) equivalent p35 gene in cell-based and plate-binding assays [72]. These studies also claim that the p35 protein not only binds the CC chemokine MCP-1, but it also competes for the same receptor binding site. M-T1 and other p35 equivalents have been shown to bind several CC and CXC chemokines; however, a greater affinity for CC chemokines has been observed. Despite this selective binding, M-T1 shows no sequence similarity with chemokine receptors and, according to database searches, has no mammalian homologue.

In order to determine the functional relevance of this chemokine-binding protein in disease, the M-T1 equivalent in rabbitpox virus was deleted. Unlike myxoma virus, rabbitpox only encodes the M-T1 equivalent of poxvirus chemokine binding proteins. In these experiments, the wild-type virus showed very little leukocyte infiltrate whereas the rabbitpox lacking the M-T1 gene showed a marked increase in leukocyte infiltrate and edema in the virus lesion which is representative of an acute inflammatory reaction [71].

Two chemokine-like seven-transmembrane receptors have been identified in poxviruses. Capripox virus contains an open reading frame designated Q2/3L [73] which shares some homology with chemokine receptors. Likewise, the swinepox virus open reading frame K2R also shares homology with chemokine receptors. Of the viral chemokine receptors, both of these receptors are more closely related to each other. These genes, however, have yet to be functionally characterized.

Concluding Remarks

As the chemokine field continues to rapidly advance, the multiple immune functions of these molecules becomes more evident. It is intriguing that so many viral groups have evolved mechanisms to selectively utilize such a complex system. While retroviral utilization of chemokine receptors for infection is well established, the role which these chemokine homologues play in herpesviruses and poxviruses is just beginning to be determined. Collectively, viral chemokines display agonist and antagonist properties; therefore, each virus may be utilizing the respective encoded chemokines disparately.

While we attempt to understand the biological function of chemokines, it appears that poxviruses and herpesviruses, by living in equilibrium with their hosts, have already understood the importance of these molecules in immune deviation and leukocyte trafficking. The fact that functional viral chemokines and chemokine receptors have been retained and optimized in these viruses suggests their importance in the viral life cycle.

Indeed viruses are still teaching us lessons in immunology. Some poxviruses encode functional soluble TNF-α and IFN-γ receptors and each has been shown to be required for viral pathogenesis [6]. Interestingly, this same concept is being utilized for development of new therapeutics. As biological data continues to mount, perhaps viral chemokines and chemokine receptors will provide the next lessons for chemokine immunology.

Acknowledgments

The authors would like to thank Alberto Mantovani, Thomas J. Schall, Daniel J. Dairaghi, Thue W. Schwartz, Marvin C. Gershengorn, and Inger Damon for generously providing unpublished information for this chapter.

References

1 Coffin JM, Hughes SH, Varmus HE (eds): Retroviruses. New York, Cold Spring Harbor Laboratory Press, 1998.
2 Spriggs MK: One step ahead of the game: Viral immunomodulatory molecules. Annu Rev Immunol 1996;14:101–130.
3 Moore PS, Chang Y: Antiviral activity of tumor-suppressor pathways: Clues from molecular piracy by KSHV. Trends Genet 1998;14:144–150.
4 Dairaghi DJ, Greaves DR, Schall TJ: Abduction of chemokine elements by herpesviruses. Semin Virol 1998;8:377–385.
5 Wells TNC, Schwartz TW: Plagiarism of the host immune system: Lessons about chemokine immunology from viruses. Curr Opin Biotechnol 1997;8:741–748.

6 Lalani AS, McFadden G: Secreted poxvirus chemokine binding proteins. J Leukoc Biol 1997;62: 570–576.
7 Baggiolini M, Dewald B, Moser B: Human chemokines: An update. Annu Rev Immunol 1997;15: 675–705.
8 Unutmaz D, KewalRamani VN, Littman DR: G protein-coupled receptors in HIV and SIV entry: New perspectives on lentivirus-host interactions and on the utility of animal models. Semin Immunol 1998;10:225–236.
9 Bonecchi R, Vianchi G, Bordignon PP, D'Ambrosio D, Lang R, Borsatt A, Sozzani S, Allavena P, Gray PW, Mantovani A, Sinigagli F: Differential expression of chemokine receptors and chemotactic responsiveness of type 1 T helper cells (Th1s) and Th2s. J Exp Med 1998;184:129–134.
10 Sallusto F, Lenig D, Mackay CR, Lanzavecchia A: Flexible programs of chemokine receptor expression on human polarized T helper 1 and 2 lymphocytes. J Exp Med 1998;187:875–883.
11 Zou YR, Kottmann AH, Kuroda M, Taniuchi I, Littman DR: Function of the chemokine receptor CXCR4 in hematopoiesis and in cerebellar development. Nature 1998;393:595–599.
12 Ransohoff RM: Chemokines in neurological disease models: Correlation between chemokine expression patterns and inflammatory pathology. J Leukoc Biol 1997;62:645–652.
13 Moore PS, Boshoff C, Weiss RA, Chang Y: Molecular mimicry of human cytokine and cytokine response pathway genes by KSHV. Science 1996;274:1730–1744.
14 Chang Y, Cesarman E, Pessin MS, Lee F, Culpepper J, Knowles DM, Moore P: Identification of herpesvirus-like DNA sequences in AIDS-associated Kaposi's sarcoma. Science 1994;265:1865–1869.
15 Cesarman E, Chang Y, Moore PS, Said JW, Knowles DM: Kaposi's sarcoma-associated herpesvirus-like DNA sequences are present in AIDS-related body cavity based lymphomas. N Engl J Med 1995;332:1186–1189.
16 Soulier J: Kaposi's sarcoma-associated herpesvirus-like DNA sequences in multicentric Castleman's disease. Blood 1995;86:1276–1280.
17 Neipel F, Albrecht JC, Fleckenstein B: Cell-homologous genes in the Kaposi's sarcoma-associated rhadinovirus human herpesvirus 8: Determinants of its pathogenicity? J Virol 1997;71:4187–4192.
18 Boshoff C, Endo Y, Collins PD, Takeuchi Y, Reeves JD, Schweichart VL, Siani MA, Sasaki T, Williams TJ, Gray PW, Moore PS, Chang Y, Weiss RA: Angiogenic and HIV-inhibitory functions of KSHV-encoded chemokines. Science 1997;278:290–294.
19 Ponath PD, Qin S, Post TW, Wang J, Wu L, Gerard NP, Newman W, Gerard C, Mackay CR: Molecular cloning and characterization of a human eotaxin receptor expressed selectively on eosinophils. J Exp Med 1996;183:2437–2448.
20 Kledal TN, Rosenkilde MM, Coulin F, Simmons G, Johnson AH, Alouani S, Power CA, Luttichau HR, Gerstoft J, Clapham PR, Clark-Lewis I, Wells TNC, Schwartz TW: A broad-spectrum chemokine antagonist encoded by Kaposi's sarcoma-associated herpesvirus. Science 1997;277 1656–1659.
21 Chen S, Bacon KB, Li L, Garcia GE, Xia Y, Lo D, Thompson DA, Siani MA, Tamamoto T, Garrison JK, Feng L: In vivo inhibition of CC and CX3C chemokine-induced leukocyte infiltration and attenuation of glomerulonephritis in Wistar-Kyoto (WKY) rats by vMIP-II. J Exp Med 1998; 188:193–198.
22 Mueller R, Bradley LM, Krahl T, Sarvetnick N: Mechanism underlying counterregulation of autoimmune diabetes by IL-4. Immunity 1997;7:411–418.
23 Rocken M, Racke M, Shevach EM: IL-4-induced immune deviation as antigen-specific therapy for inflammatory autoimmune disease. Immunol Today 1996;17:225–231.
24 Karp CL, Wysocka M, Wahl LM, Ahearn JM, Cuomo PJ, Sherry B, Trinchieri G, Grifin DE: Mechanism of suppression of cell-mediated immunity by measles virus. Science 1996;273:228–231.
25 Actor JK, Shirai M, Kullberg MC, Buller RM, Sher A, Berzofsky JA: Helminth infection results in decreased virus-specific CD8+ cytotoxic T-cell and Th1 cytokine responses as well as delayed virus clearance. Proc Natl Acad Sci USA 1993;90:948.
26 Cesarman E, Nador RG, Bai F, Bohenzky RA, Russo JJ, Moore PS, Chang Y, Knowles DM: Kaposi's sarcoma associated herpesvirus contains G protein-coupled receptor and cyclin D homologs which are expressed in Kaposi's sarcoma and malignant lymphoma. J Virol 1996;70:8218–8223.

27 Guo HG, Browning P, Nicholas J, Hayward GS, Tschachler E, Jiang JW, Sadowska M, Raffeld M, Colombini S, Gallo RC, Reitz MS Jr: Characterization of a chemokine receptor-related gene in human herpesvirus 8 and its expression in Kaposi's sarcoma. Virology 1997;228:371–378.
28 Arvanitakis L, Gera-Raaka E, Vrma A, Gershengorn MC, Cesarman E: Human herpesvirus KSHV encodes a constitutively active G-protein-coupled receptor linked to cell proliferation. Nature 1997; 385:347–350.
29 Geras-Raaka E, Varma A, Ho H, Clark-Lewis I, Gershengorn MC: Human interferon-γ-inducible protein 10 (IP-10) inhibits constitutive signaling of Kaposi's sarcoma-associated herpesvirus G protein-coupled receptor. J Exp Med 1998;188:405–408.
30 Bais C, Santomasso B, Coso O, Arvanitakis L, Geras-Raaka E, Gutkind JS, Asch AS, Cesarman E, Gershengorn MC, Mesri EA: G-protein-coupled receptor of Kaposi's sarcoma-associated herpesvirus is a viral oncogene and angiogenesis activator. Nature 1998;391:86–89.
31 Nicholas J, Cameron KR, Honess RW: Herpesvirus saimiri encodes homologues of G protein-coupled receptors and cyclins. Nature 1992;355:362–365.
32 Meinl E, Hohlfeld R, Wekerle H, Fleckenstein B: Immortalization of human T cells by herpesvirus saimiri. Immunol Today 1995;16:55–58.
33 Albrecht JC, Nicholas J, Biller D, Cameron KR, Biesinger B, Newman C, Wittman S, Craxton MA, Coleman H, Fleckstein B, Honess RW: Primary structure of the herpesvirus saimiri genome. J Virol 1992;66:5047–5058.
34 Ahuja SK, Murphy PM: Molecular piracy of mammalian interleukin-8 receptor type B by herpesvirus saimiri. J Biol Chem 1993;268:20691–20694.
35 Geras-Raaka E, Arvanitakis L, Gais C, Cesarman E, Mesri EA, Gershengorn MC: Inhibition of constitutive signaling of Kaposi's sarcoma-associated herpesvirus G protein-coupled receptor by protein kinases in mammalian cells in culture. J Exp Med 1998;187:801–806.
36 Fossiez F, Djossou O, Chomarat P, Flores-Romo L, Ait-Yahia S, Maat C, Pin JJ, Garrone P, Garcia E, Saeland S, Blanchard D, Gaillard C, Das Mahapatra B, Rouvier E, Golstein P, Banchereau J, Lebecque S: T cell interleukin-17 induces stromal cells to produce proinflammatory and hematopoietic cytokines. J Exp Med 1996;183:2593–2603.
37 Birkenbach M, Josefsen K, Yalamanchili R, Lenoir G, Kieff E: Epstein-Barr virus-induced genes: First lymphocyte-specific G protein-coupled peptide receptors. J Virol 1993;67:2209–2220.
38 Yoshida R, Imai T, Hieshima K, Kusuda J, Baba M, Kitaura M, Nishimura M, Kakizaki M, Nomiyama H, Yoshi O: Molecular cloning of a novel human CC chemokine EBI1-ligand chemokine that is a specific functional ligand for EBI1, CCR7. J Biol Chem 1997;272:13803–13809.
39 Sunil-Chandra NP, Arno J, Fazakerley J, Nash AA: Lymphoproliferative disease in mice infected with murine gamma-herpesvirus 68. Am J Pathol 1994;145:818–826.
40 Weck KE, Barkon ML, Yoo LL, Speck SH, Virgin HW: Mature B-cells are required for acute splenic infection, but not for establishment of latency, by murine gamma-herpesvirus 68. J Virol 1996;70:6775–6780.
41 Telford EA, Watson MS, Aird HC, Perry J, Davidson AJ: The DNA sequence of equine herpesvirus 2. J Mol Biol 1995;249:520–528.
42 Chee MS, Satchwell SC, Preddie E, Weston KM, Barrell BG: Human cytomegalovirus encodes three T protein-coupled receptor homologues. Nature 1990;344:774–777.
43 Gao JL, Murphy PM: Human cytomegalovirus open reading frame US28 encodes a functional beta-chemokine receptor. J Biol Chem 1994;269:28539–28542.
44 Billstrom MA, Johnson GL, Avdi NJ, Worthen GS: Intracellular signaling by the chemokine receptor US28 during human cytomegalovirus infection. J Virol 1998;72:5535–5544.
45 Pleskoff O, Treboute C, Brelot A, Heveker N, Seman M, Alizon M: Identification of a chemokine receptor encoded by human cytomegalovirus as a cofactor for HIV-1 entry. Science 1997;276: 1874–1878.
46 Pleskoff O, Treboute C, Alizon M: The cytomegalovirus-encoded chemokine receptor US28 can enhance cell-cell fusion mediated by different viral proteins. J Virol 1998;72:6389–6397.
47 Margulies BJ, Browne H, Gibson W: Identification of the human cytomegalovirus G protein-coupled receptor homologue encoded by UL33 in infected cells and enveloped virus particles. Virology 1996; 225:111–125.

48 Rawlinson WD, Farrell HE, Barrell BG: Analysis of the complete DNA sequence of murine cytomegalovirus. J Virol 1996;70:8833–8849.
49 Davis-Poynter NJ, Lynch DM, Vally H, Shellam GR, Rawlinson WD, Barrell BG, Farrell HE: Identification and characterization of a G protein-coupled receptor homolog encoded by murine cytomegalovirus. J Virol 1997;71:1521–1529.
50 MacDonald MR, Li XY, Virgin HW IV: Late expression of a beta-chemokine homolog by murine cytomegalovirus. J Virol 1997;71:1671–1678.
51 Yamanishi K, Okuno T, Shiraki K, Takahashi M, Kondo T, Asano Y, Kurata T: Identification of human herpesvirus-6 as a causal agent for exanthem subitum. Lancet 1988;i:1065–1067.
52 Soldan SS, Berti R, Salem N, Secchiero P, Flamand L, Calabresi PA, Brennan MB, Maloni HW, McFarland HF, Lin HC, Patnaik M, Jacobson S: Association of human herpes virus 6 (HHV-6) with multiple sclerosis: Increased IgM response to HHV-6 early antigen and detection of serum HHV-6 DNA. Nat Med 1997;3:1394–1397.
53 Singh N, Carrigan DR: Human herpesvirus-6 in transplantation: An emerging pathogen. Ann Intern Med 1996;124:1065–1071.
54 Salahuddin SZ, Ablashi DV, Markham PD, Josephs SF, Sturzenegger S, Kaplan M, Halligan G, Biberfeld P, Wong-Staal F, Kramarksy B: Isolation of a new virus, HBLV, in patients with lymphoproliferative disorders. Science 1986;234:596–601.
55 Takahashi K, Sonoda S, Higashi K, Kondo T, Takahashi H, Takahashi M, Yamanishi K: Predominant CD4 T-lymphocyte tropism of human herpesvirus 6-related virus. J Virol 1989;63:3161–3163.
56 Levy JA, Ferro F, Lennette ET, Oshiro L, Poulin L: Characterization of a new strain of HHV-6 (HHV-6SF) recovered from the saliva of an HIV-infected individual. Virology 1990;178:113–121.
57 He J, McCarthy M, Zhou Y, Chandran B, Wood C: Infection of primary human fetal astrocytes by human herpesvirus 6. J Virol 1996;70:1296–1300.
58 Levy JA, Ferro F, Greenspan D, Lennette ET: Frequent isolation of HHV-6 from saliva and high seroprevalence of the virus in the population. Lancet 1990;335:1047–1050.
59 Gompels UA, Nicholas J, Lawrence G, Jones M, Thomson BJ, Martin ME, Efstathiou S, Craxton M, Macaulay HA: The DNA sequence of human herpesvirus-6: Structure, coding content, and genome evolution. Virology 1995;209:29–51.
60 Isegawa Y, Ping Z, Nakano K, Sugimoto N, Yamanishi K: Human herpesvirus 6 open reading frame U12 encodes a functional beta-chemokine receptor. J Virol 1998;72:6104–6112.
61 Ablashi DV, Berneman ZN, Kramarsky B, Asano Y, Choudhury S, Pearson GR: Human herpesvirus-7 (HHV-7). In Vivo 1994;8:549–554.
62 Nicholas J: Determination and analysis of the complete nucleotide sequence of human herpesvirus. J Virol 1996;70:5975–5989.
63 Porter CD, Blake NW, Cream JJ, Archard LC: Molluscum contagiosum virus. Mol Cell Biol Hum Dis Ser 1992;1:233–257.
64 Gottlieb SL, Myskowski PL: Molluscum contagiosum. Int J Dermatol 1994;33:453–461.
65 Senkevich TG, Bugert JJ, Sisler JR, Koonin EV, Darai G, Moss B: Genome sequence of a human tumorigenic poxvirus: Prediction of specific host response-evasion genes. Science 1996;273:813–816.
66 Krathwohl MD, Hromas R, Brown DR, Broxmeyer HE, Fife KH: Functional characterization of the C-C chemokine-like molecules encoded by molluscum contagiosum virus types 1 and 2. Proc Natl Acad Sci USA 1997;94:9875–9880.
67 Damon I, Murphy PM, Moss B: Broad-spectrum chemokine antagonistic activity of a human poxvirus chemokine homolog. Proc Natl Acad Sci USA 1998;95:6403–6407.
68 Clark-Lewis I, Kim KS, Rajarathnam K, Gong JH, Dewald B, Moser B, Baggiolini M, Sykes BD: Structure-activity relationships of chemokines. J Leukoc Biol 1995;57:703–711.
69 McFadden G, Graham K: Modulation of cytokine networks by poxviruses: The myxoma virus model. Semin Virol 1994;5:421–429.
70 Upton C, Mossman K, McFadden G: Encoding of a homologue of the IFN-γ receptor by myxoma virus. Science 1992;258:1369–1372.

71 Graham KA, Lalani AS, Macen JL, Ness TL, Barry M, Liu LY, Lucas A, Clark-Lewis I, Moyer RW, McFadden G: The T1/35kDa family of poxvirus-secreted proteins bind chemokines and modulate leukocyte influx into virus-infected tissues. Virology 1997;229:12–24.
72 Smith CA, Smith TD, Smolak PJ, Friend D, Hagen H, Gerhart M, Park L, Pickup DJ, Torrance D, Mohler K, Schooley K, Goodwin RG: Poxvirus genomes encode a secreted, soluble protein that preferentially inhibits beta-chemokine activity yet lacks sequence homology to known chemokine receptors. Virology 1997;236:316–327.
73 Cao JX, Gershon PD, Black DN: Sequence analysis of HindIII Q2 fragment of capripoxvirus reveals a putative gene encoding a G-protein-coupled chemokine receptor homologue. Virology 1995;209:207–212.

Johnny T. Stine, ICOS Corporation, 22021 20th Ave SE, Bothell, WA 98021 (USA)
Tel. +1 425 485 1900/ext 4419, Fax +1 425 485 1961, E-Mail jstine@icos.com

Mantovani A (ed): Chemokines.
Chem Immunol. Basel, Karger, 1999, vol 72, pp 181–201

Strategies to Interfere with the Chemokine Network in Disease

Timothy N.C. Wells, Amanda E.I. Proudfoot, Christine A. Power

Serono Pharmaceutical Research Institute, Geneva, Switzerland

Chemokines were originally isolated based on their ability to selectively attract and activate different populations of leukocytes. From early on, it was seen that being able to interfere with the way in which these proteins can act on cells could offer a means to finding novel classes of selective anti-inflammatory compounds. In 1996, chemokine receptors were identified as the coreceptors for fusion of HIV strains with human cells, and therefore chemokine mimetics could also play a role in the pathology of HIV infection and AIDS, thus widening the disease perspective. The fact that chemokine receptors belong to the seven-transmembrane G-protein-coupled family completely revolutionized the interest in the chemokine area from the perspective of the pharmaceutical industry. The seven-transmembrane family of receptors have been a very fruitful area in terms of finding small molecule inhibitors which can modify the course of disease – many of the classic drugs of the 1970s and 1980s work by binding to structurally similar receptors. In this review we discuss the data supporting the idea that molecules which bind to chemokine receptors may lead to a change in disease status in inflammation or viral infection, and some of the different methods that have been used to find antagonists.

Chemokine Receptors and Their Ligands

Chemokines or chemoattractant cytokines are a large family of small proteins that are involved in both the routine leukocyte trafficking, and in the activation and recruitment of specific cell populations during disease. Ten years ago, little was known about the factors which might act as the traffic controllers to regulate cell recruitment to sites of inflammation. The purification of these proteins by classical methods led initially to the identification of interleukin-8 (IL-8) [1] and subsequently monocyte chemotactic protein-1 (MCP-1) [2]. It turned out that these proteins are very similar, in fact the three-dimensional structures are almost superimposable [3, 4]. Sequencing of the amino terminal ends showed different patterns of cysteine residues. In IL-8 the residues are separated by a single amino acid to form a CXC motif whereas in MCP-1 they are adjacent, and form a CC motif. This allowed their classification into two main subclasses depending on the spacing of the first two cysteines: the CXC or α-subclass and the CC or β-subclass. Recently two new subclasses have been identified, each with a single member to date: the C chemokine, lymphotactin [5], and the CX_3C chemokine, named either fractalkine [6] or neurotactin [7] by the groups who identified it. For a long time it was thought that the two main subclasses had separate activities, since the α-subclass principally activates neutrophils whilst the β-subclass activates the other leukocyte types such as T cells, eosinophils, monocytes/macrophages, basophils and dendritic cells. Thus the α-chemokines were thought to be associated with acute inflammation which is of short duration and is characteristically accompanied by plasma fluid exudates and neutrophil accumulation. Chronic inflammation is of longer duration and is characterized by a dense cellular infiltrate comprised of lymphocytes, eosinophils and monocytes/macrophages, and is thus associated with the β-chemokines. However, as studies on chemokine biology are elaborated, this rule is beginning to show deviations – the identification of the CXC receptor CXCR3 highly expressed on activated T cells [8], suggesting a potentially important role for CXC chemokines in chronic inflammation.

The chemokine family has exploded in complexity over the last few years. In the early years, new members of the family were purified from cell culture media by classical protein chemistry. Later, standard cDNA cloning techniques were used. More recently there has been a dramatic increase in the member of chemokines caused by the identification of chemokine-like sequences in expressed sequence tag collections. These are large numbers of DNA sequences obtained by sequencing clones at random from a cDNA library. The availability of this data over the World Wide Web, combined with the fact that chemokine open reading frames are typically around 100 amino acids, and ESTs are typically 300–500 bases long, has led to a rapid increase in the number of chemokines [9]. Currently some 26 CC chemokines, 17 CXC chemokines, 1 C chemokine as well as a CX_3C chemokine have been identified [see 10 for a review]. One problem with such a fast-moving field is that lists and alignments of chemokines are invariably out of date before they are even published.

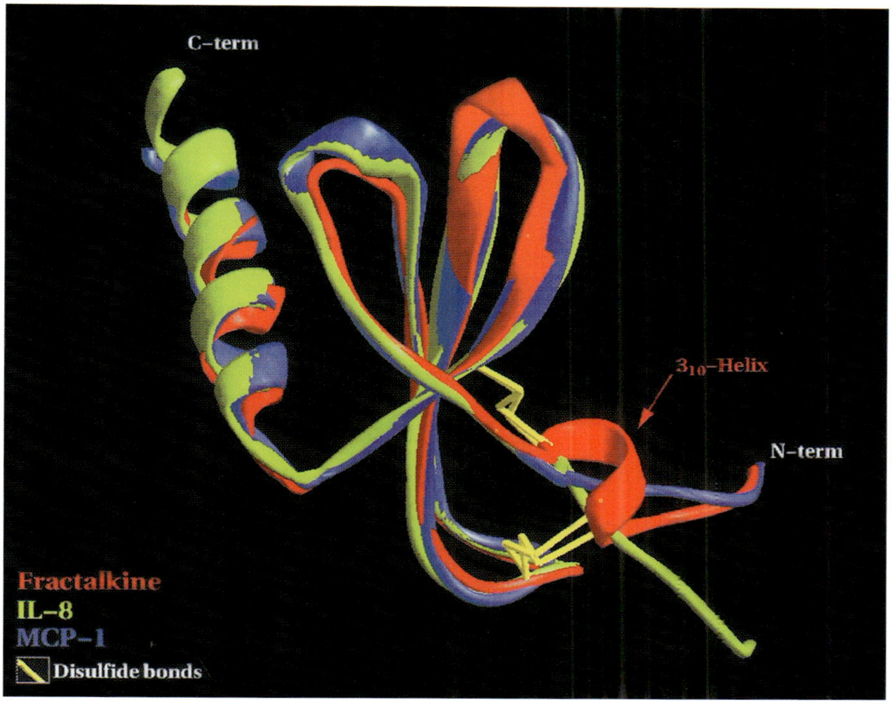

Fig. 1. Three-dimensional (3D) overlay of IL-8, MCP-1 and fractalkine. The similarity in these 3D structures is remarkable despite the low level of sequence identity. Comparison of the 3D structures of human IL-8 (green), MCP-1 (blue) and fractalkine (from the EST Z44443). The IL-8 structure is taken from the PDB entry 1IL-8 and the MCP-1 structure is from a model based on the NMR structure for MIP-1β (PDB entry 1HUM). The intrachain disulfide bonds are shown in yellow. A model for the chemokine domain of fractalkine was built using the Swiss-Model server. As can be seen, the three structures show a large degree of conservation of the overall fold of the monomeric protein. The additional amino acids in fractalkine are accommodated as a 3_{10}-helix between the two N-terminal cysteine residues. The model-building software, Swiss-model can also be accessed via the World Wide Web at http://www.expasy.ch/swissmod/swiss-model.html (see Wells and Peitsch [9] for details).

An automated web server in Japan (http://cytokine.medic.kumamoto-u.ac.jp/CFC/CK/chemokine.html) gives a regularly updated list of sequences along with their accession numbers, and also their genomic localization if known. The structural identity of the different chemokines is remarkable (see fig. 1), even though there is often less than 20% sequence identify the overall structure of the protein in three dimensions is conserved. The protein similarities of chemokines are shown in figure 2.

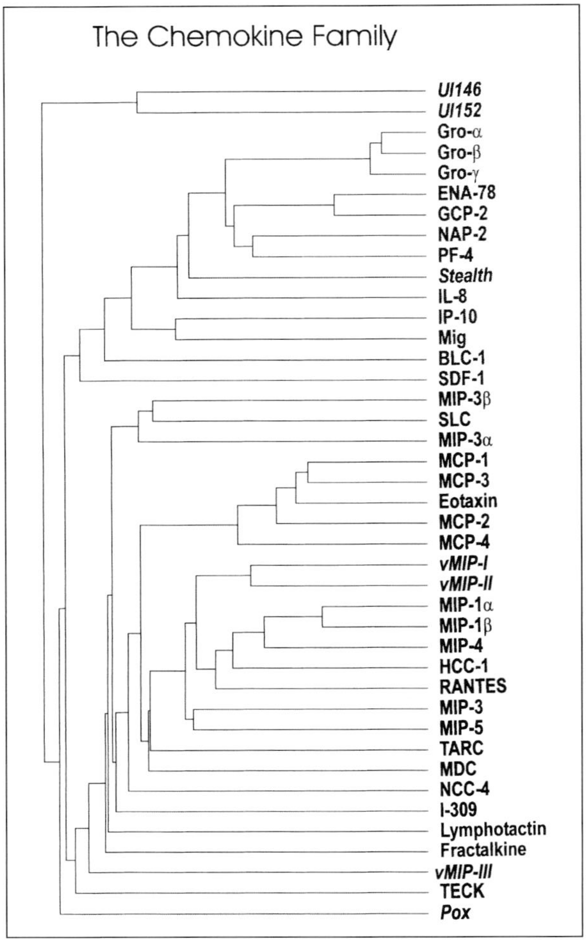

Fig. 2. The chemokine family: dendrogram showing the similarities between the human and virally encoded chemokine protein sequences. The sequences cluster in terms of the level of identity pairs of amino acids. The further to the right that the branch points are shown on the diagram, the more similar the two proteins are.

The availability of many more new ligands over the past four years has meant that a number of new receptors have now been formally identified. Many cDNAs which code for molecules similar to chemokine receptors were cloned during the early 1990s using reverse transcriptase-PCR strategies, with degenerate primers. The challenge over the past few years has been to identify the correct ligand. The pharmacology of the receptors has been reviewed extensively and elsewhere in this book – but at the time of writing there are

Table 1. Human chemokine receptors identified to date

Receptor	Ligands	Main cell type	Accession code (human)	Reference	Accession code (murine)
CXCR1	IL-8	Neutrophils	P25024	Holmes et al., 1991	
CXCR2	IL-8, NAP-2, Groα, ENA-78	Neutrophils	P25025	Murphy et al., 1991	P35343
CXCR3	IP-10 MIG, I-TAC	Activated T cells (TH1)	P49682	Loetscher et al., 1996; Cole et al., 1998	AF045146
CXCR4	SDF	Naive T cells, B cells	P30991	Bleul et al., 1996; Oberlin et al., 1996	P70658
CCR1	MCP-3, RANTES, MIP-1α	Activated T cells, monocytes, eosinophils, DCs	P32446	Neote et al., 1993; Gao et al., 1993	P51675
CCR2	MCP-1, -2, -3, -4, -5	Monocytes, macrophages, activated T cells	P41597	Charo et al., 1994	P51683
CCR3	Eotaxin, MCP-3, -4 RANTES	Eosinophils, basophils, activated T cells (TH2)	P51677	Ponath et al., 1996	P51676
CCR4	TARC, MDC, MIP-1α, RANTES, MCP-1	Activated T cells (TH2), basophils, platelets	P51679	Power et al., 1995; Imai et al., 1997	P51680
CCR5	MIP-1β, RANTES, MIP-1α	Activated T cells, monocyte/macrophages, DCs	P51681	Samson et al., 1996	P51682
CCR6	MIP-3α	DCs, T cells	P51684	Baba et al., 1997; Power et al., 1997; Greaves et al., 1997	
CCR7	MIP-3β, SLC	B cells T cells	P32248	Yoshida et al. 1997; Campbell et al., 1998	P47774
CCR8	I-309	Monocytes, macrophages	P51685	Tiffany et al., 1997	P56484
CCR9	CC chemokines	T, macrophages, monocyte	Y12815	Nibbs et al., 1998	Y12879
Duffy antigen	IL-8, Groα, RANTES, MCP-1	Erythrocytes	Q16300	Neote et al., 1993	
CX_3CR1	Fractalkine (neurotactin)	NK cells, CD8 T cells	P49238	Imai et al., 1997	
XCR1	Lymphotactin	T cells	P46094	Yoshida et al., 1998	

published reports of 5 human CXC chemokine receptors, 9 CC chemokine receptors, the CX3C chemokine receptor, Duffy antigen, and various murine and virally encoded chemokine receptors. (The reader is referred to Wells et al. [10] for a recent review; the data are summarized in table 1).

The Problem of Selectivity

One of the initial hopes for the use of chemokine antagonists in inflammatory disease was that they would be able to selectively control the activation of individual groups of leukocytes – and therefore offer a distinct advantage over currently available therapy. As more and more receptors have been identified, then the number of chemokines which can be bound by each receptor has also increased. This has led to the suggestion by some groups that in fact there is simply too much redundancy in the chemokine network. That is to say that since for the majority of the players any one chemokine can bind several receptors, and most receptors bind several chemokines, then the disruption of any particular ligand pair interaction will have very little effect on a given inflammatory disease state.

This is still an overly pessimistic viewpoint for a number of reasons. First, most of the ligand binding data that is discussed is obtained from in vitro experiments, where receptors are expressed at very high levels on the surface, often 10–100 times higher than is actually seen in primary cell types. Little data is available as to how this overexpression effects selectivity. Second, the cell context may well be important – since it defines which G-proteins are present, and they in turn may alter the conformation of the receptor. Different cell backgrounds have in fact given conflicting results, as is well demonstrated by the ligand binding profile of one of the CC receptors, CCR4. When this receptor was originally cloned in our laboratory and expressed in oocytes, it was activated by RANTES, MIP-1α and MCP-1 [11]. RANTES and MIP-1α were shown to bind to CCR4 when expressed in HL60 cells [12]. Recently other laboratories have shown that CCR4 is in fact the receptor for TARC [13] and MDC. Third, although a seven-transmembrane receptor may bind several ligands with equal potency in equilibrium binding assays, there may still be one ligand which is capable of competing away all the others [14, 15]. One explanation of this phenomenon requires a slow conformational change of the receptor ligand complex. Data showing similar effects has been reported in the chemokine area [T. Schwartz, pers. commun.], but since there are relatively few groups doing all of the homologous and heterologous competition experiments, the data in this area are still relatively limited. Fourth, although in vitro the receptor and ligand may bind, in vivo they have to be expressed in the same place and at the same time. Thus it is clear that the control of both the ligand and receptor expression is extremely important, and at least for the receptors this question has largely been neglected. However, the pioneering work of Loetscher et al. [16], showing that CCR1 and CCR2 were upregulated in the presence of IL-2, clearly demonstrated the importance that cytokines play in the chemokine system. Another example is that the proinflammatory cytokine IFNγ, upregulates the CC chemokine receptors CCR1 and CCR3 on neutrophils, a cell type previously thought to only be activated by CXC chemokines [17]. Furthermore it is not well defined in vivo how much presentation by glycosaminoglycans alters the pharmacokinetics of the formation and destruction of chemokine gradients, but these are essential questions and are the subject of much active research. The work in this area is discussed below. Finally, although chemokine antagonists (or agonists) need to be potent, and selective in the sense that they do not bind to other distantly related seven-transmembrane receptors, it is far from clear what the optimal receptor binding profile for a chemokine therapeutic in any given disease area is. For example, in asthma it may be better to have a single compound which can antagonize both CCR3 and CCR1, both of which are expressed in the eosinophil, the cell type believed to play a major role in the pathology of this disease.

Validation of Chemokines as Targets

One of the key questions in drug discovery is to make sure that as far as possible the target is validated – in other words that there is sufficient data to support the idea that altering the particular receptor/ligand interaction would alter the progression of a disease. In many cases it may be clear that a particular receptor/ligand system plays a role in the development of the disease process or an animal model of disease. However, it is still important to have as much information as possible that modifying a target will actually have an effect on the progression of the disease. Clearly, this process of validation has many levels, the ultimate being that of testing a potential molecule in patients with the disease (the so-called 'proof of principle in man'). However, before attaining this level of validation, it is important to obtain as much information as possible in vivo from animal models that are relevant to the diseases being studied. In the chemokine area there is now much data which strongly suggests that chemokines are valid targets to interfere with the development of pathology. The first step is to clearly demonstrate that the chemoattractant effects of chemokines that are observed in vitro, can also be seen in vivo. For example, the eosinophil chemoattractant eotaxin, which was originally purified from BAL of allergen-sensitized animals, causes eosinophil migration in chemotaxis assays and also to the site of injection into guinea pig skin in vivo [18]. However, although RANTES is clearly an eosinophil chemoattractant in vitro, injection intradermally does not always result in recruitment of eosinophils to the site of injection in nonsensitized animals, but requires presensitization of the animals [19]. In man, intradermal injections of RANTES into nonallergic and allergic patients showed significant eosinophil recruitment occurring only in allergic patients 6 h after injection [20]. Similar results can also be produced using mice that have been genetically manipulated to overexpress a chemokine. Here the pattern of tissue distribution directed by the expression vector is important in determining the pathology. Mice overexpressing MCP-1 in several organs show specific monocyte infiltration [21]. However, when MCP-1 expression was directed to the pancreas, although the mice developed a chronic monocytic infiltrate, insulinitis did not progress. MCP-1 on its own appears to be sufficient to elicit cellular migration, but not inflammation [22].

A second line of validation can come from animals in which the gene either for the chemokine or the receptor has been deleted. This type of study addresses the question of redundancy in vivo – the fear that blockade of a particular chemokine/receptor pair will be ineffective because there are other molecules which can carry the 'inflammatory signal' so to speak. Deletion of the CXCR2 homologue in mice showed impaired neutrophil recruitment upon infection [23]. Deletion of CCR1 again had a normal phenotype, although the mice showed disordered myeloid progenitor cell distribution and trafficking [24]. However, these mice showed impaired immune responses when stressed by exposure to pathogens. A human equivalent to the murine deletion experiments exists in approximately 1% of the population, who carry a 32 base pair deletion in the CCR5 gene. This deletion, Δ32-CCR5, prevents any functional surface expression of the receptor, and their 'phenotype' appears very normal, without any immune defects, and with an added inestimable advantage of being highly resistant to HIV infection.

In most fields of cytokine biology, validation of the importance of a given receptor in a disease model may also come from studies using blocking monoclonal antibodies in various animal models of disease. In the chemokine area, work has been limited by the availability of good blocking monoclonal antibodies – seven-transmembrane receptors are notoriously difficult to raise antibodies against since they have very little protein exposed on the extracellular surface. Such antibodies are now becoming available – so we should expect to see more antibody validation data over the next couple of years. Antibodies have the main advantage that they mimic therapy much more closely – since they are given as a therapeutic injection. It can always be argued with receptor knockout mice that they have adjusted their chemokine network to make up for the lack of the particular receptor. Clearly, in the future, knockout mice with inducible promoters will be much more important in the study of disease pathology. In the absence of antibodies, much of our understanding of the role of breaking the chemokine network may have on the progression of a given disease model comes from studies with modified chemokines – these are discussed below.

Searching for Small Molecules – Classic Receptor Blockade

Searching for small molecule antagonists of chemokine receptors has been a highly active area of pharmaceutical research in the last few years. The approaches taken by many groups are similar – using solid phase assays with recombinant receptors, radiolabelled chemokines and automated assay systems [25]. Using receptors present in membranes from cells which express functional chemokine receptors at high levels, it is possible to screen some 10,000 molecules per day to look for inhibition of binding. There has been a lot of debate about the type of molecules that are screened in this manner. Early screening experiments used compounds which had been shown to be inactive in other assays – a random approach, which is only possible in organizations having relatively large collections of compounds. Even in large companies, this approach may prove to be self-limiting, since radioligand binding assays typically cost USD 1–2 per sample, which limits the number of compounds which can be screened purely on economic grounds. The development of combinatorial chemistry in the early 1990s meant that focused sets of molecules could be screened. Focused sets of molecules can be made based on templates or chemical themes, which are known to occur in small molecules which are active against seven-transmembrane receptors – for example benzodiazepines or diphenylmethylenes. This approach has been far more successful, although it does raise the philosophical question as to where novel templates will arise from in the future.

Within the cytokine world there has been much debate as to whether small molecule antagonists of cytokine receptors would ever be found [26]. For cytokines such as IL-1, IL-2 and IL-5, large high throughput screening campaigns were run in the early 1990s by a number of different companies using several different formats, but with disappointingly few results, none of which have so far been reported to have clear activity in cell-based assays. The best explanation for this failure is that when a cytokine and a receptor bind, the interaction surface between the two proteins is relatively large [27]. Unfortunately, the molecules screened typically have a molecular weight of <500 (which is generally a requirement if the molecule is to be orally available). Such small molecules are unlikely to be able to cover all of the receptor/ligand binding surface on a receptor. Under these circumstances, success or failure will depend on just how localized the key residues in the receptor involved in ligand binding really are. Recent progress in search for cytokine antagonists and agonists supports this analysis. Dimeric peptides which can agonize and antagonize cytokine receptors have been found with nanomolar potency, but relatively high molecular weight ($>2,000$) [28, 29]. More recently, small molecule mimetics of granulocyte colony-stimulating factor (G-CSF) have been found with micromolar potency, in a reasonably small molecule [30].

With this relatively difficult history in mind, there was much excitement when the first real small molecule inhibitors of the IL-8 receptor, CXCR2, were reported [31]; the patents had appeared earlier, and are reviewed in Ponath [32]. SB 225002 is a urea-based inhibitor of CXCR2, which has nanomolar potency, and also a high degree of selectivity over CXCR1. According to the SmithKline group, it is selectively able to block neutrophil margination in rabbit models of inflammation, suggesting that CXCR2 plays a key role in this process. These data are somewhat at odds with previous data in this model, which suggest CXCR1 as the key receptor [33] – however, it does serve to highlight how useful selective small molecule antagonists are going to be in dissecting out the molecular mechanisms of many inflammatory diseases.

Other groups have produced peptides which have biological activity in blocking the binding of IL-8 to its receptor, however, their usefulness as starting points in drug design are limited. A report of the peptide AcRRWWWCR-NH2 [34] has been published, although this sequence is full of amino acids which are known to bind strongly to membranes, and therefore the effect is not likely to be specific. As discussed in the review by Ponath [32], a 15 amino acid peptide based on IL-8 has also been shown to have limited activity, but this is much less attractive as a starting point for small molecule design than the urea series published by SmithKline.

There are three reports of antagonists for CXCR4 – one of the coreceptors for HIV-1: AMD3100, a bicyclam, blocks infection of PBMC by T-tropic strains, and is a competitive inhibitor for SDF-1α [35, 36]; a molecule isolated from *Limulus polyphemus*, which also has HIV-1 inhibitory activity [37], and another peptide derivative acting through CXCR4 was identified through its antiviral activity [38]. However, the data that individuals carrying the homozygous Δ32-CCR5 allele are relatively resistant to infection, and at least the heterozygotes have a longer survival time [39], implies that the key receptor to block to prevent disease progression in HIV infection may well be CCR5. This conclusion is tempered by the fact that once Δ32-CCR5 individuals are infected, progression to death is more rapid [40]. The debate as to which is the key receptor to block in HIV infection will of course finally only be solved in the clinic. Recent reports presented at the World AIDS Conference (Geneva 1998), indicated that AMD3100 is in early clinical testing; however, there is still no publicly available data on small molecule antagonists of CCR5.

The only data on small molecule antagonists of CC chemokine receptors comes from the patent literature, and so far no data has appeared in peer reviewed literature. Takeda has claimed nanomolar inhibitors of CCR1 [32]. The compounds are based on diphenylmethylene scaffolds, a motif found in many molecules binding tightly to seven-transmembrane receptors. It will be interesting to see how selective these compounds are – whether they also bind to CCR3 – which is closely related to CCR1 in terms of primary sequence. It is also important to point out that there is no clear consensus on what receptor binding profile is needed for a molecule to be potentially useful in any given disease area. The work on modified chemokines suggests that being able to selectively bind more than one type of chemokine receptor may be an advantage.

Lessons from Modified Chemokines

Whilst searching for small molecule inhibitors of chemokine receptors, the field had a useful helping hand in understanding their potential pharmacology. Many groups showed that modification of the amino terminus of some chemokines could lead to a change in their activity, leading to partial agonists and even antagonists.

Truncation of RANTES, MCP-1 and MCP-3 results in proteins that have lost their capacity to activate their receptors, but are still able to bind to the receptors, thus generating receptor antagonists that compete with the active proteins thereby inhibiting their action [41]. Removal of 8 residues from the amino terminal region of MCP-1 forms an antagonist protein [42]. Administration of the MCP-1(9-76) protein to mice which have a genetic predisposition to an arthritic condition very similar to human rheumatoid arthritis causes a significant reduction in the onset of arthritis, joint swelling and the histopathology that typifies this condition [43]. Administration of the antagonist even 12 days after disease onset still causes a reduction in joint swelling. The macrophage is thought to be a major player in arthritic inflammation, along with the T cell which is involved in all inflammatory processes. MCP-1 is certainly believed to be a major chemokine for the activation of this cell type, and acts through CCR2, suggesting that blocking CCR2 is the most effective means of preventing the cellular infiltration responsible for the arthritic inflammatory condition.

When we expressed RANTES in the bacterial host *Escherichia coli*, the initiating methionine was retained, and the resultant protein, Met-RANTES, is a functional antagonist of RANTES receptors with nanomolar potency in its ability to inhibit both RANTES and MIP-1α-induced effects in vitro [44]. In vitro Met-RANTES will prevent the recruitment and activation of a variety of cell types. In vivo, the results are also impressive. Met-RANTES treatment in the collagen-induced murine model of arthritis causes delay in the disease onset, reduction of severity and the number of affected paws, but this protective effect is only achieved if the antagonist is administered prior to the onset of the arthritic condition [45]. Another autoimmune inflammatory condition, glomerulonephritis, is also associated with macrophage accumulation, as is arthritis, both of which are T-cell-mediated. Lloyd et al. [46] have performed a comparative study using the receptor antagonist Met-RANTES and a monoclonal anti-MCP-1 antibody. This study showed that whilst Met-RANTES caused a significant decrease in macrophage and T-cell infiltration, as did the anti-MCP-1 antibody, only the latter was able to prevent the fibrosis typical of this disease.

We have also shown that administration of a receptor antagonist can have even more profound effects [47]. In the ovalbumin-sensitized murine model of airways inflammation that is very reminiscent of human asthma, treatment with Met-RANTES almost totally abrogates cellular accumulation in the airways. This is achieved with low doses of antagonist, with a dose of 1 μg per mouse (0.04 mg/kg) resulting in greater than 95% inhibition of eosinophil accumulation. Similarly the accumulation of T cells is reduced by 80–90% of the control animals. Even more striking though is the inhibition of broncho-hyperreactivity and mucus secretion – both hallmarks of asthma. The sensitized animals show a marked hyperactivity when challenged with methacholine, as is the case in human asthmatic patients, whereas the Met-RANTES-treated animals were far less reactive. Blockage of the airways with mucus in asthmatics is often fatal, and the sensitized mice secrete significant amounts of mucus as a result of their induced inflammation – again a dose of 1 μg per mouse completely inhibited this process. This contrasts with work using administration of monoclonal antibodies which neutralize chemokine ligands in models of airways inflammation and which significantly reduce (by approximately 50–70%) but do not eliminate eosinophil recruitment into the lungs. When Met-RANTES was used in comparison with neutralizing antibodies against chemokines that were demonstrated as being upregulated in this model, the treatment with Met-RANTES caused the greatest inhibition of eosinophil recruitment [48]. Which receptor is blocked by the Met-RANTES is not clear at this stage – since it has pleiotropic effects – working on CCR1, CCR3, CCR4 and CCR5, but the protein has had clear effects both in lung and skin models of allergy [49].

Taken together, these results lend support to the notion that despite the apparent redundancy in the chemokine family with an alarming large number of ligands, a relatively small number of receptors and a large amount of promiscuity as determined by receptor binding studies, receptor antagonism yields impressive results in eliminating inflammation. However, there still remains a considerable amount of work to precisely identify which receptors are upregulated and on which cell type and in which inflammatory disease – a formidable task that requires the availability not only of animal models, but of human biopsies from diseased tissues and suitable reagents for their analyses.

Chemokine Receptors and the HIV Connection

As has been reviewed elsewhere in this book – in the spring of 1996 the chemokine world was taken by surprise as it found itself inexorably fused with a hitherto unrelated domain – HIV virology (for more extensive information the reader is referred to Berger [50] for a review). Whilst the absolute requirement for cell surface expression of CD4 for the recognition of the HIV-1 virus for its host target cell had been irrefutably proven for over a decade, it was equally irrefutably proven that this molecule was not sufficient for viral fusion and cell entry. Following the observation that RANTES, MIP-1α and MIP-1β inhibited HIV infection [51], and the cloning of CXCR4 as the T-tropic virus coreceptor, CCR5 was identified as the coreceptor used by M-tropic strains [52]. For certain strains the chemokine receptor alone is sufficient for fusion which can occur in the absence of CD4 [53].

Once the chemokine receptors had been identified as being essential for HIV infectivity, their possibility as a target for therapeutic intervention stimulated research in most pharmaceutical companies as well as numerous academic laboratories. Two theories of how to interfere with the HIV virus/chemokine receptor interaction were proposed. First, an agonist that induces receptor internalization thereby removing the receptor from the cell surface thus eliminating the possibility of receptor usage for fusion and infection. Second, that the ligands simply sterically block the virus/receptor interaction as a competitive receptor antagonist [54]. The first scenario is supported by the fact that the CCR5 ligands prevent infection by M-tropic HIV-1, and that the CXCR4 ligand, SDF-1α, prevents infection by T-tropic strains [55, 56]. However, there have been reports of increased infectivity in the presence of RANTES [57]. Evidence that the second hypothesis was correct came from the result that the chemokine receptor antagonists RANTES(9-68), Met-RANTES and AOP-RANTES, a chemically modified form of RANTES, were capable of inhibiting HIV infectivity [58, 59]. However only AOP-RANTES was more potent in preventing infection than RANTES itself and moreover, it was capable of preventing the infection of primary macrophages [59].

Initially the potency of AOP-RANTES was thought to be due to its increased affinity for the CCR5 receptor, and although this may still remain essentially true, it has recently been observed to have another mode of action – inhibition of receptor recycling [60]. Several reports have appeared correlating receptor downregulation with inhibition of HIV infectivity, lending strength to the first hypothesis emitted above for the inhibition of HIV cell entry. SDF-1α has been shown to induce downregulation of CXCR4 [61, 62] as has RANTES for CCR5. Surprisingly the receptor antagonists RANTES(9-68) [61] and AOP-RANTES [60] also induce receptor downregulation. These antagonist proteins have been reported to be devoid of receptor activation resulting in chemotaxis, yet since receptor internalization requires the interaction of an agonist with the receptor, these proteins must still be capable of triggering the endocytic signalling pathway. The capacity of chemokine receptors to endocytose does not appear to be directly linked to their role as functioning as coreceptors for viral entry since mutations in the receptor that abrogate internalization do not prevent them from functioning as coreceptors [61]. Taken together, it appears that both mechanisms, competitive inhibition that prevents the virus from binding to the chemokine receptor, and the removal of the receptor from the cell surface, play a role in preventing viral infection.

Glycosaminoglycans – Blocking the Presentation of Chemokines

As we discussed above, the large number of chemokines, and receptors, and the way in which an individual receptor binds many overlapping chemokines, raises the question of whether there is too much redundancy in the chemokine system. From a drug design perspective this question is critical – since if the consequence of one receptor being blocked, is that another receptor type can take over the same role, then chemokine receptors would cease to be interesting therapeutic targets. However, there are several levels of control in the body which result in a greater degree of specificity: oligomerization on cell surfaces may be one of these. It is a well-known fact that chemokines bind to glycosaminoglycans (GAGs) [63, 64], a property that has been used extensively in their purification on heparin Sepharose columns. This property of binding to GAGs would certainly be essential for their immobilization on endothelial cells lining the vessel walls. This is one place where they presumably create the chemotactic gradient in order to fulfill their principal role, directing cellular trafficking of leukocytes. The binding of chemokines to heparin induces oligomerization [65]. The K_D for this oligomerization ranged from 1 to 25 nM, for the four chemokines tested, RANTES, MIP-1α, MCP-1 and IL-8, indicating a sensitive mechanism of creating elevated localized concentrations. Furthermore, it has been shown that chemokines display a selectivity for different GAGs [64], and that certain chemokines such as RANTES show two orders of magnitude difference in their K_D values for GAGs such as heparin and chondroitin sulfate [66]. This selectivity in the binding of chemokines to GAGs could thus introduce a level of control whereby oligomerization on GAGs could specifically favor an elevated local concentration of a certain chemokine. In inflammatory disorders this could contribute to the recruitment of certain leukocytes since cell surface expression of GAGs can be modified. An example is the increased cell surface chondroitin sulfate on atherosclerotic plaque tissues [67, 68]. Thus, whilst in solution, where the dissociation constants for ligand dimerization are several log units above the concentrations required for biological activity and receptor binding [69, 70], the association constants on the surface of cells may well be in the physiological range. This opens up another possible way of getting small molecules to interfere with the chemokine system. If a small molecule can be made which interferes with the binding of chemokines to GAGs, the immobilized gradient of oligomerized chemokine, which drives the directed migration of the cell, would disappear. Although no such molecules have been found to date, two further lines of evidence support the concept. First, the observation that among its many activities in the clinic, low-molecular-weight heparin is indeed used as an anti-inflammatory. Second, we have shown that molecules as small as disaccharides can interfere with the binding of chemokines to GAGs, and that this binding is not absolutely dependent on the number of charged interactions [71].

Did the Viruses Get to the Ideas First?

In their attempts to evade the host immune system, and create a better environment for themselves, mammalian viruses have evolved a wide range of strategies. These have included the expression of many cytokines, chemokines and chemokine receptors (recently reviewed in Wells and Schwartz [72]). The attempts to understand the mode of action of these virally encoded cytokines will clearly enhance our understanding of immunology, and may lead to therapeutic molecules.

Viral chemokine receptors were first identified in human cytomegalovirus – where the US28 open reading frame was shown to be a functional receptor for CC chemokines but not CXC chemokines, such as IL-8 [73]. Links with the expression of the viral receptor in disease such as atherosclerosis [74] remain speculative, although attractive hypotheses. However, studies on murine herpesviruses indicate that the virally encoded seven-transmembrane receptors may have important roles in the life cycle of the virus in vivo. Deletion of the M33 gene, which encodes for a chemokine receptor-like orphan, shows that it plays an important role in the dissemination and growth of the virus in the salivary glands [75] – which are clearly important in the viral life cycle. The case of cytomegalovirus emphasizes the importance of working with primary strains of virus. Sequencing of the Toledo strain revealed a DNA segment of 13 kb, which was not present in other strains of the virus. This segment contains 19 open reading frames – some of which encode chemokines [76].

One hypothesis is that these genes are necessary for the ability of the virus to survive in vivo, but are not so important in vitro and therefore can be eliminated without altering viability.

The most intensely studied viral chemokines to date are those from Herpesvirus 8 [77, 78] which encoded three chemokines that show the highest similarity to human MIP-1α. Interestingly, the vMIP-II has been shown to be relatively promiscuous binding to both CC and CXC chemokine receptors. The protein is able to block infection of cells by HIV, but is most potent when CCR3 is being used as the coreceptor. In some assays, such as monocyte migration, vMIP-II has been shown to be a partial agonist [79], and on eosinophils appears to be a full agonist [78].

One final twist in the viral chemokine story is the identification of a soluble protein capable of binding chemokines with picomolar affinity, termed p35 protein [80]. This is presumably involved in antagonizing the activity of chemokines during viral infection, but in addition may offer insights into how small molecules that bind to chemokines, and inactivate them, may be designed. Clearly, if the virus uses both chemokine binding and chemokine mimetic strategies to evade and modulate the immune system, this indicates that both small molecule pharmaceuticals that attempt to alter both binding and modulate activity, may be useful. Direct use of either the p35 protein or the vMIP proteins in disease may be precluded by their inherent antigenicity. Although they are optimized to avoid stimulating a host antigenic response, these proteins could be likely to stimulate a response, upon repeated injection.

Conclusion

The recent increase in the number of chemokine receptors and ligands identified means that we are much closer now to having a complete picutre of the players that could be involved in the control of the immune system both in routine immunosurveillance and in inflammation. The availability of antibodies and engineered mice lacking key receptors, is now giving us clearer ideas about which receptors are important in which disease processes. Whilst we are refining these ideas, the typical pharmaceutical industry lead discovery laboratories are busy identifying small molecule antagonists, which so far have been shown to have effects mainly in vitro. Over the next few years, we should see an increase in the number of experiments reported where groups put these two strands of chemokine research together – and show activity of chemokine receptor agonist or antagonist in an animal model of disease. The work that we and others have reported using modified chemokines as protein receptor antagonists, and partial agonists, is already giving a flavor of what the future will look like.

Acknowledgments

We thank all our colleagues both in Geneva and elsewhere for helpful suggestions, and Nicole Gullu, and Marie-Christine Vuargnier for help in the final formatting.

References

1 Yoshimura T, Matsushima K, Tanaka S, Robinson EA, Appella E, Oppenheim JJ, Leonard EJ: Purification of a human monocyte-derived neutrophil chemotactic factor that has peptide sequence similarity to other host defense cytokines. Proc Natl Acad Sci USA 1987;84:9233.

2 Matsushima K, Larsen CG, DuBois CC, Oppenheim JJ: Purification and characterization of a novel monocyte chemotactic and activating factor produced by a human myelomonocytic cell line. J Exp Med 1989;169:1485.

3 Clore GM, Appella E, Yamada M, Matsushima K, Gronenborn AM: Three-dimensional structure of interleukin-8 in solution. Biochemistry 1990;29:1689.

4 Lubkowski J, Bujacz G, Boque L, Domaille PJ, Handel TM, Wlodawer A: The structure of MCP-1 in two crystal forms provides a rare example of variable quaternary interactions. Nat Struct Biol 1997; 4:64.

5 Kelner GS, Kennedy J, Bacon KB, Kleyensteuber S, Largaespada DA, Jenkins NA, Copeland NG, Bazan JF, Moore KW, Schall TJ: Lymphotactin: A cytokine that represents a new class of chemokine. Science 1994;266:1395.

6 Bazan JF, Bacon KB, Hardiman G, Wang W, Soo K, Rossi D, Greaves DR, Zlotnik A, Schall TJ: A new class of membrane-bound chemokine with a CX_3C motif. Nature 1997;385:640.

7 Pan Y, Lloyd C, Zhou H, Dolich S, Deeds J, Gonzalo JA, Vath J, Gosselin M, Ma J, Dussault B, Woolf E, Alperin G, Culpepper J, Gutierrez-Ramos JC, Gearing D: Neurotactin, a membrane-anchored chemokine upregulated in brain inflammation. Nature 1997;387:611.

8 Loetscher M, Gerber B, Loetscher P, Jones SA, Piali L, Clark-Lewis I, Baggiolini M, Moser B: Chemokine receptor specific for IP10 and mig: Structure, function, and expression in activated T-lymphocytes. J Exp Med 1996;184:963.

9 Wells TN, Peitsch MC: The chemokine information source: Identification and characterization of novel chemokines using the World Wide Web and expressed sequence tag databases. J Leukoc Biol 1997;61:545.

10 Wells TNC, Power CA, Proudfoot AEI: Definition, function and pathophysiological significance of chemokine receptors. Trends Pharmacol Sci 1998;19:376.

11 Power CA, Meyer A, Nemeth K, Bacon KB, Hoogewerf AJ, Proudfoot AE, Wells TN: Molecular cloning and functional expression of a novel CC chemokine receptor cDNA from a human basophilic cell line. J Biol Chem 1995;270:19495.

12 Hoogewerf A, Black D, Proudfoot AE, Wells TN, Power CA: Molecular cloning of murine CC CKR-4 and high affinity binding of chemokines to murine and human CC CKR-4. Biochem Biophys Res Commun 1996;218:337.

13 Imai T, Baba M, Nishimura M, Kakizaki M, Takagi S, Yoshie O: The T cell-directed CC chemokine TARC is a highly specific biological ligand for CC chemokine receptor 4. J Biol Chem 1997;272:15036.

14 Leff P, Scaramellini C, Law C, McKechnie K: A three-state receptor model of agonist action. Trends Pharmacol Sci 1997;18:355.

15 Maggi CA, Schwartz TW: The dual nature of the tachykinin NK1 receptor. Trands Pharmacol Sci 1997;18:351.

16 Loetscher P, Seitz M, Baggiolini M, Moser B: Interleukin-2 regulates CC chemokine receptor expression and chemotactic responsiveness in T lymphocytes. J Exp Med 1996;184:569.

17 Bonecchi R, Polentarutti N, Luini W, Borsatti A, Bernasconi S, Locati M, Power CA, Proudfoot AEI, Wells TNC, Mackay C, Mantovani A, Sozzani S: Upregulation of CCR1 and CCR3 and induction of chemotaxis to CC chemokines by interferon γ in human neutrophils. J Immunol 1999; 162:474–479.

18 Jose PJ, Griffiths-Johnson DA, Collins PD, Walsh DT, Moqbel R, Totty NF, Truong O, Hsuan JJ, Williams TJ: Eotaxin: A potent eosinophil chemoattractant cytokine detected in a guinea pig model of allergic airways inflammation. J Exp Med 1994;179:881.

19 Meurer R, van Riper G, Feeney W, Cunningham P, Hora D Jr, Springer MS, MacIntyre DE, Rosen H: Formation of eosinophilic and monocytic intradermal inflammatory sites in the dog by injection of human RANTES but not human monocyte chemoattractant protein 1, human macrophage inflammatory protein 1 alpha, or human interleukin 8. J Exp Med 1993;178:1913.

20 Beck LA, Dalke S, Leiferman KM, Bickel CA, Hamilton R, Rosen H, Bochner BS, Schleimer RP: Cutaneous injection of RANTES causes eosinophil recruitment: Comparison of nonallergic and allergic human subjects. J Immunol 1997;159:2962.

21 Rutledge BJ, Rayburn H, Rosenberg R, North RJ, Gladue RP, Corless CL, Rollins BJ: High level monocyte chemoattractant protein-1 expression in transgenic mice increases their susceptibility to intracellular pathogens. J Immunol 1995;155:4838.

22 Grewal IS, Rutledge BJ, Fiorillo JA, Gu L, Gladue RP, Flavell R, Rollins BJ: Transgenic monocyte chemoattractant protein-1 (MCP-1) in pancreatic islets produces monocyte-rich insulitis without diabetes: Abrogation by a second transgene expressing systemic MCP-1. J Immunol 1997;159:401.

23 Cacalano G, Lee J, Kikly K, Ryan AM, Pitts-Meek S, Hultgren B, Wood WI, Moore MW: Neutrophil and B cell expansion in mice that lack the murine IL-8 receptor homolog. Science 1994;265:682.

24 Gao JL, Wynn TA, Chang Y, Lee EJ, Broxmeyer HE, Cooper S, Tiffany HL, Westphal H, Kwon CJ, Murphy PM: Impaired host defense, hematopoiesis, granulomatous inflammation and type 1-type 2 cytokine balance in mice lacking CC chemokine receptor 1. J Exp Med 1997;185:1959.

25 Mellor GW, Fogarty SJ, O'Brien MS, Congreve M, Banks MN, Mills KM, Jefferies B, Houston JG: Searching for chemokine receptor binding antagonists by high throughput screening. J Biomolec Screen 1997;2:153.

26 McKinnon M, Proudfoot AEI, Wells TNC, Solari R: Strategies for the discovery of cytokine receptor antagonists. Drug News Perspect 1996;9:389.

27 Wells JA, De Vos AM: Hematopoietic receptor complexes. Annu Rev Biochem 1996;65:609–634.

28 Wrighton NC, Farrell FX, Chang R, Kashyap AK, Barbone FP, Mulcahy LS, Johnson DL, Barrett RW, Jolliffe LK, Dower WJ: Small peptides as potent mimetics of the protein hormone erythropoietin. Science 1998;273:458.

29 Cwirla SE, Balasubramanian P, Duffin DJ, Wagstrom CR, Gates CM, Singer SC, Davis AM, Tansik RL, Mattheakis LC, Boytos CM, Schatz PJ, Baccanari DP, Wrighton NC, Barrett RW, Dower WJ: Peptide agonist of the thrombopoietin receptor as potent as the natural cytokine. Science 1997;276:1696.

30 Tian S, Lamb P, King AG, Miller SG, Kessler L, Luengo JI, Averill LL, Johnson RK, Gleason JG, Pelus LM, Dillon SB, Rosen J: A small, nonpeptidyl mimic of granulocyte-colony-stimulating factor. Science 1998;281:257.

31 White JR, Lee JM, Young PR, Hertzberg RP, Jurewicz AJ, Chaikin MAW, Foley JJ, Martin LD, Griswold DE, Sarau HM: Identification of a potent, selective non-peptide CXCR2 antagonist that inhibits interleukin-8-induced neutrophil migration. J Biol Chem 1998;273:10095.

32 Ponath PD: Chemokine receptor antagonists: Novel therapeutics for inflammation and AIDS. Exp Opin Invest Drugs 1998;7:1–18.

33 Quan JM, Martin TR, Rosenberg GB, Foster DC, Whitmore TGR: Antibodies against the N-terminus of IL-8 receptor A inhibit neutrophil chemotaxis. Biochem Biophys Res Commun 1996;219:405.

34 Hayashi S, Kurdowska A, Miller EJ, Albright ME, Girten BE, Cohen AB: Synthetic hexa- and heptapeptides that inhibit IL-8 from binding to and activating human blood neutrophils. J Immunol 1995;154:814.

35 Schols D, Struyf S, Van DJ, Este JA, Henson G, De CE: Inhibition of T-tropic HIV strains by selective antagonization of the chemokine receptor CXCR4. J Exp Med 1997;186:1383.

36 Donzella GA, Schols D, Lin SW, Este JA, Nagashima KA, Maddon PJ, Allaway GP, Sakmar TP, Henson G, De Clercq E, Moore JP: AMD3100, a small molecule inhibitor of HIV-1 entry via the CXCR4 co-receptor. Nat Med 1998;4:72.

37 Murakami T, Nakajima T, Koyanagi N, Tachibana K, Fujii N, Tamamura H, Yoshida N, Waki M, Matsumoto A, Yoshie O, Kishimoto T, Yamamoto N, Nagasawa T: A small molecule CXCR4 inhibitor that blocks T cell line-tropic HIV-1 infection. J Exp Med 1997;186:1389.

38 Doranz BJ, Grovit FK, Sharron MP, Mao SH, Goetz MB, Daar E, Doms RW, Brien WA: A small-molecule inhibitor directed against the chemokine receptor CXCR4 prevents its use as an HIV-1 coreceptor. J Exp Med 1997;186:1395.

39 Paxton WA, Martin SR, Tse D, O'Brien TR, Skurnick J, VanDevanter NL, Padian N, Braun JF, Kotler DP, Wolinsky SM, Koup RA: Relative resistance to HIV-1 infection of CD4 lymphocytes from persons who remain uninfected despite multiple high-risk sexual exposure. Nat Med 1996;2:412.

40 Garred P, Eugen-Olsen J, Iversen AK, Benfield TL, Svejgaard A, Hofmann B: Dual effect of CCR5 delta 32 gene deletion in HIV-1-infected patients. Copenhagen AIDS Study Group. Lancet 1997; 349:1884.

41 Gong JH, Uguccioni M, Dewald B, Baggiolini M, Clark-Lewis I: RANTES and MCP-3 antagonists bind multiple chemokine receptors. J Biol Chem 1996;271:10521.

42 Gong JH, Clark-Lewis I: Antagonists of monocyte chemoattractant protein 1 identified by modification of functionally critical NH_2-terminal residues. J Exp Med 1995;181:631.

43 Gong JH, Ratkay LG, Waterfield JD, Clark LI: An antagonist of monocyte chemoattractant protein 1 (MCP-1) inhibits arthritis in the MRL-lpr mouse model. J Exp Med 1997;186:131.

44 Proudfoot AEI, Power CA, Hoogewerf AJ, Montjovent MO, Borlat F, Offord RE, Wells TN: Extension of recombinant human RANTES by the retention of the initiating methionine produces a potent antagonist. J Biol Chem 1996;271:2599.

45 Plater-Zyberk C, Hoogewerf AJ, Proudfoot AE, Power CA, Wells TN: Effect of a CC chemokine receptor antagonist on collagen induced arthritis in DBA/1 mice. Immunol Lett 1997;57:117.

46 Lloyd CM, Minto AW, Dorf ME, Proudfoot A, Wells TN, Salant DJ, Gutierrez-Ramos JC: RANTES and monocyte chemoattractant protein-1 (MCP-1) play an important role in the inflammatory phase of crescentic nephritis, but only MCP-1 is involved in crescent formation and interstitial fibrosis. J Exp Med 1997;185:1371.

47 Coyle AJ, Kips J, Hoogewerf AJ, Pauwels R, Tyers MD, Chvatchko Y, Power CA, Proudfoot AEI, Wells TNC: Upregulation of chemokine receptors in the airways after allergen provocation: Inhibition of airway inflammation and altered airway responsiveness by Met-RANTES, a chemokine receptor antagonist. J Clin Invest (submitted).

48 Gonzalo JA, Lloyd CM, Wen D, Albar JP, Wells TN, Proudfoot A, Martinez-A C, Dorf M, Bjerke T, Coyle AJ, Gutierrez-Ramos JC: The coordinated action of CC chemokines in the lung orchestrates allergic inflammation and airway hyperresponsiveness. J Exp Med 1998;188 157–167.

49 Teixeira MM, Wells TC, Lukacs NW, Proudfoot AI, Kunkel SL, Williams TJ, Hellewell PG: Chemokine-induced eosinophil recruitment – Evidence of a role for endogenous eotaxin in an in vivo allergy model in mouse skin. J Clin Invest 1997;100:1657.

50 Berger EA: HIV entra and tropism: The chemokine receptor connection. AIDS 1997;11:S3–S16.

51 Cocchi F, DeVico AL, Garzino-Demo A, Arya SK, Gallo RC, Lusso P: Identification of RANTES, MIP-1-alpha, and MIP-1-beta as the major HIV-suppressive factors produced by CD8– T cells. Science 1995;270:1811.

52 Clapham PR: HIV and chemokines: Ligands sharing cell-surface receptors. Trends Cell Biol 1997; 7:264–268.

53 Endres MJ, Clapham PR, Marsh M, Ahuja M, Turner JD, McKnight A, Thomas JF, Stoebenau-Haggarty B, Choe S, Vance PJ, Wells TN, Power CA, Sutterwala SS, Doms RW, Landau NR, Hoxie JA: CD4-independent infection by HIV-2 is mediated by fusin/CXCR4. Cell 1996;87:745.

54 Wells TN, Proudfoot AE, Power CA, Marsh M: Chemokine receptors – The new frontier for AIDS research (review). Chem Biol 1996;3:603.

55 Oberlin E, Amara A, Bachelerie F, Bessia C, Virelizier JL, Arenzana-Seisdedos F, Schwartz O, Heard JM, Clark-Lewis I, Legler DF, Loetscher M, Baggiolini M, Moser B: The CXC chemokine SDF-1 is the ligand for Lestr/fusin and prevents infection by T-cell-line-adapted HIV-1. Nature 1996;382:833.

56 Bleul CC, Farzan M, Choe H, Parolin C, Clarklewis I, Sodroski J, Springer TA: The lymphocyte chemoattractant sdf-1 is a ligand for lestr/fusin and blocks HIV-1 entry. Nature 1996;382:829.

57 Schmidtmayerova H, Sherry B, Bukrinsky M: Chemokines and HIV replication. Nature 1996;382:767.

58 Arenzana-Seisdedos F, Virelizier JL, Rousset D, Clark-Lewis I, Loetscher P, Moser B, Baggiolini M: HIV blocked by chemokine antagonist. Nature 1996;383:400.

59 Simmons G, Clapham PR, Picard L, Offord RE, Rosenkilde MM, Schwartz TW, Buser R, Wells TC, Proudfoot AEI: Potent inhibition of HIV-1 infectivity in macrophages and lymphocytes by a novel CCR5 antagonist. Science 1997;276:276.
60 Mack M, Luckow B, Nelson PJ, Cihak J, Simmons G, Clapham PR, Signoret N, Marsh M, Stangassinger M, Borlat F, Wells TN, Schlondorff D, Proudfoot AE: Aminooxypentane-RANTES induces CCR5 internalization but inhibits recycling: A novel inhibitory mechanism of HIV infectivity. J Exp Med 1998;187:1215.
61 Amara A, Legall S, Schwartz O, Salamero J, Montes M, Loetscher P, Baggiolini M, Virelizier JL, Arenzanaseisdedos F: HIV coreceptor downregulation as antiviral principle – SDF-1-alpha-dependent internalization of the chemokine receptor CXCR4 contributes to inhibition of HIV replication. J Exp Med 1997;186:139.
62 Signoret N, Oldridge J, Pelchen MA, Klasse PJ, Tran T, Brass LF, Rosenkilde MM, Schwartz TW, Holmes W, Dallas W, Luther MA, Wells TN, Hoxie JA, Marsh M: Phorbol esters and SDF-1 induce rapid endocytosis and down modulation of the chemokine receptor CXCR4. J Cell Biol 1997;139:651.
63 Rot A: Neutrophil attractant/activation protein-1 (interleukin-8) induces in vitro neutrophil migration by haptotactic mechanism. Eur J Immunol 1993;23:303.
64 Witt DP, Lander AD: Differential binding of chemokines to glycosaminoglycan subpopulations. Curr Biol 1994;4:394.
65 Hoogewerf AJ, Kuschert GS, Proudfoot AE, Borlat F, Clark LI, Power CA, Wells TN: Glycosaminoglycans mediate cell surface oligomerization of chemokines. Biochemistry 1997;36:13570.
66 Kuschert GS, Coulin F, Hubbard RE, Power CA, Wells TNC, Hoogewerf AJ: Soluble glycosaminoglycans interact selectively with chemokines and inhibit 7-transmembrane chemokine receptor binding and cellular responses. Biochemistry (submitted).
67 Marquezini MV, Strunz CM, Dallan LA, Toledo OM: Glycosaminoglycan distribution in atherosclerotic saphenous vein grafts. Cardiology 1995;86:143.
68 Wasty F, Alavi MZ, Moore S: Distribution of glycosaminoglycans in the intima of human aortas: Changes in atherosclerosis and diabetes mellitus. Diabetologia 1993;36:316.
69 Paolini JF, Willard D, Consler T, Luther M, Krangel MS: The chemokines IL-8, monocyte chemoattractant protein-1, and I-309 are monomers at physiologically relevant concentrations. J Immunol 1994;153:2704.
70 Burrows SD, Doyle ML, Murphy KP, Franklin SG, White JR, Brooks I, McNulty DE, Scott MO, Knutson JR, Porter D: Determination of the monomer-dimer equilibrium of interleukin-8 reveals it is a monomer at physiological concentrations. Biochemistry 1994;33:12741.
71 Kuschert GS, Hoogewerf AJ, Proudfoot AEI, Chung CW, Cooke R, Hubbard RE, Wells TNC, Sanderson PN: Identification of a glycosaminoglycan binding surface on human interleukin-8. Biochemistry 1998;37:11193.
72 Wells TC, Schwartz TW: Plagiarism of the host immune system – Lessons about chemokine immunology from viruses. Curr Opin Biotechnol 1997;8:741.
73 Gao JL, Murphy PM: Human cytomegalovirus open reading frame US28 encodes a functional beta-chemokine receptor. J Biol Chem 1994;269:28539.
74 Persoons MC, Daemen MJ, Bruning JH, Bruggeman CA: Active cytomegalovirus infection of arterial smooth muscle cells in immunocompromised rats. A clue to herpesvirus-associated atherogenesis? Circ Res 1994;75:214.
75 Davis-Poynter NJ, Lynch DM, Vally H, Shellam GR, Rawlinson WD, Barrell BG, Farrell HE: Identification and characterization of a G-protein-coupled receptor homolog encoded by murine cytomegalovirus. J Virol 1997;71:1521.
76 Cha TA, Tom E, Kemble GW, Duke GM, Mocarski ES, Spaete RR: Human cytomegalovirus clinical isolates carry at least 19 genes not found in laboratory strains. J Virol 1996;70:78.
77 Kledal TN, Rosenkilde MM, Coulin F, Simmons G, Johnsen AH, Alouani S, Power CA, Luttichau HR, Gerstoft J, Clapham PR, Clarklewis I, Wells TNC, Schwartz TW: A broad-spectrum chemokine antagonist encoded by Kaposi's sarcoma-associated herpesvirus. Science 1997;277:1656.
78 Boshoff C, Endo Y, Collins PD, Takeuchi Y, Reeves JD, Schweickart V, Siani MA, Sasaki T, Williams TJ, Gray PW, Moore PS, Chang Y, Weiss RA: Angiogenic and HIV-inhibitory functions of KSHV-encoded chemokines. Science 1997;278:290.

79 Sozzani S, Luini W, Bianchi G, Allavena P, Wells TNC, Napolitano M, Bernardini G, Vecchi A, D'Ambrosio D, Mazzeo D, Sinigaglia F, Santoni A, Maggi E, Romagnani S, Mantovani A: The viral chemokine macrophage inflammatory protein-II is a selective Th2 chemoattractant. Blood 1998;92:4036–4039.
80 Alcami A, Symons JA, Collins PD, Williams TJ, Smith GL: Blockade of chemokine activity by a soluble chemokine binding protein from vaccinia virus. J Immunol 1998;160:624.
81 Yoshida T, Imai T, Kakizaki M, Nishimura M, Takagi S, Yoshie O: Identification of single C motif-1/lymphotactin receptor XCR1. J Biol Chem 1998;273:16551–16554.

Timothy N.C. Wells, Serono Pharmaceutical Research Institute,
14 Chemin des Aulx, CH-1228 Plan-les-Ouates, Geneva (Switzerland)
Tel. +41 22 706 9930, Fax +41 22 7948507, E-Mail Tim.wells@serono.com

Author Index

Subject Index